SENILE DEMENTIA:
OUTLOOK FOR THE FUTURE

MODERN AGING RESEARCH

Series Editors

Richard C. Adelman
Jay Roberts
George T. Baker III
Vincent J. Cristofalo

Volume 1: Neural Regulatory Mechanisms During Aging, Richard C. Adelman, Jay Roberts, George T. Baker III, Steven I. Baskin, and Vincent J. Cristofalo, *Editors*

Volume 2: Aging and Human Visual Function, Robert Sekuler, Donald Kline, and Key Dismukes, *Editors*

Volume 3: Intervention in the Aging Process, William Regelson and F. Marott Sinex, *Editors*. Published in two volumes. Part A: Quantitation, Epidemiology, and Clinical Research. Part B: Basic Research and Preclinical Screening.

Volume 4: Comparative Pathobiology of Major Age-Related Diseases: Current Status and Research Frontiers, Dante G. Scarpelli and George Migaki, *Editors*

Volume 5: Senile Dementia: Outlook for the Future, Jean Wertheimer and Maurice Marois, *Editors*

SENILE DEMENTIA: OUTLOOK FOR THE FUTURE

Proceedings of the International Conference
"Senile Dementia in the Course of the Next Two Decades"
Sponsored by the Institut de la Vie
Held in Lausanne, Switzerland
May 2–4, 1983

Editors

Jean Wertheimer
President of Pro Senectute Vaud
Director of Service Universitaire de
Psycho-Gériatrie
Prilly, Switzerland

Maurice Marois
President and Founder of the
Institut de la Vie
Professor at the
Medical Faculty of Paris
Paris, France

Alan R. Liss, Inc., New York

Address all Inquiries to the Publisher
Alan R. Liss, Inc., 150 Fifth Avenue, New York, NY 10011

Printed in the United States of America.

Second Printing, October 1984

Senile dementia.

(Modern aging research; v. 5)
Bibliography: p.
Includes index.
1. Senile dementia—Congresses. I. Wertheimer, Jean.
II. Marois, M. (Maurice), 1922- . III. Series.
[DNLM: 1. Dementia, Senile—Congresses. W1 M0117
v.5 / WT 150 S4775 1983]
RC524.S47 1984 618.97689'83 84-3952
ISBN 0-8451-2305-X

Contents

Contributors

Sami Abdel-Al, Department of Gerontological Brain Research, Pharmaceutical Division, Sandoz Ltd, CH-4002 Basel, Switzerland **[125]**

Theodor Abelin, Department of Social and Preventive Medicine, University of Berne, Finkenhubelweg 11, CH-3012 Berne, Switzerland **[395]**

Luigi Amaducci, Department of Neurology, University of Florence, Viale Morgagni 85, Florence, Italy 50134 **[21]**

Gary R. Andrews, Department of Community and Geriatric Medicine, University of Sydney, Westmead Centre, Westmead, N.S.W. 2145, Australia **[479]**

Tom Arie, Professor of Health Care of the Elderly, University of Nottingham, Hucknall Road, NG5 1PD Nottingham, England **[201]**

Gil Assal, Department of Neuropsychology and Speech Pathology, CHUV Lausanne, 1011 Lausanne, Switzerland **[279]**

Walter M. Beattie, Jr., School of Social Work, Syracuse University, Syracuse, NY 13210 **[159]**

D. Behrens, Department of Geriatrics, University of Basel, CH-4031 Basel, Switzerland **[269]**

Stig Berg, Departments of Geriatric and Long-Term Care Medicine and Psychiatry, University of Göteborg, Göteborg, Sweden **[405]**

Simon Bergman, School of Social Work, University of Tel Aviv, 69978 Tel Aviv, Israel **[467]**

L. Bizzini, Service Universitaire de Psychiatrie Gériatrique, University of Geneva, Geneva, Switzerland **[253]**

Jacob A. Brody, Associate Director for Epidemiology Demography, and Biometry Program, NIH, 7550 Wisconsin Avenue, Bethesda, MD 20205 **[383]**

Robert N. Butler, Department of Geriatrics and Adult Development, Mount Sinai Medical Center, 1 Gustave L. Levy Place, New York, NY 10029 **[83]**

Richard I. Carp, Department of Virology, New York State Institute for Basic Research in Developmental Disabilities, 1050 Forest Hill Road, Staten Island, NY 10314 **[31]**

Jorge Cervós-Navarro, Institute of Neuropathology, Free University Berlin, Hindenburgdamm 30, 1000 Berlin 45, Federal Republic of Germany **[113]**

Donna Cohen, Departments of Psychiatry, Medicine, and Neuroscience, Montefiore Medical Center, 111 East 210th Street, Bronx, NY 10467 **[221]**

Jean Constantinidis, Department of Psychiatry, University of Geneva, 1225 Geneva, Switzerland **[55]**

Daniel Coquoz, Service Universitaire de Psycho-Gériatrie, Hôpital Psycho-Gériatrique, 1008 Prilly, Switzerland **[427]**

The boldface number in brackets indicates the opening page of the contributor's article.

Peter S. Cross, Center for Geriatrics and Gerontology, Columbia University and the New York State Office of Mental Health, 100 Haven Avenue, New York, NY 10032 **[327]**

David Danon, Center for the Biology of Aging, The Weizmann Institute of Science, Rehovot 76100, Israel **[3]**

Ann Harris Davidson, Department of Community and Health Medicine, University of Sydney, Westmead Centre, Westmead, N.S.W. 2145, Australia **[479]**

J. Deboise, Physician Responsible on the National Level of the U.C.C.M.A., Paris, France **[177]**

P. Droz, Service Universitaire de Psychiatrie Gériatrique, University of Geneva, Geneva, Switzerland **[253]**

Carl Eisdorfer, Department of Psychiatry and Neuroscience, Montefiore Medical Center, 111 East 210th Street, Bronx, NY 10467 **[221]**

Marco Ermini, Pharmaceutical Division, Sandoz Ltd, 4002 Basel, Switzerland **[365]**

Charles J. Fahey, Third Age Center, Fordham University, 113 West 60th Street, New York, NY 10023 **[445]**

Claire Favre, Department of Neuropsychology and Speech Pathology, CHUV Lausanne, 1011 Lausanne, Switzerland **[279]**

Michel Gaillard, Service Universitaire de Psycho-Gériatrie, 1008 Prilly, Switzerland **[411]**

Pierre Gilliand, Professeur à la Faculté de Sciences Sociales et Politiques, Université de Lausanne, Cité Devant 2, Lausanne, Switzerland **[167]**

A. Gommers, Centre d'Etudes Gérontologiques, Faculté de Médecine, Université de Louvain, 1200 Bruxelles, Belgique **[189]**

C.G. Gottfries, Department of Psychiatry and Neurochemistry, St. Jörgen's Hospital, S-422 03 Hisings Backa, Sweden **[69]**

Barry J. Gurland, Center for Geriatrics and Gerontology, Columbia University and the New York State Office of Mental Health, 100 Haven Avenue, New York, NY 10032 **[327]**

A.M. Hew-Winzeler, Department of Geriatrics, University of Basel, CH-4031 Basel, Switzerland **[269]**

Theodore Hovaguimian, Department of Radiology, University of Geneva, Geneva, Switzerland **[317]**

Lissy F. Jarvik, Department of Psychiatry and Biobehavioral Sciences, University of California, Los Angeles, 760 Westwood Plaza, Los Angeles, CA 90024 **[283]**

Jean-Pierre Junod, Department of Radiology, University of Geneva, Geneva, Switzerland **[317]**

W. Douglas Knowles, Department of Physical Sciences, IBM T.J. Watson Research Center, Yorktown Heights, NY 10598 **[291]**

Solomon Laurian, Department of Psychiatry, University of Lausanne, CH-1008 Prilly, Switzerland **[305]**

Peter D. Leathwood, Department of Research, Nestlé Products Technical Assistance Co. Ltd, CH-1814 La Tour de Peilz, Switzerland **[9]**

Alastair Macdonald, Institute of Psychiatry, Denmark Hill, SE5 London, England **[327]**

George L. Maddox, University Council on Aging and Human Development, Duke University, Durham, NC 27710 **[339]**

Philippe Magistretti, Department of Radiology, University of Geneva, Geneva, Switzerland **[317]**

Ebba Mahler, Department of Radiology, University of Geneva, Geneva, Switzerland **[317]**

Anthony H. Mann, Deparment of Psychiatry, Royal Free Hospital, Pond Place, NW3 London, England **[327]**

Rudolf Markstein, Pharmaceutical Division, Sandoz Ltd, 4002 Basel, Switzerland **[365]**

Maurice Marois, Institut de la Vie, Tour Maine-Montparnasse, 75755 Paris, Cedex 15, France **[xvii,xxiii].**

Steven S. Matsuyama, Department of Psychiatry and Biobehavioral Sciences, University of California, Los Angeles, 760 Westwood Plaza, Los Angeles, CA 90024 **[283]**

Jean Mauron, Department of Research, Nestlé Products Technical Assistance Co. Ltd, CH-1814 La Tour de Peilz, Switzerland **[9]**

W. Meier-Ruge, Department of Gerontological Brain Research, Pharmaceutical Division, Sandoz Ltd, CH-4002 Basel, Switzerland **[125]**

George S. Merz, Department of Pathological Neurobiology, New York State Institute for Basic Research in Developmental Disabilities, 1050 Forest Hill Road, Staten Island, NY 10314 **[31]**

Lars Nilsson, Departments of Geriatric and Long-Term Care Medicine and Psychiatry, University of Göteborg, Göteborg, Sweden **[405]**

Akim I. Oifa, All-Union Research Center of Mental Health, Academy of Medical Sciences of the USSR, Moscow, USSR **[107]**

Diana D. Orlovskaya, All-Union Research Center of Mental Health, Academy of Medical Sciences of the USSR, Moscow, USSR **[107]**

Timothy A. Pedley, Department of Neurology, Neurological Institute, 710 West 168th Street, New York, NY 10032 **[291]**

Göran Persson, Departments of Geriatric and Long-Term Care Medicine and Psychiatry, University of Göteborg, Göteborg, Sweden **[405]**

Silvia Piacentini, Department of Neurology, University of Florence, Viale Morgagni 85, Florence, Italy 50134 **[21]**

Alphonse Probst, Department of Pathology, University of Basel, Schonbeinstrasse 40, CH-4003 Basel, Switzerland **[151]**

Franco Regli, Department of Neurology, CHUV Lausanne, 1011 Lausanne, Switzerland **[279]**

J. Richard, Service Universitaire de Psychiatrie Gériatrique, University of Geneva, Geneva, Switzerland **[253]**

Sir Martin Roth, Professor of Psychiatry, University of Cambridge School of Clinical Medicine, Cambridge, England **[493]**

Alfred Sauvy, Institut National d'Etudes Démographiques, 27 Rue du Commandeur, 75675 Paris, Cedex 14, France **[455]**

Arnold B. Scheibel, Departments of Anatomy and Psychiatry, UCLA Medical Center, Los Angeles, CA 90024 **[137]**

Pierre Schwed, Médecin Directeur-Adjoint, Hôpital Psycho-Gériatrique, 1008 Prilly, Switzerland **[211]**

W.O. Seiler, Department of Geriatrics, University of Basel, CH-4031 Basel, Switzerland **[269]**

Sandro Sorbi, Department of Neurology, University of Florence, Viale Morgagni 85, Florence, Italy 50134 **[21]**

H.B. Stähelin, Department of Geriatrics, University of Basel, CH-4031 Basel, Switzerland **[269]**

Alvar Svanborg, Departments of Geriatric and Long-Term Care Medicine and Psychiatry, University of Göteborg, Göteborg, Sweden **[405]**

Roger D. Traub, Department of Physical Sciences, IBM T.J. Watson Research Center, Yorktown Heights, NY 10598 **[291]**

Jurg Ulrich, Department of Pathology, University of Basel, Schönbeinstrasse 40, CH-4003 Basel, Switzerland **[125,151,269]**

Jean Wertheimer, Directeur du Service Universitaire de Psycho-Gériatrie, Hôpital de Prilly, 1008 Prilly, Switzerland **[xiii,xv,93]**

Henryk M. Wisniewski, Department of Pathological Neurobiology, New York State Institute for Basic Research in Developmental Disabilities, 1050 Forest Hill Road, Staten Island, NY 10314 **[31]**

Masaki Yoshikawa, Professor Emeritus, University of Tokyo, Tokyo, Japan 102 **[239]**

Margaret Zinder, Department of Psychology, Hôpital de Psycho-Gériatrie, 1008 Prilly, Switzerland **[353]**

Conference Sponsors

Communauté Suisse de Recherche sur les Problèmes de la Vieillesse, Berne
Pro Senectute Suisse
Société Suisse de Gérontologie

Organizing Committee

D. Girardet, Directeur du Comité Vaudois de Pro Senectute, Lausanne
R. Guisan, Secrétaire Générale de l'Institut de la Vie, Membre du Conseil de Direction du Comité Vaudois de Pro Senectute, Lausanne
J. Wertheimer, Président du Comité Vaudois de Pro Senectute, Lausanne

Honorary Committee

T. ABELIN, Président de la Communauté Suisse de Recherche sur les Problèmes de la Vieillesse, Berne
P. BINSWANGER, Président du Comité de Direction de la Fondation pour la Vieillesse Pro Senectute, Zurich
C. BRIDEL, Recteur de l'Université de Lausanne
M. CEVEY, Médecin Cantonal, Lausanne
U. FREY, Directeur de l'Office Fédéral de la Santé Publique, Berne
N. GENTON, Doyen de la Faculté de Médecine, Lausanne
J.P. JUNOD, Professeur à la Faculté de Médecine de Genève
M. MAROIS, Président Fondateur de l'Institut de la Vie, Paris
P.R. MARTIN, Syndic de la Ville de Lausanne
J. MAURON, Directeur de la Société d'Assistance Technique pour Produits Nestlé S.A., Vevey
C. PEREY, Conseiller d'Etat, Chef du Département de l'Intérieur et de la Santé Publique, Lausanne
A. SCHUELER, Directeur de l'Office Fédéral des Assurances Sociales, Berne
H.B. STAEHELIN, Directeur du Centre de Gériatrie, Bâle
P. SCHWED, Président de la Société Suisse de Gérontologie, Lausanne
J. WERTHEIMER, Directeur du Service Universitaire de Psycho-Gériatrie, Prilly

FOREWORD

Jean Wertheimer

Professeur
Service Universitaire de Psycho-gériatrie
1008 Prilly - Suisse

A year ago, when Professor Marois suggested to Pro Senectute Switzerland the creation in our country of an international Centre dealing with problems concerning old age, the idea occurred to begin by organizing a conference on to-day's topic. It appeared at that time that the most urgent problem was senile dementia. This disease, which concerns about 10% of the people aged 65 and more, and 20% of those aged 80 and more, has become a real challenge to humanity. By disturbing deeply the intellectual faculties, the affectivity and the personality, it gives rise to innumerable human dramas. It involves deeply the whole family, which looses the permanent and secure image of the father or mother, now affected by this disease. On the social level, it brings about an increasing need for hospital beds, for ambulatory and intermediate services, and for support organisations, needs that the Public Health Services have to coordinate and which have to be found rational and economic answers. As the growing older of the population can be foreseen in the next decades, it is time to pay attention to this affliction. Time to pay attention to this problem on a worldwide level, as the increase of the proportion and of the absolute number of old people will concern the industrialised countries as well as the countries of the third world, that one may call countries of the multitude.

Paradoxically, the alarming increase of patients affected by senile dementia is the contribution of the progresses of medecine, which has rendered very small the infantile mortality and has given us weapons against the infectious diseases. The development of the medical technology together with that of a more attentive clinical observation help the research to make real progresses in the study of senile dementia. What are the hopes ? Towards which aim will the representatives of the fundamental, clinical and social sciences direct their efforts? These are the main topics of this meeting.

AVANT-PROPOS

Jean Wertheimer

Professeur
Service Universitaire de Psycho-gériatrie
1008 Prilly - Suisse

Lorsque le Professeur Marois suggéra il y a plus d'une année à Pro Senectute Suisse de constituer dans notre pays un Centre international s'occupant des problèmes de la vieillesse, l'idée vint de commencer par l'organisation d'une conférence dédiée à un sujet d'actualité. Or, il a paru que le thème le plus brûlant était celui de la démence sénile. Cette maladie qui affecte environ 10% des gens de 65 ans et plus et 20% de ceux de 80 ans et plus, constitue un véritable défi à l'humanité. En altérant profondément les facultés intellectuelles, l'affectivité et la personnalité de celui qui en est atteint, elle est à l'origine d'innombrables drames personnels. Elle entraîne en outre dans son tourbillon la famille qui ne retrouve plus l'image permanente et sécurisante du père ou de la mère maintenant malade. Sur le plan de la société, elle est à l'origine d'une demande croissante conduisant à la création de lits, de services ambulatoires et intermédiaires, d'organismes de soutien, que les services de santé publique doivent s'efforcer de rationaliser et de coordonner. Etant donné le vieillissement prévisible des populations au cours des prochaines décennies, il est temps de se préoccuper maintenant de la nature de ce fléau. Il en est temps à l'échelle planétaire, puisque ce vieillissement démographique sera le lot aussi bien des pays industrialisés que de ceux en voie de développement, ceux que l'on pourrait appeler les pays de la multitude.

Paradoxalement, l'augmentation alarmante du nombre de sujets affectés par la démence sénile est le tribu des progrès de la médecine, qui a rendu minimes les risques de mortalité infantile et qui a fourni les armes contre les maladies infectieuses. Le développement de la technologie médicale, allant de pair avec une observation clinique plus attentive permettent à la recherche de faire de réels progrès dans l'étude de la démence sénile. Quels sont les espoirs? Dans quelles directions les représentants des sciences fondamentales, de la clinique, des sciences sociales vont-ils diriger leurs efforts? Telles sont les questions que nous nous posons au moment d'ouvrir ce séminaire.

OPENING ADDRESS

PROFESSOR MAURICE MAROIS

Professor at the Medical Faculty of Paris
Founder and President of the Institut de la Vie
Tour Maine-Montparnasse, 33 avenue du Maine,
Case 183, 75755 PARIS CEDEX 15, FRANCE

In opening this meeting, I would like to read to you the following message by Nobel prizewinner Sir John Eccles :

"Please convey to the members of the conference my great interest in the scientific study of this terrible disease, which is such a profound threat to humans, destroying their mental and social life. I am confident that at this conference there will be ideas generated on the nature of the disease and of its scientific treatment. I wish this most important conference every success."

In the name of the Institut de la Vie I join in Professor Wertheimer´s courteous welcome of the participants of this congress. Coming from Australia, Japan, the United States, the Soviet Union, Sweden, Great Britain, the Federal Republic of Germany, Italy, Belgium, Israel, France, they have been friendly enough to accept our invitation to join the best Swiss specialists and representatives of international organisations to share their special knowledge and their future outlook on senile dementia.

And here once more I contemplate this kind of joyous endeavour in cooperation, generosity, devotion and intelligence in the service of the only cause that really counts : human life. An endeavour which is, perhaps, a miracle of the Institut de la Vie. Certainly it is the miracle of a female personality to whom I want publicly to acknowledge, in front of her people, in her own town and country, and at the risk of offending her feelings : Madame Michèle Guisan. It is to you, Madame, that I render my first homage. On September 16, 1976, I had the honour of meeting you : it was at Brussels, at a congress on gerontology - do you remember ? Since then, what a way we have come! There is no end in telling what our institution owes you, like having obtained the privilege to establish its world headquarters in Switzerland and its chancellery in the house of General Guisan in Pully. If it were in my power, I would place this meeting under your gracious and sensitive patronage. For you are the heart and soul of this enterprise, just as you have been the soul of the Institut de la Vie.

Many heartfelt thanks are also due to your stalwart and loyal companion, Mrs. Hélène Bircher.

We thank the organisations who have constituted a committee for the patronage, many thanks to all the personalities who constitute the honorary committee. These organisations and these personalities bring the force of their authority and proof of the wholehearted participation of Switzerland. We thank the benefactors whose moral and material support has made this congress possible. Thanks go to Daniel Girardet, whose subtle determination joined enthusiasm to efficiency. Most heartfelt thanks to my dear colleague and dear friend Professor Wertheimer. When I presented the project of assembling the world committee of the Institut de la Vie on the theme of ageing to the members of the Pro Senectute council of Zürich, you immediately understood the importance of such a meeting. Thanks to the dynamism of the canton of Vaud this project could be realized here. You have insisted on presenting the cause on the move by proposing a definite subject, and it is you who chose the theme : "Senile dementia during the course of the next two decades". It is you who knew how to obtain the magnificent contribution of Swiss science and medicine. L'Institut de la Vie is proud to have brought you the participation of foreign scientific and medical authorities who unanimously and immediately answered to its appeal.

The theme of ageing has long been worked on by the Institut de la Vie. In September 1975, in January and December 1976 it convened international committees in Paris which then prepared the conference of Vichy in April 1977. 230 participants from 25 countries have widened the bonds of our knowledge in the biological, medical, psychological, psychiatric, demographic, administrative and socio-economic domains. 1200 pages in three volumes give an account of the proceedings; they have been published by the Oxford University Press under the auspices of the Institut de la Vie and the European office of WHO. The editors are the Professors Beattie Jr., Birren and Shock of the United States, Piotrowski of Poland, Danon of Israel, Thomae of the Federal Republic of Germany, Munnichs of the Netherlands, Svanborg of Sweden, Gilmore of Great Britain, and myself. Moreover in 1978 the Institut de la Vie organized at the headquarters of the United Nations in New York the first conference on ageing dedicated to the Developing Countries. This conference, incepted by Dr. Tarek Shuman, was inspired and realized by Professor Beattie Jr.

At the Institut de la Vie's congress in Vienna, in July 1979, under the title of "Science at the Service of Life", the theme of ageing was treated by the Professors Junod and Wertheimer. In 1980, during the international conference on gerontology held in Tokyo, Professor Yoshikawa reunited the executive council of our world committee on ageing.

The meeting on aged people, organized in 1982 by the United Nations in Vienna, heavily underlined the necessity of interdisciplinary exchanges. This re-enforced our determination, affirmed in 1977, to create a world office, and I greatly hope to see created in Switzerland, maybe even here in Lausanne, an international centre of the Institut de la Vie on senile dementia.

This present conference is of great scientific, medical, social, economic and human importance. It is also of symbolic significance, since our theme is the menace on our brain, our brain which makes us fully human.

Founded 23 years ago, the Institut de la Vie is historically the first institution to have chosen life as its central theme, and having perceived it under all theoretical and practical aspects, fundamental and applied. This institution has united 2000 scientists, with 50 Nobel prizewinners among them, from 60 countries. It has acquired a universal diplomatic confidence. Its 3 themes are : Science, evidence of the greatness of the spirit, beneficial Science, Science as power and wisdom. The Institut works under the triple heading of science, life and hope. It proposes a philosophy and an ethic. It proclaims the value of life. It respects man in his dignity. It awakens the spirit of a responsibility growing in freedom. The Institut de la Vie has organized 60 international conferences on the mechanisms of life (from theoretical physics to biology), on the protection of chromosomes against environmental chemical substances, mutagenic and cancerogenic, on parasitical maladies, on ageing, concerning the needs and resources of humanity and the methods of prognostication, concerning life in towns, concerning the consequences of scientific and technical discoveries for man and society. The institution has established permanent commissions and sets up regional and world offices. Its international juries of the highest level of representativity have awarded 16 prizes of 250 000 to 300 000 FF each to personalities or institutions who have great merits for either defending life or having defined it.

And now the Institut de la Vie is preparing a major event : a world conference on LIFE.

Coming to the end of my address, let me express my emotion about being welcomed in this city : for it was in Lausanne that the 20th Anniversary Ceremony of the Institut de la Vie took place, held on October 11, 1980, under the presidency and in the presence of Federal Councillor Georges André Chevallaz, then president of the Swiss Confederation. It was on this occasion that we announced at the Palais Beaulieu our initiative for a world conference on life, aiming to raise hope, to break the fatal circle of the perils of war, to affirm the exigencies of conscience and to challenge the highest stake in life, the radiant face of peace. In the spirit of Pierre Elliott Trudeau, Prime Minister of Canada, this meeting should allow the scientific community to make its mark in questions of worldwide interest and to deliberate on the means of putting science and technology at the service of life. During the course of the congress on "Biology and the Future of Humanity" which preceeded the 20th Anniversary Ceremony, Nobel prizewinner Professor Arber of Basel and myself presented the project of our centre for the protection of life, a kind of Red Cross of which the canton of Vaud could become the haven.

We refuse to accept the pessimistic view which considers all civilization as mortal. We want to give voice to an irrepressible hope. We have forged great civilisations. Their partial triumphs make us impatient with what has not been achieved. Their new accomplishments must enhance a passionate zest for a life that wants to live and to flourish. We affirm our attachment to human life. This affirmation is inseparable from the proclamation of the highest standards that give it a reason to be, and a meaning. The future of life is entrusted to the liberty of man. To open the path for the future, we intend to develop the attention to life in all human domains. Facing death, we want to engage mankind in a dynamic of life. This is our challenge.

In the name of all men on earth who have the will to live in common, in our own name, in the name of "human love and understanding" we celebrate life, we see life as the main stake today and for the millions of centuries to come.

ALLOCUTION D'OUVERTURE

PROFESSEUR MAURICE MAROIS,

Professeur à la Faculté de Médecine de Paris
Président-Fondateur de l'Institut de la Vie
Tour Maine-Montparnasse, 33 avenue du Maine,
Case 183, 75755 PARIS CEDEX 15, FRANCE.

En ouvrant cette conférence, je tiens à vous lire le message suivant de Sir John Eccles, Prix Nobel :

"Please convey to the members of the conference my great interest in the scientific study of this terrible disease, which is such a profound threat to humans, destroying their mental and social life. I am confident that at this conference there will be ideas generated on the nature of the disease and of its scientific treatment. I wish this most important conference every success".

Au nom de l'Institut de la Vie, je m'associe aux si courtois propos de bienvenue à l'intention des congressistes, prononcés par le Prof. Wertheimer. Venus d'Australie, du Japon, des Etats-Unis, d'Union Soviétique, de Suède, de Grande-Bretagne, d'Allemagne fédérale, d'Italie, de Belgique, d'Israël, de France, ils nous ont fait l'amitié de répondre à notre invitation pour partager avec les meilleurs spécialistes helvétiques et les représentants d'organisation internationales leurs connaissances et leurs vues d'avenir sur la démence sénile.

Et voici qu'une fois encore je contemple de mes yeux cette sorte d'émulation joyeuse dans la coopération, la générosité, le dévouement, l'intelligence et l'élégance au service de la seule cause qui vaille : la vie humaine. Miracle peut-être, de l'Institut de la Vie. Miracle sûrement d'une personnalité féminine à qui je veux publiquement, devant les siens, dans sa ville et dans son pays, rendre témoignage, au risque, je le sais, d'offusquer sa délicatesse : Madame Michèle Guisan C'est à vous Madame, que je rends le premier hommage. Le 16 septembre 1976, j'ai eu l'honneur de vous rencontrer : c'était à Bruxelles, dans un congrès déjà de gérontologie - vous en souvient-il ? Depuis quel chemin parcouru ! Je n'en finirai pas de dire ce que vous doit notre institution, et d'abord, d'avoir obtenu le privilège de pouvoir fixer son siège mondial en Suisse et le siège de sa chancellerie dans la maison du Général Guisan à Pully. Si j'en avais le pouvoir, c'est sous votre gracieux patronage, souriant et sensible que je placerais cette manifestation. Car vous êtes l'âme de cette entreprise comme vous avez été l'âme de l'Institut de la Vie.

Merci à votre vaillante compagne, Madame Hélène Bircher.

Merci aux organisations qui ont constitué le comité de patronage, merci à toutes les personnalités qui ont constitué le comité d'honneur. Ces organisations et ces personnalités apportent la caution de leur haute autorité et témoignent de la participation plénière de la Suisse. Merci aux bienfaiteurs dont le soutien moral et matériel a rendu possible ce congrès. Merci à Daniel Girardet dont la détermination subtile marie l'enthousiasme à l'efficacité. Merci enfin, de très grand coeur à vous cher Collègue et cher ami, cher Prof. Wertheimer. Lorsque j'ai présenté à Zürich devant les membres du conseil de Pro Senectute le projet de réunir le comité mondial de l'Institut de la Vie sur le vieillissement vous avez immédiatement perçu l'importance d'une telle rencontre. Grâce au dynamisme du canton de Vaud, c'est ici que ce projet se réalise. Mais vous avez tenu à démontrer le mouvement en marchant, en proposant un sujet concret et c'est vous qui avez choisi le thème : "La démence sénile au cours des deux prochaines décennies". C'est vous qui avez su obtenir la magnifique contribution de la science et de la médecine suisses. L'Institut de la Vie est fier de vous avoir apporté la participation de hautes autorités scientifiques et médicales étrangères qui ont répondu unanimement et immédiatement à son appel.

L'Institut de la Vie avait de longue date et profondément labouré le champ du vieillissement. En septembre 1975, janvier et décembre 1976, il avait rassemblé à Paris des comités internationaux qui ont préparé la conférence de Vichy d'avril 1977. 230 participants de 25 pays ont fait le point de nos connaissances dans les domaines biologiques, médicaux, psychologiques, psychiatriques, démographiques, administratifs, socio-économiques. 1200 pages en 3 volumes en rendent compte ; ils viennent d'être publiés par Oxford University Press sous les auspices de l'Institut de la Vie et du bureau régional pour l'Europe de l'OMS. Les éditeurs sont les Professeurs Beattie Jr., Birren, Shock des Etats-Unis, Piotrowski de Pologne, Danon d'Israël, Thomae de la République fédérale d'Allemagne, Munnichs des Pays-Bas, Svanborg de Suède, Gilmore de Grande-Bretagne et moi-même. Puis, l'Institut de la Vie a organisé au siège des Nations-Unies à New-York, la première conférence sur le vieillissement consacrée aux pays en voie de développement en 1978. Cette conférence, voulue par le Dr. Tarek Shuman a été inspirée et réalisée par le Professeur Beattie Jr.

Au congrès de l'Institut de la Vie à Vienne : "La science au service de la vie" de juillet 1979, le thème du vieillissement fut traité par les Prof. Junod et Wertheimer. En 1980, au cours de la conférence internationale de gérontologie tenue à Tokyo, le Prof. Yoshikawa a réuni le conseil exécutif de notre comité mondial sur le vieillissement.

L'Assemblée sur les personnes âgées organisée en 1982 à Vienne par les Nations-Unies a souligné la nécessité des échanges interdisciplinaires. Ainsi se trouve renforcée notre détermination affirmée en 1977 de créer un office mondial. Dès aujourd'hui, je forme le souhait de voir naître en Suisse, à Lausanne peut-être, un centre international de l'Institut de la Vie sur la démence sénile.

La présente conférence a une grande importance scientifique, médicale, sociale, économique, humaine. Elle a aussi une signification symbolique puisque notre sujet est la menace sur notre cerveau, notre cerveau qui nous fait pleinement homme.

Fondé il y a 23 ans, l'Institut de la Vie est historiquement la première institution qui ait choisi la vie comme thème central et qui l'ait appréhendée sous tous les aspects théoriques et pratiques, fondamentaux et appliqués. L'institution a réuni 2 000 hommes de science de 60 pays dont 50 Prix Nobel. Elle a acquis une confiance diplomatique universelle. Ses 3 thèmes sont : la Science, témoin de la grandeur de l'esprit, la Science bienfaisante, Science, puissance et sagesse. Elle se place sous le triple signe de la science, de la vie, de l'espoir. Elle propose une philosophie et une éthique. Elle proclame la valeur de la vie. Elle respecte l'homme dans sa dignité. Elle éveille sa liberté à la responsabilité. L'Institut de la Vie a organisé 60 conférences internationales sur les mécanismes de la vie (de la physique théorique à la biologie), sur la protection des chromosomes contre les substances chimiques de l'environnement, mutagènes et cancérigènes, sur les maladies parasitaires, sur le vieillissement, sur les besoins et les ressources de l'humanité et les méthodes de prévision, sur la vie dans la ville, sur les conséquences pour l'homme et la société des découvertes scientifiques et techniques. L'institution a établi des commissions permanentes ; elle met en place des organes régionaux et mondiaux. Ses jurys internationaux du plus haut niveau de représentativité ont décerné 16 prix de 250 000 à 300 000 FF chacun à des personnalités ou des institutions qui ont bien mérité de la vie soit pour l'avoir défendue, soit pour l'avoir illustrée.

Et voici, que l'Institut de la Vie prépare un événement majeur : une conférence mondiale de la Vie.

Au moment de conclure, je voudrais dire mon émotion d'être accueilli dans cette ville : car c'est à Lausanne que s'est tenue sous la présidence et en présence de Monsieur le Conseiller fédéral, Georges-André Chevallaz, alors Président de la Confédération, la cérémonie du XXème anniversaire de l'Institut de la Vie, le 11 octobre 1980. C'est en cette circonstance que nous avons annoncé au Palais de Beaulieu notre initiative de la conférence mondiale de la Vie, pour donner les raisons de l'espoir, rompre le cercle fatal du péril guerrier, affirmer les exigences de la conscience et lancer le pari de la vie, visage radieux de la paix. Dans l'esprit de Pierre Elliot Trudeau, Premier Ministre du Canada, ce sommet devrait permettre à la communauté scientifique de faire le point sur les questions d'intérêt mondial et de délibérer sur les moyens de mettre la science et les techniques au service de la vie. Au cours du congrès : "Biologie et avenir humain" qui a précédé la cérémonie du XXème anniversaire, le Professeur Arber, Prix Nobel de Bâle, et moi-même, avons présenté le projet de notre centre de protection de la vie, sorte de Croix-Rouge de l'espèce dont la terre d'accueil pourrait être le canton de Vaud.

Nous refusons la vue pessimiste qui considère toute civilisation comme mortelle. Nous voulons donner une voix à l'irrépressible espoir. Nous avons forgé de grandes civilisations. Leurs triomphes partiels redoublent en nous l'impatience de l'inaccompli. Leurs nouveaux accomplissements doivent plus encore donner droit à la revendication passionnée de la vie qui veut vivre et s'épanouir. Nous affirmons notre attachement à la vie humaine. Cette affirmation est indissociable de la proclamation des plus hautes valeurs qui lui donnent une raison d'être et un sens. L'avenir de la vie est confié à la liberté de l'homme. Pour ouvrir les voies de l'attention à la vie. Face à la mort, nous voulons engager l'humanité dans une dynamique de vie. Tel est notre défi.

Au nom de tous les hommes de la terre qui ont en commun le vouloir vivre, en notre nom propre, au nom de la "tendresse humaine", nous célébrons la vie, nous la proposons comme enjeu majeur aujourd'hui et pour les millions de siècles à venir.

I. INTRODUCTION

Senile Dementia: Outlook for the Future, pages 3–6

BIOLOGY OF AGING FOR NON-BIOLOGISTS

David Danon, M.D.
Director, Center for the Biology of Aging
The Weizmann Institute of Science,
Rehovot 76100, Israel

About one hundred years ago several important events took place in the scientific community, mainly in Europe. These started a new era in the thinking and development of life sciences in general and medicine in particular. Claude Bernard pioneered experimental medicine. He said, among other important things: "Cells live together-they die alone". Pasteur dispelled the myth of spontaneous generation of living things, initiating the aseptia and preventive medicine. Koch contributed the basic idea that a particular organism causes a particular disease. Ehrlich has set the foundations of modern bacteriology. Mechnikof discovered the macrophages and microphages. Dastre, the physiologist and philosopher formulated that "Life is a harmony of cells and systems". At the same period, a man of a completely different discipline, not a biologist, not a physiologist or a physician, not a philosopher, a german general by the name of Bismarck campaigning for his election as a chancellor of Germany, said: "If I am elected, the men will stop working at the age of 65 and the women at the age of 60." Since that time, one hundred years ago, we still consider this as the official "old age" in many countries.

At that time in Europe as well as in the United States only about 3% of the population were "old".

The first years after these milestones did not show dramatic developments. Thus in World War I the therapy consisted of arsenicals and carbolic acid. In World War II we see the german sulfa (french sto - varsol) and towards the end british penicillin. And one more important progress the decision of the American Congress to fight "One more war – the war against disease". They created the National Institutes of Health (NIH).

During 100 years the biomedical sciences were directed almost exclusively to eliminating diseases or curing them. As a result of a certain amount of success, the number of people reaching an advanced age has markedly increased. The probability of becoming old is very high, especially in the developed countries. It reaches now 10% of the population in developed countries and in some parts of old cities even 20% or more. The question is, "how old is old"?.

This question may relate to the number of months, or years, that must pass for an animal to be considered "old". However, it may also be related to how an old animal becomes "old". The answer to the first aspect of the query, based on observation and statistics, varies in humans according to country, civilization, and an accepted norm.

The attempt to answer the second form of the question has preoccupied many scientists. Initially, research was devoted to quantitation of physiological and anatomical changes occurring with the passage of years. From these studies we have learned that the efficiency of important functions, such as the vital capacity of lungs, cardiac pumping, or renal filtration, declines with age by about one quarter to one third. The normal levels of sugar and other important components in the blood are maintained if exaggerated challenges are avoided. In a second phase of research, scientists tried to formulate "theories" of aging, relating all symptoms of senescence to one general cause. One theory, for example, attributed aging to chemical and physical changes taking place in the connective tissue with increasing chronological age. Another claimed that aging is due to molecular alterations caused by ionizing radiation. There was also a theory suggesting that the deterioration of physiological functions could be ascribed to the accumulation of waste materials in cells while yet another one proposed, that aging is due to an accumulation of errors in molecules that are involved in the production of other molecules. Thus, the probability of more errors increases with age, until a "catastrophe" of errors causes senescence and death. Additionally, the immunological theory of aging claims that symptoms of aging are due to diminished immunological defence. It has also been proposed that aging is programmed and controlled by the pituitary gland.

It is now clear that we should retain only the experimental results of all those studies and put aside any attempt to place the totality of the phenomena of aging under one common denominator.

Aging is not a disease, it is not a syndrome caused by one pathogenic agent.

A third phase in biological research on aging can be characterized by the passage from the systemic and tissue level to the cellular levels. The discovery twenty years ago, that cells in tissue culture have a limited capacity for doubling their population, opened up the possibilities of test tube experiments in cellular aging. Organ cultures and the study of cells (of limited life span) in the living animal, have enabled scientists to close the gap between extracorporal experiments and those in living animals. The remarkable progress of biochemical and biophysical methods of research have made possible the intensive study of aging in molecular and structural terms.

As we age, we witness the escape of more and more functional parts of the body from the general control system. Some cells multiply less; others divide too rapidly. Some tissues degenerate; others proliferate. While the "over-design" of most our cells and functions enables the continuation of life under favourable conditions, extreme conditions may result in failure. For example, the retarded response in correcting sugar levels in blood, typical of old age, may be due to a diminished number of cells secreting stored insulin, or to the insufficiency of cells that should synthesize the insulin. It may be that structural alteration in the sensors for the sugar level made the sensor less sensitive; and finally, as some results indicate, the retarded response may be due to an excess of antagonistic hormones.

The number of structural and molecular changes that can take place in even more complex systems (i.e. the immune or nervous system) is practically endless in view of the number and complexity of cells and extracellular molecules participating in the processes inherent in these systems. It is not difficult to realize that changes in the number of cells or their structural components do not take place identically or even similarly in all animals or in all people. This fact in itself is indicative of the need to separate the symptoms that might, together, create the accepted image of senescence and to identify in each case the cause of its appearance or not appearance.

Behavioral alterations that occur in young as well as in old age, were approached for a long time in terms of changes in the soul.

Professor Morel, my teacher of psychiatry in Geneva, about 30 years ago, devoted a considerable effort in search of anatomical changes in the central nervous system of patients who suffered from dementia.

It is hard to think of an alteration in behaviour without alteration in the communication between cells in the central and peripheral nervous system.

The early anatomical and histological discoveries led to ultrastructural discoveries of changes in neurons and dendrites. Molecules have been identified as responsible for transmission of impulses across synapses from one nerve end to another. Let us keep in mind that molecules react to molecules or with molecules. Alterations in behaviour should be sooner or later expressed in terms of ultrastructural and molecular alterations. These may be either qualitative or quantitative, or both. The probability of finding one single cause for alterations of behaviour in advanced age, is as poor as finding one theory that will explain all the phenomena associated with advanced age.

Concentration on the study of the separate phenomena of aging will increase the probability of a better understanding of the mechanisms of their occurrence, greatly improve the probability of controlling them and justify the hope for their prevention.

II. CEREBRAL BIOCHEMISTRY AND SENILE DEMENTIA

Presided by C.G. Gottfries (Göteborg)

Senile Dementia: Outlook for the Future, pages 9–19

LECITHIN AND SENILE MEMORY LOSS IN ANIMALS

Peter D. Leathwood, Ph.D. and Jean Mauron, Ph.D.

Nestlé Products Technical Assistance Co.Ltd.
Research Department, P.O. Box 88
CH-1814 La Tour de Peilz (Switzerland)

For nearly 100 years, therapy for Parkinson's disease depended on the use of relatively inefficient anticholinergic agents. However, in the 1950's, it was shown that reserpine (which depletes brain dopamine) produced Parkinsonian-like side-effects. This was followed by observations of marked deficits in striatal dopamine in Parkinsonian patients and led to tests of L-Dopa (a precursor of dopamine which can readily cross the blood-brain barrier) in the treatment of Parkinson's disease. The first clinical trials were not very convincing, and only after what, at the time, were considered to be massive oral doses of Dopa did Cotzias, Van Woert and Schiffer (1967) note an appreciable improvement in 8 out of 16 patients with Parkinson's disease.

The success of this "neurochemical" approach led to the hope that administration of neurotransmitter precursors would be useful in the treatment of other debilitating nervous system diseases. In particular, it has been suggested that the acetylcholine precursor, phosphatidyl choline (often called lecithin), could be used to treat senile memory loss and perhaps senile dementia of the Alzheimer's type. We will review the evidence for this hypothesis that can be supplied from animal studies.

It is now well-established that there is often a decrease in cholinergic function in elderly animals.

Several different criteria can be used to assess cholinergic status. The most popular, measuring the activity of choline acetyl transferase in the brain, has produced contradictory results (see Bartus, Dean, Beer and Lippa, 1982 for review), but it is also of doubtful physiological significance since the enzyme is unsaturated in vivo and unlikely to control acetylcholine (ACh) function. More direct measures (Gibson, Peterson and Jenden, 1981) have demonstrated an age-related decrease in the rate of acetylcholine synthesis in 2 strains of mouse.

There have also been consistent reports of decreases in the density of cortical, hippocampal and striatal muscarinic binding sites with increasing age (Bartus et al., 1982).

Lastly, patients with Alzheimer's disease show profound deficits (greater than 75 %) in cholinergic neurones in the nucleus basalis of Meynert (Whitehouse, Struble, Clark, Coyle and Delong, 1982) and a reduction in presynaptic markers for acetylcholine in the hippocampus and cerebral cortex.

Many animal species also show age related deficits in learning ability. Elderly monkeys show deficits in short term memory (Bartus, Fleming and Johnson, 1978). In mice, the ability to learn an active avoidance response in the shuttle-box decreases with age (Bovet, Bovet-Nitti and Oliverio, 1969; Leathwood, Heck and Mauron, 1982). Passive avoidance learning decreases with advancing age in both rats (Lippa, Pelham, Beer, Critchett, Dean and Bartus, 1980) and mice (Bartus, Dean, Goas and Lippa, 1980). In the multiple T-maze, error scores and trials to learn the maze increase markedly in elderly mice (Golczewski, Hiramoto and Ghanta, 1982). Lastly, difficulty in remembering recent events is a common problem in elderly people (Drachman and Leavitt, 1972).

Thus the phenomenon of senile memory loss is well documented although analysis of its causes is only just beginning. A multitude of factors can be involved, but several lines of evidence suggest that the memory deficits (particularly for recent events) are often closely linked to inadequate central cholinergic function. The patterns of deficits in memory storage and cognitive function in the elderly are surprisingly similar to those produced by giving young people scopolamine, an acetylcholine antagonist (Drachman and Leavitt, 1974). Furthermore, the cholinergic agonist, physostigmine, improves scores both in the elderly (Drachman and Sahakian, 1980) and in young people pretreated with scopolamine (Drachman and Leavitt, 1974). Analysis is complicated by the extreme variability in individual responses to physostigmine and Bartus et al. (1982) have suggested that improvement only occurs within a very narrow dose range and this optimum range differs dramatically among individuals.

Unfortunately, cholinergic drugs produce unpleasant side effects, such as tachycardia and intestinal hypermotility, so even when they do help to improve cognitive function they are therapeutically impractical. More recently, Wurtman and his colleagues (Wurtman, Hefti and Melamed, 1981) have suggested an alternative means of increasing cholinergic function. They showed that large doses of phosphatidyl choline (PCh) can increase synthesis of acetylcholine in the brain (Hirsch and Wurtman, 1978). Several laboratories were unable to repeat this finding (Flentge and Van den Berg, 1982), but this may have happened because the extent to which cholinergic neurones respond to elevated choline concentrations varies with their firing frequency (Wurtman et al., 1980). This has been clearly demonstrated using the rat phrenic nerve preparation, where adding 30 μM choline to the medium produced no significant change in acetylcholine release when the nerve was at rest, but a 35 % increase ($p < 0.01$) after electrical stimulation (Bierkamper and Goldberg, 1980). More indirect evidence for a similar relationship between firing frequency and precursor responsiveness within the brain was obtained by unilaterally destroying some striatal cholinergic neurones with kainic acid. After this treatment, systemic choline administration did not change acetylcholine levels in the intact striatum but it doubled them in the lesioned side (London and Coyle, 1978).

The first animal study using short-term treatment with choline to attenuate senile memory loss in rats did not produce very encouraging results (Bartus, 1980). Choline chloride (100 mg/kg/day) administered for 1 week prior to passive avoidance retention testing in aged rats produced no significant improvement in performance (Fig. 1). Later studies (see below) suggest that this dose level may have been too low. Furthermore, as retention by the older animals had already fallen to less than 10 % of the level observed in younger rats (Lippa et al., 1980), it is also possible that the old animals were beyond improvement.

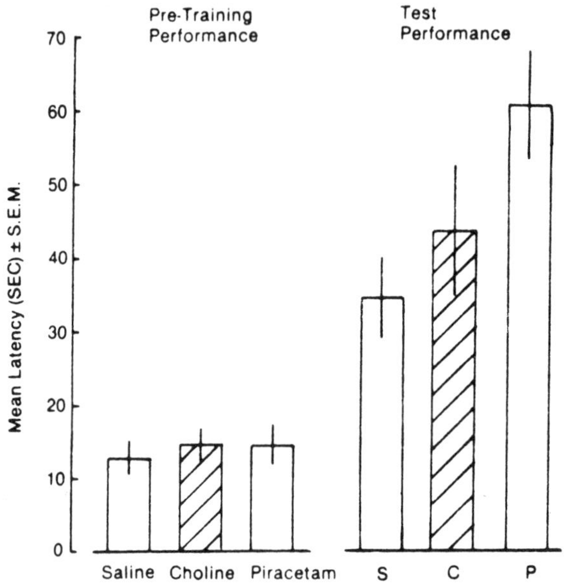

Fig. 1. Effects of choline chloride (100 mg/kg), piracetam (100 mg/kg) and saline administered for 1 week prior to testing on passive avoidance retention in 2-year-old Fischer 344 rats (Bartus, 1980. Copyright : American Psychological Association. Reprinted with permission).

We carried out a dose-response test of the effects of phosphatidyl choline on avoidance learning in mice (Leathwood et al., 1982). Young (6 month old) and elderly (17 month old) male SEC/1ReJ mice were fed 0, 2, 4 or 8 % phosphatidyl choline in the diet (the level of choline intake was approximately 0, 0.3, 0.6 or 1.2 g/kg/day). These diets were fed for 10 days, beginning 4 days before, and continuing throughout the period of avoidance training.

Mice were given 5 daily avoidance sessions of 100 trials each in the shuttle-box. In each trial the conditioning stimulus (a 10 W light) preceded by 5 sec the unconditioned stimulus (US) and overlapped with it for 2 sec. The unconditioned stimulus was an a.c. shock (35v, fed through a 30KΩ resistance and scrambled by a silicon rectifier). The shock was switched off at the beginning of the next trial. Passage of the mouse from one side of the cage to the other was recorded by a micro- switch tripped by movement of the cage floor. A condi- tioned response (CR) was recorded if the mouse avoided the shock by running into the adjacent compartment within 5 sec after the light was switched on.

Avoidance acquisition in young mice was rapid. High performance levels were reached by all groups and the learning curves for control and treated groups were practically identical (Fig. 2). The older mice given no phosphatidyl choline supplement acquired the avoidance response more slowly and the final level of performance reached was lower. The decrease in performance with advancing age was significant ($p < 0.01$; Mann-Whitney "U" test). It is unlikely that the low performance was due to physical handicap as all the older mice actively explored the shuttle-box, and the 5 sec delay between US and CS provided ample time to pass from one side of the box to the other (the response latency was usually less than 2 sec). There was also a marked increase in the variability of results in older mice with the animals tending to separate into high and low performers. This means that non-parametric statistics are more appropriate for analysis of the results.

In the younger mice, phosphatidyl choline had no effect at all, and performance levels in all groups were remarkably similar. Comparison of the 0 % and 8 % phosphatidyl choline groups at 17 months old showed that those given 8 % PCh reached significantly higher levels of avoidance performance ($p < 0.05$; Mann-Whitney "U" test, one-sided comparison). Mean performance levels for the intermediate groups, although higher than control values, were not significantly different from them.

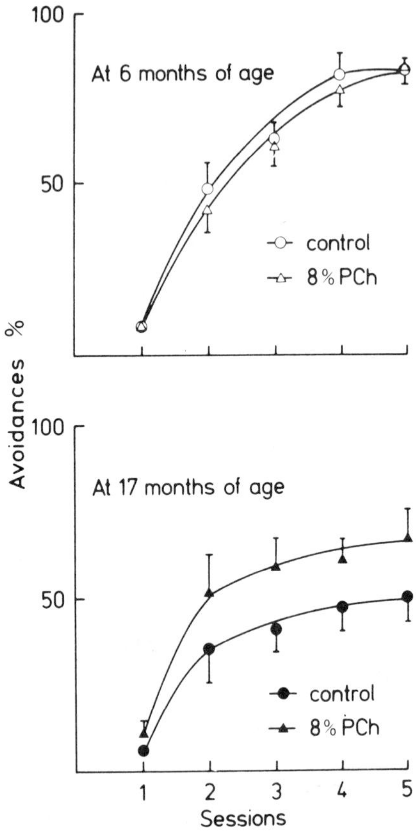

Fig. 2. Avoidance performance of male SEC/1ReJ mice during 5 daily sessions of 100 trials each. Each point represents the mean (± SEM) for 8 mice (Leathwood et al., 1982. Copyright : Pergamon Press Ltd. Reprinted with permission).

This study illustrates some of the problems involved in designing and interpreting experiments with elderly animals. The original design provided for larger groups at 17 months, but not all the animals survived to be tested. On avoidance testing the older animals did show deficits in performance and an increase in variability of performance. This, coupled with the smaller number of animals surviving to be tested makes analysis of phosphatidyl choline effects rather difficult. The process of aging inevitably includes a heterogenous pattern of physical and functional degeneration. Thus the factors leading to the different levels of performance deficit are unlikely to be exactly the same for each animal. This means that we cannot expect all the animals to respond in the same way to any one treatment, and implies that the most logical analysis is to compare the proportions of high and low performers in the treatment and control groups. Using 60 % CR as the cut-off and comparing the 0 % and 8 % PCh supplement, there was a significant increase in the proportion of high performers in the 8 % PCh group ($p < 0.05$, one-sided comparison).

In a subsequent study, Golczewski et al. (1982) measured learning in a multiple T-maze of 23-31 month old C57BL/6 mice fed a 25 % lecithin diet (estimated choline intake $\sim$ 1 g/kg/day) from 4 days before behavioural testing began. They observed significant improvements in error scores and in the number of trials to learn the maze.

These three sets of results are consistent with the idea that impaired cholinergic mechanisms may be partly responsible for the memory deficits associated with advancing age, and PCh acts by ameliorating this impairment. We cannot at present rule out the possibility that PCh also acts by other neurochemical mechanisms, especially as it may influence membrane function or interact with other neurotransmitter systems. The results also show that, for short-term therapy at least, very large intake levels of phosphatidyl choline are needed before behavioural effects can be seen.

Using a rather different approach, Bartus et al. (1980) reasoned that, though it may be difficult to reverse existing age-related neurochemical deficits with choline or lecithin, it might be possible to retard the onset of these changes by feeding choline from early middle age through into old age. They tested this hypothesis by feeding C57Bl/6j mice approximately 1 g/kg/day choline beginning at the age of 8.5 months. As can be seen from fig. 3, at 13 months, rentention scores in a passive avoidance test were significantly better than those of control (consuming about 100 mg/kg/day of choline) or choline deficient mice (<50 mg/kg/day). This study offers the tantalizing suggestion that prolonged feeding of acetylcholine precursors may delay the onset of mental degeneration.

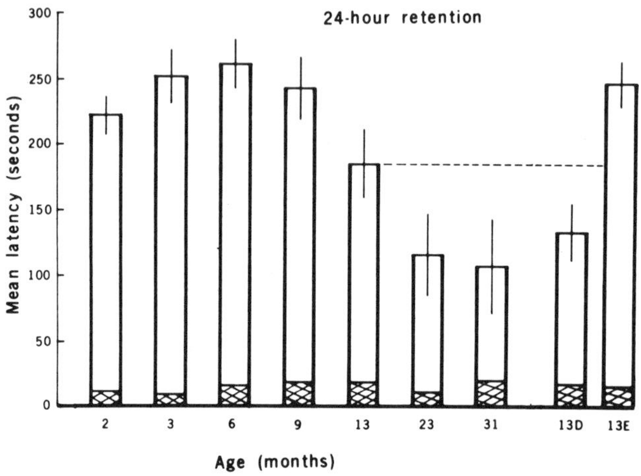

Fig. 3. Latencies to enter the shock chamber 24 hours after training in C57Bl/6j mice (hatched bars show latencies on the test day). The two right-hand bars depict the latencies of 13-month-old mice maintained either on diets deficient (13 D) or enriched (13 E) in choline for 4.5 months. The 13-month-old choline deficient mice performed as poorly as 23-month-old controls, while with choline enrichment, performance was no worse than in 6-month-old controls. (From Bartus et al., 1980. Copyright : American Association for the Advancement of Science. Reprinted with permission).

Several clinical trials have now been carried out to test the effects of choline or phosphatidyl choline on senile memory loss or senile dementia of the Alzheimer's type. The hope was that, in a manner equivalent to the actions of L-Dopa on Parkinson's disease, the treatment would slow down or reverse the degenerative changes.

At first sight the results are disappointing. Of the 17 studies reviewed by Bartus et al. (1982), only one found substantial improvement (in 60 % of the patients) while a second reported no further degeneration; the others were ambiguous or negative. However, in comparison to the minimum effective dose found in the animal studies (∿1.0 g/kg/day of choline) almost all the clinical trials have used very small levels of choline (0.1-0.2 gm/kg/day). It is perhaps significant that the two studies with positive results (Christie, Blackburn, Glen, Zeisel, Shering and Yates, 1979; Vroulis, Smith, Brinkman, Schoolar and Gordon, 1981) used the highest doses of lecithin (∿1 g/kg/day) and continued treatment for the longest period (2-3 months).

As Bartus et al. (1982) suggested, the predominance of negative results with precursor therapy may have occurred because the functional disturbance in the aged brain is at the receptor level, so that increasing the rate of acetylcholine synthesis is of little use. Comparison with the results of animal studies described above suggests an additional possibility : that in most of the clinical trials carried out so far, the levels of choline administration were insufficient to influence brain acetylcholine. A very recent study (Levy, Little, Chuaqui and Reith, 1983), in which patients with Alzheimer's disease showed significant improvements when treated with high doses of phosphatidyl choline for long periods, tends to support this suggestion.

In conclusion, there seems to be fairly convincing evidence that cholinergic deficits play an important rôle in senile memory loss and senile dementia of the Alzheimer's type. As with the treatment of Parkinson's disease, the first clinical trials using precursor therapy have been disappointing, but the approach has not failed entirely. It is possible that the doses of lecithin required to influence brain acetylcholine will be so large as to be impracticable, and either an alternative source, more rich in choline, should be sought, or combinations of drug and precursor therapy should be tried. Finally, if the results of Bartus et al. (1980) using long-term therapy are confirmed, it may ultimately be more useful to aim at identifying and treating "at risk" individuals before severe degeneration sets in.

Bartus RT (1980). Cholinergic drug effects on memory and cognition in animals. In : LW Poon (ed) Aging in the 1980s : Psychological issues. Am Psychol Assn Washington DC, p 163.
Bartus RT, Dean RL, Beer B, Lippa AS (1982). The cholinergic hypothesis of geriatric memory dysfunction. Science 217:408.
Bartus RT, Dean RL, Goas JA, Lippa AS (1980). Age related changes in passive avoidance retention and modulation with chronic dietary choline. Science 209:301.
Bartus RG, Fleming D, Johnson HR (1978). Aging in the rhesus monkey : effects on short-term memory. J Gerontol 33:858.
Bierkamper GG, Goldberg AM (1980). Release of acetylcholine from the vascular perfused phrenic nerve-hemidiaphragm. Brain Res 202:234.
Bovet D, Bovet-Nitti F, Oliverio A (1969). Genetic aspects of learning and memory in mice. Science 163:139.
Christie JE, Blackburn IM, Glen AIM, Zeisel S, Shering A, Yates GM (1979). Effects of choline and lecithin on CSF choline levels and on cognitive function in patients with presenile dementia of the Alzheimer type. In : A Barbeau, JH Growden and RJ Wurtman (eds) "Nutrition and the Brain" volume 5, Raven NY,.
Cotzias GC, Van Woert MH, Schiffer LM (1967). Aromatic amino acids and modification of parkinsonism. New Engl J Med 276:379.
Drachman DA, Leavitt JL (1972). Memory impairment in the aged - storage versus retrieval deficit. J Exp Psychol 93:302.
Drachman DA, Leavitt JL (1974). Human memory and the cholinergic system. A relationship to aging ? Arch Neurol 30:113.
Drachman DA, Sahakian GH (1980). Memory and cognitive function in the elderly. A preliminary trial of physostigmine. Arch Neurol (Chicago) 37:674.
Flentge F, Van Den Berg CJ (1982). Choline precursors and Alzheimer's disease. Lancet ii:1472.
Gibson GE, Peterson C, Jenden DJ (1981). Brain acetylcholine synthesis declines with senescence. Science 213: 674.
Golczewski JA, Hiramoto RN, Ghanta VK (1982). Enhancement of maze learning in old C57BL/6 mice by dietary lecithin.
Hirsch MJ, Wurtman RJ (1978). Lecithin consumption elevates acetylcholine concentrations in rat brain and adrenal gland. Science 207:223.

Leathwood PD, Heck E, Mauron J (1982). Phosphatidyl choline and avoidance performance in 17 month old SEC/1ReJ mice. Life Sci 30:1065.

Levy R, Little A, Chuaqui P, Reith M (1983). Early results from double blind, placebo controlled trial of high dose phosphatidyl choline in Alzheimer's disease. Lancet ii: 987.

Lippa A, Pelham RW, Beer B, Critchett DJ, Dean RL, Bartus RT (1980). Brain cholinergic dysfunction and memory in aged rats. Neurobiol of Aging 1:13.

London ED, Coyle JT (1978). Pharmacological augmentations of acetylcholine levels in kainate-lesioned rat striatum. Biochem Pharmacol 27:2962.

Vroulis GA, Smith RC, Brinkman S, Schoolar J, Gordon J (1971). The effects of lecithin on memory in patients with senile dementia of the Alzheimer's type. Psychopharmacol Bull 17:127.

Whitehouse PJ, Price DL, Struble RG, Clark AW, Coyle JT, Delong MR (1982). Alzheimer's disease and senile dementia : loss of neurons in the basal forebrain. Science 215:1237.

Wurtman RJ, Hefti F, Melamed E (1981). Precursor control of neurotransmitter synthesis. Pharmacol Rev 32:315.

Senile Dementia: Outlook for the Future, pages 21–29

ENERGY METABOLISM IN AGING AND DEMENTIA

Sandro Sorbi, M.D., Silvia Piacentini, M.D., Luigi Amaducci, M.D.
Department of Neurology, Univ. of Florence
V.le Morgagni 85, Florence, Italy

Aging of the brain and dementia are very complicated process characterized by functional, morphological, and biochemical alterations of the brain. A decline in higher cognitive functions in old age and in dementias might be related to a variety of biochemical and anatomical abnormalities of the brain.

Two well documented sets of abnormalities occur in dementias: abnormalities in neurotransmitter systems (Amaducci et al., 1982, 1983; Bird et al.,1974, 1977; Blass 1980; Blass et al. 1980; Bowen et al. 1976, 1979; Davies and Maloney 1976; Perry et al. 1978; Sorbi et al. 1979, 1980, 1982, 1983; Sims et al. 1982) and decreases in cerebral metabolic rate (Blass 1980; Quastel 1932; Gibson et al. 1981; Sokoloff 1966; Sorbi et al. 1983; Perry et al. 1980).

For Alzheimer type dementias marked reductions have been found by several groups in the brain at autopsy in choline acetyltransferase (CAT) activity, a marker of cholinergic system (Davies and Maloney 1976; Bird 1977; Bowen et al. 1976; Sorbi et al. 1979, 1983). CAT activity was reduced in cortical (Davies and Maloney 1976; Bird 1977; Bowen et al. 1976) and subcortical areas (Sorbi et al. 1979; Whitehouse et al. 1982). A significant decrease in the activity of this cholinergic marker and in acetylcholine synthesis has been also found in biopsy cortical specimens from Alzheimer patients (Sims et al. 1982). In Alzheimer brain alterations in catecholamines (Adolfsson et al. 1979; Bondareff et al. 1981) and in immunoreactive somatostatine (Davies and Terry 1981) have been reported. Abnormalities in central neurotransmitter systems have been also observed in alcoholic dementia (Antuono et al. 1980), Huntington disease (Bird et al. 1974, 1977; Sorbi et al. 1983) and Creutzfeldt-Jakob disease (Sorbi and Amaducci 1980).

Abnormalities in cerebral metabolic rate, cerebral oxygen consumption, cerebral blood flow, and cerebral glucose utilization have been among the earliest and best documented alterations in dementias (Quastel 1932; Sokoloff 1966). They do not appear to be specific for any particular type of dementia (Blass et al. 1980). They occur in multi-infarct dementias, Alzheimer type dementias, as well as in toxic and deficiency states associated with dementias (Blass 1980; Blass et al. 1980).

The modifications in neurotransmitter enzymes and other biochemical markers probably indicate a vulnerability of particular type of cells in the aging of the brain and in dementias, but they do not tell why and how the cells die.

Recently some studies have indicated modifications in activities of enzymes of carbohydrate energy metabolism in Alzheimer type and other dementias. Two groups have observed a significant decrease of the pyruvate dehydrogenase complex activity in the affected areas of Alzheimer (Perry et al. 1980; Sorbi et al. 1983) and Huntington brain (Sorbi et al. 1983). In an extensive study Bowen and colleagues (1979) observed that 19 of 37 neuroconstituents examined were reduced in Alzheimer post-mortem brain. Among them the most marked decrease was in the activity of phosphofructokinase (PFK), a key enzyme in glycolysis that may be the rate limiting enzyme in cerebral glucose utilization (Lowrey and Passanneau 1964). Iwangoff et colleagues (1980) have also reported declines of PFK activity with age and a marked decrease (90% of age matched control values) in Alzheimer cerebral cortex. The abnormality in PFK observed in post-mortem brain seems to be present and persist in cultured skin fibroblasts from some Alzheimer patients even after several passages (Sorbi and Blass 1983). Studies on cultured skin fibroblasts have also shown abnormalities in PDHC and PFK activities in C-21 trisomy Down patients (Sorbi et al. 1983; Sorbi and Blass 1983) who are at very high risk to develop Alzheimer changes in the brain if they live long enough. Modifications in glucose metabolism in the brain have been also observed by positron emission tomography and ^{18}F-labeled 2-deoxy-D-glucose in C-21 trisomy Down Syndrome (Schwartz et al. 1983).

These findings of deficient activities of carbohydrate energy metabolism related enzymes in post-mortem brain and in skin cultured fibroblasts from Alzheimer patients are of particular interest since even mild impairement of carbohydrate oxidation impairs cognitive functions (Blass et al. 1980; Gibson et al. 1981). Cholinergic system and other neuronal systems have been shown to be impaired as well by impairements of glucose utilization (Ksiezak and Gibson 1981, Gibson et al. 1981).

Several data suggest that the two set of alterations which are related of aging of the brain and dementias - abnormalities in cerebral oxidative metabolism and abnormalities in neurotransmitter systems - may be linked mechanistically.

The nervous system shows a marked dependance on glucose oxidation than does any other organ. Pyruvate derived from glucose is quantitatively the major oxidative substrate of brain and therefore the major source of electron for the electron transport chain. Recently it has been reported (Magilen et al. 1981; Morgan and Routtenberg 1980; Browing et al. 1981) that the phosphorilation state of a 41,000 dalton α- peptide of PDHC plays an important role in synaptic plasticity and that its phosphorilation pitch changes with training or habituation. PDHC is a critical enzymes complex for carbohydrate oxidation, present in minimal excess in human brain (Sorbi et al. 1983) and closely related to neurotransmitters metabolism. PDHC is the major source of the acetyl group of acetyl choline (Blass et al. 1980; Tucek 1978). A close correlation between CAT and PDHC activities in human brain has been reported by Perry and colleagues (1980) and Sorbi and colleagues (1983). Indeed, cholinergic system appears to be extremely sensitive to conditions which impair pyruvate oxidation, and the resulting deficits in acetylcholine synthesis seem to be functionally important (Gibson et al. 1981). Thus even mild reduction of PDHC in cholinergic neurons can reduce the synthesis of their major neurotransmitter and perhaps their ability to repair and renew their membranes and other cellular constituents.

The finding of a marked decrease of the glycolitic key enzyme PFK in autopsy brain from

Alzheimer (Bowen et al. 1979; Iwangoff et al. 1980) and Huntington (Bird et al. 1977) patients and of a small but significant decrease of PFK in cultured skin fibroblasts from some patients with Alzheimer type dementia (Sorbi and Blass 1983) agrees whith the suggestion that impairements of the intrinsic oxidative machinary of the brain are involved in the pathophysiology of dementias. Indeed, deficiencies of several other glycolitic and oxidative markers have been found in Alzheimer brain (Bowen et al. 1979).

Impairement of oxidative metabolism severe enough to reduce ATP levels kills neurons (Pusinelli et al. 1981), and it is reasonable that insults which impair the oxidation of glucose would lead to more or less widespread abnormality in function of nerve cells. It has been proposed (Lassen 1957) that the decreases in cerebral blood flow, glucose utilization, and oxygen consumption, common to many dementias result from abnormalities of brain structure with a high oxidative capacity. The observed abnormalities in PDHC, PFK and other oxidative and glycolitic markers agree with that suggestion.

Adolfsson R, Gottfries CG, Roos BE, Winblad B (1979). Changes in brain catecholamines in patients with dementia of the Alzheimer type. Br J Psychiatry 135:216.

Amaducci L, Bracco L, Sorbi S (1982). Dementia as a primarily subcortical disease. In Terry RD, Bolis CL, Toffano G (Eds):"Neuronal Aging and its Implications in Human Neurological Disease", New York: Raven Press, p143.

Amaducci L, Bracco L, Sorbi S (1983). Cholinergic system and cognitive functions in man: A possible relationship. In Algeri S, Samuel D (Eds): "The Aging of the Brain", New York: Raven

Press, p 221.

Amaducci L, Bracco L, Sorbi S (1983). Energy metabolism and neurotransmitters in the aging brain. In Crepaldi G, Fellin R, Olsson AG, Toffano G (Eds):"Arteriosclerotic Brain Disease", New York; Raven Press, in press.

Antuono P, Sorbi S, Bracco L, Fusco T, Amaducci L (1980). A discrete sampling technique in senile dementia of the Alzheimer type and alcoholic dementia: Studies of the cholinergic system. In Amaducci L, Antuono P, Davison AN (Eds):"Aging of the Brain and Dementia", New York: Raven Press, p 151.

Bird ED, Iversen LL (1974). Huntington's chorea. Post-mortem measurements of glutamic acid decarboxylase, choline acetyltransferase and dopamine in basal ganglia. Brain 97:539.

Bird ED, Gale JS, Spokes EG (1977). Huntington's chorea: post-mortem activity of enzymes involved in cerebral glucose metabolism. J Neurochem 29:539.

Bird ED (1977). The clinical significance of disturbance in the central GABA system. In VanPraag HM, Bruinvels J (Eds):"Neurotransmission and Disturbed Behavior", Bohn: Utrecht, p 140.

Blass J (1980). Metabolic dementias. In Amaducci L, Antuono P, Davison AN (Eds):"Aging of the Brain and Dementia", New York: Raven Press, p 261.

Blass JP, Gibson GE, Shimada M, Kihara T, Watanaba M, Kurinioto K (1980). Brain carbohydrate metabolism and dementias. In Roberts PJ (Ed):"Biochemistry of Dementias", Boston: John Wiley and Sons Ltd, p 121.

Bondareff W, Mountjoy CQ, Roth M (1981). Selective loss of neurons of origin of adrenergic projection to cerebral cortex (nucleus locus coeruleus) in senile dementia. Lancet 1:783.

Bowen DM, Smith AB, White P, Davison AN (1976). Neurotransmitter related enzymes and indeces of hypoxia in senile dementia and other abiotrophies. Brain 99:459.

Bowen DM, White P, Spillane JA, Goodhart MJ, Curzon G, Iwangoff P, Mayer-Ruge W, Davison AN (1970). Accelerated aging or selective neuronal loss as an important cause of dementia? Lancet 1:11.

Browing M, Pondy M, Benet W et al. (1981). Phosphorilation changes in pyruvate dehydrogenase activity influence pyruvate-supported calcium accumulation by brain mitochondria. J Neurochem 36:1932.

Davies P, Maloney AJF (1976). Selective loss of central cholinergic neurons in Alzheimer's disease. Lancet 2:1403.

Davies P, Terry RD (1981). Cortical somatostatin-like immunoreactivity in cases of Alzheimer's disease and senile dementia of the Alzheimer type. Neurobiol Aging 2:9.

Gibson GE, Pulsinell WA, Blass JP, Duffy TE (1981). Brain dysfunction in mild to moderate hypoxia. Amer J Med 70:1247.

Gibson GE, Peterson C, Sansone J (1981). Decrease in amino acid and acetylcholine metabolism during hypoxia. J Neurochem 37:192.

Iwangoff P, Armbruster R, Enz A, Mayer-Ruge W (1980). Glycolitic enzymes from human autopsy brain cortex: normal aged and demented cases. Mech Ageing Dev 14:203.

Ksiezak H, Gibson GE (1981). Oxygen dependance of glucose and acetylcholine metabolism in slices and synaptosomes from rat brain. J Neurochem 37:305.

Lassen NA, Munck O, Tottey ER (1957). Mental

function and cerebral oxygen consumption in organic dementia. Arch Neurol Psychiat 77:126.

Lowrey OH, Passanneau J (1964). The relations between substrates and enzymes of glycolisis in brain. J Biol Chem 139:31.

Magilen DG, Gordon A, Au A et al. (1981). Identification of a mitochondrial phosphorilation in brain synaptic membrane preparations. J Neurochem 36:1861.

Morgan DG, Routtenberg (1980). Evidence that a 41,000 dalton brain phosphoprotein is Pyruvate dehydrogenase. Biochem Biophys Res Comm 95:569.

Perry EK, Tomlinson BE, Blassed G, Bergman K, Gibson PH, Perry RH (1978). Correlation of cholinergic abnormalities with senile plaques and mental test scores in senile dementia. Br Med J 2:1457.

Perry EK, Perry RH, Tomlinson BE, Blessed G, Gibson PH (1980). Coenzyme A acetylating enzymes in Alzheimer's disease: Possible cholinergic "compartments" of pyruvate dehydrogenase. Neurosci Lett 18:105.

Pulsinelli W, Brierly J, Duffy T, Levy D, Plum F (1981). J CBF Metab 1:166.

Quastel JH (1932). Biochemistry and mental disorders. Lancet 2:1417.

Schwartz M, Duara R, Haxby J, Grady C, White BJ, Kessler RM, Kay AD, Cutler NR, Rapaport SI (1983). Down's syndrome in adults: Brain metabolism. Lancet 2:781.

Sims NR, Bowen DM, Davison AN (1982). Acetylcholine syntesis and glucose metabolism in aging and dementia. In Giacobini E (Ed):"The Aging Brain: Cellular and Molecular Mechanisms of Aging in the Nervous System", New York: Raven Press, p 153.

Sokoloff L (1966). Cerebral circulatory and metabolic changes associated with aging. Res

Publ Assoc Res Nerv Mental Dis 41:237.

Sorbi S, Amaducci L (1979). Is dementia primarily a subcortical disease? Riv Pat Nerv Mental 100:200.

Sorbi S, Antuono P, Amaducci L (1980). Choline acetyltransferase and acetylcholinesterase abnormalities in senile dementia: importance of biochemical measurements in human post-mortem brain specimens. Ital J Neurol Sci 2:75.

Sorbi S, Amaducci L (1980). Enzymatic changes in Creutzfeldt-Jakob disease. Arch Sui Neurol Neuroch Psych 127:253.

Sorbi S, Amaducci L, Blass JP, Bird ED (1982). Pyruvate dehydrogenase complex and choline acetyltransferase in aging and dementia. In Giacobini E (Ed):"The Aging Brain: Cellular and Molecular Mechanisms of Aging in the Nervous System", New York:Raven Press, p 223.

Sorbi S, Bird ED, Blass JP (1983). Decreased pyruvate dehydrogenase in Huntington and Alzheimer brain. Ann Neurol 13:72.

Sorbi S, Blass JP (1983). Fibroblasts phosphofructokinase in Alzheimer's disease and Down's syndrome. Banbury Rep 15:297.

Tucek S (1978). Acetylcholine Synthesis in Neurons. London: Chapman and Hall.

Whitehouse PJ, Clark AW, Coyle JT, De long MR, (1982). Alzheimer's disease and senile dementia: loss of neurons in the basal forebrain. Science 215:1237.

Senile Dementia: Outlook for the Future, pages 31–54

TRANSMISSION OF UNCONVENTIONAL SLOW VIRUS DISEASES AND THE RELEVANCE TO AD/SDAT TRANSMISSION STUDIES

Richard I. Carp, V.M.D., Ph.D.
George S. Merz, Ph.D.
Henryk M. Wisniewski, M.D., Ph.D.

N.Y.S. Institute for Basic Research in Developmental Disabilities
Staten Island, NY 10314

INTRODUCTION

The cause of Alzheimer's disease and senile dementia of the Alzheimer's type (AD/SDAT) remains unknown. One suggestion has been that AD/SDAT is a transmissible disease caused by an infectious agent, probably a virus, specifically an unconventional virus similar to those that cause some slow infections. In the following report we analyze a number of critical issues relating to this possibility. In the first section, we detail the similarities between AD/SDAT and the known human infectious diseases caused by unconventional viruses and suggest that the commonality of characteristics points to a similar cause. In the second section, the most thoroughly studied unconventional slow infectious disease, scrapie is described. Its relevance as a model for AD/SDAT is outlined with special emphasis on the genetically controlled differences in histopathological manifestations; these differences span the spectrum of histopathological changes seen in both the known (Kuru, Creutzfeldt-Jakob disease (CJD)) and some of the putative unconventional slow infections of man (e.g., AD/SDAT). In the third section we note that transmission of known unconventional slow infections to a new species often occurs with low incidence on initial passage and that in a number of instances, animals will fail to show any clinical disease but will have other manifestations of the disease process (e.g., typical histopathological changes in brain). Also in this section the limited extent of past attempts at AD/SDAT transmission in non-primate hosts is noted. In the fourth section, we describe problems that have arisen in transmission studies with known and putative unconventional slow infections. These problems relate to either unreproducible readings of a specific parameter or potential cross-contamination. The fifth section poses the question of the laboratory setting in which transmission studies should be done: Should it be a laboratory with experience in studying slow infection processes or a "naive" setting? The advantages and disadvantages of both surroundings are outlined. In the last section we suggest guidelines for AD/SDAT transmission studies with stress on three points: (1) Exclusion of cross-contamination; (2) Biohazard considerations and (3) A suggested protocol to insure both unbiased evaluation of results and absence of cross-contamination.

I. A RATIONALE FOR DOING TRANSMISSION IN AD/SDAT

The concept of slow infections was introduced by Sigurdsson in 1954 to characterize a group of diseases that occur in sheep. Two of the criteria that he established have stood the test of time: (1) A long incubation period between exposure to the virus and the beginning of clinical manifestations and (2) A protracted clinical course, usually ending in serious illness and death. In the context of AD/SDAT transmission studies, diseases caused by the unconventional agents are of particular interest. This group includes two well characterized animal diseases (scrapie, found naturally in sheep and goats, and transmissible mink encephalopathy (TME) and two known human diseases (Kuru and CJD)). There are a number of parameters which place these diseases into a common group:

A. The Characteristics of the Agents

Each disease is caused by agents that have unusual characteristics which include remarkable resistance to a number of physical and chemical treatments that inactivate most viruses, the failure of the agents to elicit any immune responses, and the inability to purify or even visualize the agents (Gajdusek 1977).

B. Clinical Features

Kuru is a chronic degenerative disease characterized by cerebellar ataxia with tremors that progress to incapacity and death. Initially there are changes in mood, with depression and periodic hyperexcitibility (Hornabrook 1979). Episodes of confusion occur. For CJD clinical signs vary but dementia, myoclonus, extra-pyramidal and pyramidal tract signs, and characteristic periodic EEG abnormalities have been reported (Brown et al 1979). Recently it was found that a similar disease called Gerstmann-Straussler Syndrome (GSS) characterized by ataxia and dementia is also caused by a transmissible unconventional agent (Masters et al 1981). For scrapie in sheep the characteristic changes are scraping and rubbing the skin, with hyperexcitibility or stupor and incoordination of gait (Stamp 1962). Although dementia is difficult to characterize in lower animals, behavioral changes are an early finding in mice injected with mouse passaged scrapie. The changes include increased times of emergence from a box, reduced activity levels, altered open field and Y-maze exploration (Heitzman, Corp 1968; McFarland et al 1980; Suckling et al 1976). It is interesting that scratching and rubbing the skin are features of scrapie in the natural host, sheep, but these signs are not apparent in experimental hosts. The earliest clinical signs in TME are behavioral, indicative of mental confusion. For example, instinctively normal habits of cleanliness disappear and an aimless circling occurs (Marsh 1976). Ataxia develops and then as the disease progresses, the animals become progressively more somnolent.

C. Histopathological Analysis

All of these diseases are characterized by an absence of inflammatory responses (Carp, Thormar 1976; Gajdusek 1977; Marsh 1976). Three of the most common changes seen are vacuolation, neuronal loss, and gliosis. There is considerable variation with regard to intensity and distribution of vacuolation (Beck, Daniel 1979; Dickinson et al 1983). In fact, there are natural and experimental examples in which there is virtually no vacuolation despite clinical disease (Dickinson et al 1983; Marsh et al 1976). Another lesion which shows differences in incidence is plaque formation of either the amyloid or neuritic types (Fraser, Bruce 1973). From the data on scrapie it would appear that there are genetic components involving both host and agent which control the development of vacuolation and plaques (Fraser, Bruce 1973; Dickinson, Fraser 1979).

In humans with Kuru, vacuolar changes are common in the

cerebellum but rare in the cerebrum. Plaques of the amyloid or "burned out" type are common and are referred to as Kuru plaques. With CJD, vacuolation in the cortex is more common than in the cerebellum, and plaques are rarely seen. For TME, vacuolation is common in the cerebral cortex, but rare in the cerebellum (Marsh 1976). Plaques have not been reported in TME. For scrapie, the intensity of vacuolation seen in various areas of the brain differs in different scrapie agent-mouse strain combinations (see later section). The presence of amyloid and neuritic plaques is also under genetic control with combinations either having no detectable plaques, having a few plaques, or having many plaques. Both plaques and vacuolation have been seen in the natural disease in sheep although there are instances in sheep in which there is virtually no vacuolation (Beck, Daniel 1965; Dickinson et al 1983).

The Gerstmann-Straussler syndrome (GSS) is a familial chronic cerebellar ataxia with dementia (Masters et al 1981). Recently, some cases with prominant vacuolation have been shown to be caused by the CJD agent (Masters et al 1981). Vacuolation was reported in 11 of 17 cases and white matter loss or degeneration in 13 of the cases. Amyloid plaques were a consistent finding and these plaques usually had an appearance similar to that of the Kuru plaque, although plaques with surrounding degenerating and dystrophic neuritic, glial and microglial reaction are also seen. This latter type is referred to as a neuritic or senile plaque and it is characteristic of AD/SDAT.

A number of other parameters (see Table 1) have been analyzed in these diseases: (1) neuronal loss is seen sporadically in each of the four diseases; (2) reductions in choline acetyltransferase have been reported in scrapie and CJD (McDermott et al 1973; Sorbi et al 1981); (3) aberrant fibrillar structures (scrapie associated fibrils - SAF) (Merz et al 1981) have been detected in scrapie, GSS and CJD, and (4) cell fusion is induced when homogenates of brain from scrapie, CJD or Kuru are added to cells in culture (Brown et al 1982; Gajdusek, Gibbs 1982).

Table 1

Comparison of AD/SDAT with Known Transmissible Encephalopathies

Parameter	Kuru	GSS	CJD	TME	Scrapie	AD/SDAT
Vacuolation	Most	Some	Most	Most	Most	Occasional
Gliosis	Yes	Yes	Yes	Yes	Yes	Yes
Neuronal Loss	Yes	Yes	Yes	Yes	Varies[d]	Yes
Amyloid Plaques	Most	All	Few	None	Varies[d]	All
Aberrant Fibrils	N.D.[b]	SAF[c]	SAF	N.D.	SAF	PHF[e]
Decrease in CAT[a]	N.D.	N.D.	Yes	N.D.	Yes, slight	Yes
Cell Fusion	Yes	N.D.	Yes	N.D.	Yes	Yes-Familial
Primary Transmission	Yes	Yes	Yes	Yes	Yes	?

a) Choline acetyltransferase

b) N.D. = ot done

c) Scrapie associated fibrils

d) Variation is genetically controlled

e) Paired helical filaments

The question that then arises is: What is the relationship of the characteristics of AD/SDAT to those seen in the known transmissible encephalopathies (Brown et al 1982c)? Clinically, AD/SDAT is characterized by progressive loss of cognitive function through a chronic course. There is myoclonus and periodic EEG aberrations but at a lower incidence than is seen in CJD. Late in the disease, movements become stereotyped and an extrapyramidal type of rigidity occurs. Since there are a number of characteristics shared with regard to the symptomatology and clinical course between CJD and AD/SDAT, it is frequently difficult to differentiate the two diseases on this basis (Brown et al 1982c).

As pointed out by Brown et al. (1982c) there are other specific similarities between CJD and AD/SDAT: similar age at onset distribution curves, overlapping duration of illness, familial occurrence in 10-15% of cases, males and females equally affected, coexistence of AD/SDAT and CJD within families and perhaps in the same individual and, lastly, conjugal occurrence.

In Table 1 data obtained in analysis of a number of parameters in AD/SDAT are compared with data obtained for the known unconventional virus encephalopathies. In all of these diseases histopathological changes are found only in the CNS. The key pathological findings in AD/SDAT are amyloid plaques, gliosis, neuronal loss and aberrant fibrillar structures termed paired helical filaments (Wisniewski, Terry 1976). Vacuolation is seen occasionally. There is a decrease in choline acetyltransferase activity and CNS homogenates from familial AD/SDAT cause cell fusion (Davies, Maloney 1976; Brown et al 1982c). The presence of amyloid plaques is of special significance. Amyloid accumulations in the form of plaques in the CNS are infrequently seen and sparsely distributed in apparently normal aged humans and animals but consistently observed in abundant quantities in AD/SDAT. The only other examples of CNS plaque formation are the consequence of infection with unconventional slow viruses (Kuru, CJD, GSS and scrapie). Furthermore, evidence has been obtained by two approaches which indicates that in scrapie, plaque formation is directly related to agent concentration (Bruce, Fraser 1981; Wisniewski et al 1981). At the conclusion of an article in which Brown et al. (1982c) detailed (1) the similarities between AD/SDAT and slow virus encephalopathies and (2) the failure to transmit AD/SDAT to primates, they stated that:

"Ample justification exists on clinical, pathological, and biological grounds for considering a similar pathogenesis for AD and the spongiform virus encephalopathies"

II. SCRAPIE AS A MODEL SYSTEM

Despite the diversity of histopathological manifestations of plaques and vacuolation seen in the human unconventional virus encephalopathies and in AD/SDAT, various scrapie agent-host combinations can serve as models for different aspects of these diseases. The differences seen in these combinations are genetically controlled. Initial findings centered on incubation period (Dickinson, Meikle 1971). The mouse gene Sinc (an acronym for scrapie incubation) controls this parameter and was originally identified by comparison of incubation periods of the scrapie strain ME7 (Dickinson, Meikle 1971). Most mouse strains are s7s7 (short incubation for ME7) but there are three mouse strains that are p7p7 (prolonged incubation for ME7) (Table 2). These three strains are called VM, IM and MB. In contrast to ME7, certain scrapie strains, such as 22A and 87V, have longer incubation periods in s7s7 strains than in p7p7 strains (Table 2). Differences in histopathological lesions are also genetically controlled. Fraser and Dickinson have

Table 2

Incubation Periods in Days and Presence of Plaques for Three Standard Scrapie Strains in C57Bl and VM Mice[a]

	Mouse Strain			
	C57BL (s7s7)		VM (p7p7)	
Scrapie Strain	Incubation Period	Plaques	Incubation Period	Plaques
ME7	153	No	300	Yes
22A	381	Yes	180	No
87V	420[b]	Yes[b]	300	Yes

[a] Injected IC with a 1% brain homogenate. Brains were obtained from mice showing clinical signs of scrapie.

[b] Data from Dr. Alan Dickinson

monitored the extent of vacuolation in nine areas of the brain which included: medulla, cerebellum, midbrain, hypothalamus, thalamus, hippocampus, paraterminal body, posterior mid-line cerebral cortex (Fraser 1979; Fraser, Dickinson 1973). In this fashion they have established lesion profiles for different scrapie agent-mouse strain combinations. These lesion profiles are sufficiently reproducible so that they function as a "signature" for the particular agent-strain combination. Agent-strain combinations also differed in the extent of amyloid plaque formation with some combinations yielding many plaques, others few, and still others none (Table 2) (Bruce, Fraser 1981; Dickinson, Fraser 1979; Fraser, Bruce 1973; Wisniewski et al 1981). The extent of genetically controlled differences in scrapie is expanding as we look at more parameters and at more agent-strain combinations. An example of the latter is shown in Table 3 in which scrapie incubation periods for a number of additional mouse strains following ME7 and 22A injection have been analyzed. All of these mouse strains are classified as s7s7 (Table 3). Special note should be taken of the ME7-SJL/J combination because this yields a considerably shorter (20-45 days) incubation period than is seen with other s7s7 strains. Another point of interest is that amyloid plaque

Table 3

Incubation Periods in Days and Plaque Formation for ME7 and 22A in Various Mouse Strains[a]

	No.	ME7 Mean±SE[b]	No.	22A Mean±SE	Plaques ME7	Plaques 22A
NZW ♂	15	158±2	15	422± 5	-	-
♀	6	164±3	4	396±15	-	-
NZB ♂	8	167±4	8	458±31	-	-
CBA/J ♀	12	167±3	6	384± 9	+[c]	+[c]
SJL/J ♀	10	123±2	5	379±14	N.D.[d]	N.D.

a) Injected IC with a 1% brain homogenate. Brains were obtained from mice showing clinical signs of scrapie

b) SE = Standard error

c) For the ME7-CBA/J combination 25% of the mice had plaques and for the 22A-CBA/J combination 100% had plaques

d) N.D. = Not done

formation is observed in a proportion (25%) of ME7-CBA/J mice. In our experience this is the shortest incubation period that yields plaques in that high a proportion of animals. Another parameter that is under genetic control is the increase in weight seen in certain agent-strain combinations in the preclinical phase of disease. Some agent-strain combinations show the weight increase, whereas the weight for mice in other agent-strain combinations during the preclinical phase was similar to that of normal mouse brain injected mice (Carp et al 1982).

Differences in histopathological manifestations are seen also in scrapie sheep and in primary isolates of sheep material in mice (Fraser 1983). In some sheep, vacuolation is prevalent, whereas in others there are virtually no spongiform changes (Dickinson et al 1983). Likewise in primary isolation in mice, in those animals with histopathological changes, it has been shown that brains from some mice develop vacuolation without plaques, others develop plaques without vacuolation, and still others are characterized by both plaques and vacuolation (Frazer 1983).

To conclude, the genetically controlled differences in histopathological manifestations seen in various scrapie agent-host combinations can encompass the full range of vacuolar and amyloid changes seen in the known human slow encephalopathies and in AD/SDAT.

III. A BRIEF HISTORY OF TRANSMISSION OF THE KNOWN SLOW VIRUS ENCEPHALOPATHIES AND WHAT HAS BEEN DONE WITH AD/SDAT

There are a number of assumptions that have arisen concerning the transmission of slow encephalopathies. In 1959, Hadlow, after observing the histopathological similarity between scrapie and Kuru, suggested that if infectivity studies were to be done with Kuru, animals should remain under observation for a long time (Hadlow 1959). Gajdusek and his colleagues subsequently demonstrated that there was an infectious agent in Kuru by reproducing a disease with similar clinical and histopathological characteristics in chimpanzees following an incubation period of 20 months (Gajdusek et al 1966). This was followed by the same group's success with material from CJD patients (Gibbs et al 1968). A few years prior to this, the scrapie agent of sheep and goats had been transmitted to mice and later to other small laboratory animals (Chandler 1963).

Further effort with these two human encephalopathies led to transmission in a variety of primate and non-primate species (Gajdusek 1977). The variety of susceptible hosts and the ease of working with the agents once they have been passaged in the experimental host has led to the first unwarranted assumption: that these agents can readily be transmitted to new hosts. In fact, not all histopathologically verified Kuru, CJD and scrapie cases have been passaged (Brown et al 1982; Dickinson et al 1983; Fraser 1983). Furthermore, for those transmitted cases of scrapie, not all injected animals develop histopathological changes, and an even lower proportion of animals develop clinical scrapie (Fraser 1983). The data shown in Table 4 summarizes the attempts of Fraser to transmit scrapie from the natural disease in Icelandic sheep to mice. In this study, 1 of 5 brain

Table 4

Primary Passage of Icelandic Sheep Scrapie into Mice[a]

	Histopathol. changes indicating transmission[b]	No Histopathol. changes[c]
Neurological signs	17[d]	26(?)[e]
No neurological signs	32	318

[a] Data were adapted from publication by Fraser (1983)

[b] Mice were killed between 372-971 days post injection

[c] Mice were killed between 164 and 1103 days post injection

[d] Number of mice

[e] Neurological signs were not typical of scrapie and probably represent "normal" senile changes

homogenates from sheep failed to cause disease in mice. For the five homogenates, 694 mice were injected into a variety of strains including both s7s7 and p7p7 genotypes. Of these mice 393 brains were suitable for histopathological examination (despite daily observation, 301 mice were found dead, their brains unsuitable for examination). Of the 393 remaining mice, 26 showed neurological signs, but histopathological examination failed to confirm a scrapie diagnosis. The neurological signs noted in these animals were probably those associated with the onset of senility. For 318 mice there was no evidence of scrapie on the basis of either clinical or histopathological criteria. Only 17 of the 393 mice showed both clinical and histopathological evidence of scrapie. An additional 32 mice showed histopathological changes indicative of scrapie but without any of the clinical signs of the disease. For one of the sheep brain homogenates used, only 1 of 86 injected mice showed evidence of scrapie and for another homogenate only 5 of 75 mice were positive. Histopathological analyses showed mice with plaques but not vacuolation, mice with vacuolation but no plaques and mice with both. In general, the p7p7 mouse strains showed a higher incidence of positive results.

These data highlight the difficulty of crossing a species barrier with a slow virus encephalopathy, point to the importance of using many animals in the search for agents and emphasize the value of using animals which can show a full spectrum of lesions. Another point that this study demonstrates is that upon primary transmission, animals may fail to show clinical disease during their lifetime, but "silent," i.e., subclinical, changes will be detectable. Similar findings have been reported for transmission of CJD to mice (Gajdusek, Gibbs 1982). In crossing the species barrier, incubation periods may exceed the life of the host. In searching for silent changes during primary transmission, the logical choice of parameters to be examined are those that are known to have the potential for change in the preclinical phase of the disease, e.g., formation of amyloid plaques, changes in blood-brain barrier (Wisniewski et al 1983), appearance of aberrant fibrils (SAF) (Merz et al 1981) and behavioral changes (Heitzman, Corp 1968; McFarland et al 1980; Suckling et al 1976). It should be noted that with the exception of amyloid plaques these parameters have been examined only with passaged agent and not on primary transmission. If the agent can replicate in the new host species, then on subsequent passages in the new host, one would predict either the development of clinical disease during the life of the animal or an increase in intensity and incidence of the change noted on primary transmission. In the cases noted above for scrapie and CJD, subsequent passages of material from mice showing histopathological changes only led to clinical disease (Fraser 1983; Gajdusek, Gibbs 1982). The increase in permeability of the blood-brain barrier seen in scrapie provides us with an important "silent" marker, since there is also evidence of similar blood-brain barrier changes in AD/SDAT (Wisniewski, Kozlowski 1982). This similarity may point to a common pathogenic mechanism.

Another assumption that has become generalized is that non-human primates are the most sensitive monitor of transmission of human slow encephalopathy diseases. The early failure to transmit Kuru to a variety of small laboratory animals, followed by success with chimpanzees and the subsequent success with other primates has led to this conclusion. In recent years, transmission of CJD to guinea pigs by the Manuelidis group and to mice by the Tateishi group have been achieved with a high rate of success (Manuelidis 1975; Tateishi et al 1981a; 1981b). Homogenates from many of the Kuru and CJD cases investigated by the NIH group have been injected into a variety of non-primate laboratory animals, e.g., guinea pigs, cats and mice. The highest rate of positive transmission occurred with primates (Brown, personal communication). In an exception to this rule, Tateishi et al (1981b) found that for one of their CJD isolates small laboratory animals were at least as susceptible as primates (Table 5). The limited number of animals injected certainly leads to a cautious appraisal of this data, however, it suggests that CJD strains vary in their capacity to cause disease in different species on primary passage. There is a hamster passaged scrapie strain, the 263K agent, which causes diseases in hamsters within 60-70 days, but fails to cause disease in mice even after two years (Kimberlin, Walker 1978). This finding points to the existence of transmissible encephalopathy agents which have a very selective host range.

Table 5

Comparative Data on Injection of Different Species with a Single CJD Brain Homogenate[a]

Species	No. Sick/No. Injected	Incubation Period in Days
Mice	2/3	320
Rats	11/13	406
Guinea Pigs	1/1	652
Squirrel Monkeys	1/1	799

[a] Data were adapted from publication by Tateishi et al (1981b)

From the above data it is clear that strains of unconventional slow viruses do not readily cross species barriers and that primates may not provide the best experimental host for a putative unconventional infectious agent from AD/SDAT. The only reported large systematic study of AD/SDAT has centered on primates (Brown et al 1982). In this work preparations from 54 cases have been injected into primates, with a few animals used per each case. The precise number of animals injected for these 54 cases has not been published at this time, however for the first 17 cases a total of 32 injected animals were tested for a sufficiently long time to be classified as negative (Goudsmit et al 1980). A transmission attempt was termed negative when the time post injection exceeded by two standard deviations the mean incubation period for CJD on primary passage in that species. Two of the 54 cases have transmitted, but there are questions concerning these results which will be explored in the next section. All other cases yielded negative results. In addition to primates, AD/SDAT brain material has been injected into more than 100 guinea pigs, as well as a few goats and cats (Brown, personal communication). None of these animals have shown clinical disease at this time.

Clearly, if primates are not the appropriate species for passage of the AD/SDAT putative agent or if a large number of animals must be injected with material from each case to provide the statistical chance for a positive transmission, then much more work with different species and modified protocols (e.g., injecting larger numbers of animals per case, increasing susceptibility of hosts, using partially purified PHF or amyloid plaques as inoculum) should be attempted.

IV. PREVIOUS PROBLEMS IN TRANSMISSION STUDIES WITH KNOWN AND PUTATIVE SLOW INFECTION DISEASES

There have been two types of problems that have arisen in transmission studies. In the first instance, difficulties in the analysis of the parameters studied gave rise to unreproducible results. This situation occurred in our attempts to transmit an agent from multiple sclerosis (MS) material (Carp et al 1972). Initially, parameters examined in this study included a wide variety of physiological and biochemical markers. Positive results were obtained in that reductions in polymorphonuclear neutrophils (PMN) were seen in both MS and scrapie injected mice but not in controls (Carp et al 1972; Licursi et al 1972). This finding was confirmed in another laboratory studying MS (where scrapie was not studied) and in a third laboratory for scrapie (where MS was not studied) (Koldovsky et al 1975; Dickinson et al 1974). The scrapie study (Dickinson et al 1974) was done double blind and the assay of blood smears performed by a member of our unit. In the above studies, the effect was noted with most MS and scrapie cases and in a large proportion of the injected animals, so that the effect was not due to a rare, putative contaminating event. However, subsequent studies from a number of laboratories and from our own failed to confirm the initial results (Brown, Gajdusek 1974; Madden et al 1977). Our difficulties with this test and the problems encountered by others have been detailed in a joint paper published by our group and the Henle group (Carp et al 1977). In this, we stated that because of the unreproducible nature of the test system, further work with the PMN change as a measure of MS transmission was not warranted. No explanation for the initial results was available then, nor is it today. This experience points to the danger of relying on a single parameter as a measure of transmission, particularly one that is not a subclinical or clinical manifestation of the disease being transmitted. It also emphasizes the importance of having a finding repeated in many laboratories.

A second source of difficulty has arisen in transmission studies because of possible cross-contamination with known slow infectious agents. In work reported by Palsson et al. in Icelandic sheep and by Field in mice, two cases of MS were said to transmit to these animals, causing a scrapie like syndrome and vacuolar changes (Field 1966; Palsson et al 1965). These results could not be repeated with a large number of other cases of MS (Carp et al 1972; H. Koprowski, personal communication). The consensus is that these original findings were related to contamination with scrapie but the precise source cannot be documented by the investigators involved. Some have suggested that the material used for the Icelandic injections was stored for a time in Great Britain in a freezer containing scrapie and that cross-contamination with scrapie could have occurred at that point. For the second case (Field 1966), the material was obtained during a stereotactic operation being performed to relieve unilateral tremors. Subsequent findings in another laboratory have detailed how improperly sterilized (for CJD agent) electrodes implanted stereotactically as a treatment for epilepsy led to the transmission of CJD from person to person (Bernoulli et al 1977). It is possible that the material obtained by Professor Field from the MS patient had already been contaminated by CJD during the surgical procedure used to secure the material.

In another study, transmission of familial AD/SDAT was reported in two instances (Gibbs, Gajdusek 1980). In a review of the situation involving these two cases, Brown et al. (1982c) noted that in one case repeated follow-up experiments with the same material have failed to confirm the original finding and that laboratory contamination cannot be ruled out. In addition to primates, the follow-up protocol included injection of two cats, two goats and seven guinea pigs (Brown, personal communication). For the second case biopsy material was used and two primates developed a spongiform encephalopathy typical of CJD. A new suspension prepared from the original biopsy material failed to cause disease in three primates. Autopsy material from this case has recently been set aside for further transmission studies. Therefore, this case is open, at the moment, with regard to potential transmission. It should be noted that these authors describe another 10 familial and 42 sporadic cases which have been classified as negative for transmission in primates.

V. IN WHAT LABORATORY SETTING SHOULD TRANSMISSION BE DONE?

There is a question of the most appropropriate place for AD/SDAT transmission studies. Should the work be done in a "naive" laboratory setting in which there has never been work on unconventional slow infections or one in which these infectious processes have been studied? The advantage of the "naive" laboratory is that the chance for contaminating infection with an unconventional agent is reduced. The disadvantage is that these laboratories would lack experience in handling and diagnosing potential transmissions. It should be pointed out that several of the reported transmissions of putative slow viral infections which were not subsequently reproduced were from "naive" laboratories (Field 1966; Koldovsky et al 1975). If the concept that an AD/SDAT infectious process is analogous to that observed with known unconventional agents is correct, then experience with these slow viral infections would be advantageous. This experience is particularly important if the changes expected in a successful primary transmission would involve "silent" or subclinical changes rather than clinical disease and death. Further, the researchers involved in analyses of slow infection processes have experience with long-term projects and are familiar with the procedures of biological containment. The retention of large quantities of material from each case ensures that positive transmission findings can be validated by repeated testing. The disadvantage of the work being done by a research team with demonstrated experience with slow infections is the possibility of contamination with an unconventional agent already being studied. This possibility can be virtually eliminated by the procedures noted in the following section.

VI. PRACTICAL GUIDELINES FOR AD/SDAT TRANSMISSION STUDIES

A. Exclusion of Known Slow Viruses

As indicated above we see no compelling reason why AD/SDAT transmission studies should be precluded by the existence of ongoing studies with other unconventional slow viruses (e.g., scrapie) in the same institution provided that the following criteria are met:

1. The area in which transmission studies are to be done (animal quarters and laboratories) should be physically separated from areas working with unconventional agents. Equipment, supplies and tissues, etc., that have been in an unconventional virus laboratory should not be permitted in this area.

2. Access to the area must be limited to those involved in the transmission studies. Lock and key or magnetic card system should be used. Those who are required to enter the area should wear disposable masks, caps, gowns and boots.

3. The area should have its own means of decontaminating its waste as well as washing and sterilizing its own equipment and supplies.

4. All AD/SDAT and control tissues to be used in the transmission studies should be stored and prepared for injection within the area.

5. Animal caretakers and transmission laboratory technicians assigned to the transmission studies should have no other animal care or laboratory responsibilities.

B. Biohazard Considerations

The assumption of the presence of a slow virus in AD/SDAT tissue infers a potential biohazard risk that is difficult to estimate. A realistic precaution would be to regard the putative agent as a Class II infectious agent (as defined by the USPHS) with the added precaution that procedures which involve the manipulation of concentrated material or aerosols of putative agent (e.g., loading or unloading centrifuge tubes containing brain fractions, sonication of brain tissue, etc.) should be confined to Type II biosafety cabinets. For a more rigorous discussion of the biosafety issue see Chatigny and Prusiner (1980).

C. Suggested Transmission Protocol

1. Prior to use, autopsy instruments should be decontaminated and sterilized according to procedures used for unconventional viruses (Brown et al 1982a; 1982b; Dickinson, Taylor 1978). At autopsy the CNS tissue for transmission studies should be removed aseptically and placed in a sterile container. This should be placed inside a second container and sealed. The tissue sample should then be transported to the transmission laboratory, assigned a brain code number and stored at -70°C pending the histopathological evaluation of the brain and the rendering of a final diagnosis.

2. If the final diagnosis indicates that the brain is inappropriate for the study (e.g., presence of CNS disease other than AD/SDAT) the sealed container and its contents should be destroyed.

3. For those brains deemed appropriate, a portion should be removed, inocula prepared and treated as described in the following paragraphs. A large portion (at least 75%) of the material should be returned to the -70°C freezer. This portion will then be available so that any positive findings can be repeated with newly prepared brain homogenate from the same case.

4. Inocula should be prepared by the transmission laboratory technician and inoculated into animals supplied by the animal caretaker (Table 6). No more than one inoculum should be prepared on a given day. After each preparation, all reusable glassware, etc., should be appropriately sterilized and disposable material incinerated. (Note that disposable material should be used whenever possible.) The transmission laboratory technician should know only the brain's code number.

Table 6

Summary of the Levels of "Blinding"

Disinterested Third Party (e.g., Administrator, Chairman of another department)	:	Keeps the master list that relates diagnosis, brain code number and cage number of test animals.
Transmission Laboratory Technician	:	Knows the brain code number of each inocula.
Animal Caretaker	:	Knows the brain code number associated with each cage number.
Evaluator(s)	:	Knows the test results and the cage number of the animal. They do not know diagnosis or brain code number of the animals they evaluate.

5. The inoculated animals should be returned to the animal rooms by the animal caretaker. He should also assign a unique, randomly generated number to each cage. Finally, he should convey the cage number and brain code number to the third party (Table 6).

6. When animals are to be evaluated (e.g., biochemical, morphological and behavioral changes) the third party should inform the animal caretaker of the number of the cages to be evaluated.

7. The evaluators should evaluate each animal. The results of the evaluations should reside with the evaluators until it is decided to collate and correlate the results. The third party should not know any of the evaluator's findings until that time.

An important aspect of this research is to passage material from both positive and negative animals to more animals of the same species. For the negative animals this "blind passage" provides the possibility for augmentation of a change that was below detectability on first passage. For those animals that show an effect on first passage, subsequent passages will establish if that effect can pass from animal to animal. If a sufficient number of serial passages of the effect are successful, the presence of a replicating agent would be proven. In performing these animal to animal passages it is important that each inoculum be prepared independently of all others. Thus, a separate set of instruments, gloves, disposable bench paper, etc., should be used for each animal.

CONCLUSION

Evidence is presented to support the concept that AD/SDAT is a slow infection caused by a transmissible, unconventional agent. The fact that relatively little has been done to test this hypothesis in non-primate species, combined with the importance of this disease from an economic and public health standpoint, would certainly warrant an intensive effort to discover a possible infectious agent. The value of scrapie as a model system is stressed and the use of subclinical changes as an indication of primary transmission is emphasized. We present protocols aimed at: (1) Reducing the potential for cross-contamination with known unconventional slow infection agents and (2) Providing for unbiased analysis of data obtained.

Positive findings would have far reaching ramifications in the areas of public health and subsequent research strategies. For this reason it is extremely important that positive findings lead to a broad-based multi-laboratory attempt to reproduce findings with material from the same case.

ADDENDUM

The authors consulted with several neurovirologists and as a result of these discussions we would like to add the following: We are aware of other potential approaches in the search for an infectious agent in AD/SDAT. Tissue culture methods, including fusion of affected cells to indicator cell lines in order to potentiate agent maturation or replication, have not been used extensively in AD/SDAT research. Another approach would entail use of molecular probes obtained from known conventional viruses. These approaches must be viewed in the context of our hypothesis that AD/SDAT is caused by an agent with characteristics similar to those of the unconventional slow agents. Thus, if this hypothesis is correct there is little hope of a tissue culture approach proving effective in detecting an agent and there is no validity in searching for protein or nucleic acids of conventional viruses. Certainly, if probes were available for the known unconventional slow infection agents, their use in AD/SDAT would be strongly indicated.

ACKNOWLEDGMENT

The authors appreciate the helpful comments and criticisms of Dr. Paul Brown and Dr. Richard Johnson.

REFERENCES

Beck E, Daniel PM (1965) Kuru and scrapie compared: Are they examples of system degeneration? In Gajdusek DC, Gibbs CJ Jr, Alpers M (eds): "Slow, Latent, and Temperate Virus Infections," Washington: NINDB Monograph No. 2, Publication No. 1378, Public Health Service, pp 85-91.

Beck E, Daniel PM (1979) Kuru and Creutzfeldt-Jakob disease: Neuropathological lesions and their significance. In Prusiner SB, Hadlow WJ (eds): "Slow Transmissible Diseases of the Nervous System," New York: Academic Press, Vol. 1, pp 253-270.

Bernoulli C, Siegfried J, Baumgartner G, Regli F, Rabinowicz T, Gajdusek DC, Gibbs CJ (1977) Danger of accidental person-to-person transmission of Creutzfeldt-Jakob disease by surgery. Lancet I:478-479.
Brown P, Cathala F, Sadowsky D, Gajdusek DC (1979) Creutzfeldt-Jakob disease in France. II. Clinical characteristics of 124 consecutive verified cases during the decade 1968-1977. Ann Neurol 6:430-437.
Brown P, Gajdusek DC (1974) No mouse PMN leukocyte depression after inoculation with brain tissue from multiple sclerosis or spongiform encephalopathies. Nature 247: 217-218.
Brown P, Gibbs CJ Jr, Amyx HL, Kingsbury DT, Rohwer RG, Sulima MP, Gajdusek DC (1982a) Chemical disinfection of Creutzfeldt-Jakob disease. New Eng J Med 306:1279-1282.
Brown P, Rohwer RG, Green EM, Gajdusek DC (1982b) Effect of chemicals, heat, and histopathologic processing on high-infectivity hamster-adapted scrapie virus. J. Inf Dis 145:683-687.
Brown, P, Salazar AM, Gibbs CJ Jr, Gajdusek DC (1982c) Alzheimer's disease and transmissible virus dementia (Creutzfeldt-Jakob disease). Ann NY Acad Sci 396:131-143.
Bruce ME, Fraser H (1981) Effect of route of infection on the frequency and distribution of cerebral amyloid plaques in scrapie mice. Neuropathol Appl Neurobiol 7:289-298.
Carp RI, Licursi PC, Merz PA, Merz GS (1972) Decreased percentage of polymorphonuclear neutrophils in mouse peripheral blood after inoculation of material from multiple sclerosis patients. J Exp Med 136:618-629.
Carp RI, Licursi PC, Merz PA, Merz GS, Koldovsky U, Koldovsky P, Henle G, Henle W (1977) Multiple-sclerosis-associated agent. Lancet II:814.
Carp RI, Sersen E, Moretz R (1982) Variations in incubation periods and in the induction of increased body weight by different scrapie strains. American Society for Microbiology Meeting, Atlanta, Georgia, Abstract.
Carp RI, Thormar H (1976) Pathogenesis of slow infections of the central nervous system. In Gaull GE (ed): "Biology of Brain Dysfunction," New York: Plenum Publishing Corp, Vol 3, pp 265-306.
Chandler RL (1963) Experimental scrapie in the mouse. Res Vet Sci 4:276-285.
Chatigny MA, Prusiner SB (1980) Biohazards of investigations on the transmissible spongiform encephalopathies. Rev Infectious Diseases 2:713-724.

Davies P, Maloney AJF (1976) Selective loss of central cholinergic neurons in Alzheimer's disease. Lancet I: 1403.

Dickinson AG, Bruce ME, Scott JR (1983) The relevance of scrapie as an experimental model for Alzheimer's disease. Banbury Report 15, in press.

Dickinson AG, Fraser H (1979) An assessment of the genetics of scrapie in sheep and mice. In Prusiner SB, Hadlow WJ (eds): "Slow Transmissible Diseases of the Nervous System," New York: Academic Press, pp 367-386.

Dickinson AG, Meikle VMH (1971) Host-genotype and agent effects in scrapie incubation: Change in allelic interaction with different strains of agent. Mol Gen Genet 112:73-79.

Dickinson AG, Taylor DM (1978) Resistance of scrapie agent to decontamination. New Eng J Med 299:1413-1414.

Dickinson AG, Taylor DM, Fraser H (1974) Depression of polymorph counts by various scrapie agents. Nature 248: 510-511.

Field EJ (1966) Transmission experiments with multiple sclerosis: An interim report. Brit Med J 2:564-565.

Fraser H (1983) A survey of primary transmission of scrapie (rida) to mice. Symposium "Virus Non Conventionnels et Affections du Systeme Nerveux Central" Paris, France, in press.

Fraser H, Bruce M (1973) Argyrophilic plaques in mice inoculated with scrapie from particular sources. Lancet I: 617-618.

Fraser H, Dickinson AG (1973) Scrapie in mice: agent strain differences in the distribution and intensity of grey matter vacuolation. J Comp Pathol 83:29-40.

Gajdusek DC (1977) Unconventional viruses and the origin and disappearance of kuru. Science 197:943-960.

Gajdusek DC, Gibbs CJ Jr (1982) Slow virus infections and aging. In Terry RD, Bolis CL, Toffano G (eds): "Neural Aging and its Implications in Human Neurological Pathology," New York: Raven Press, Aging Vol 18, pp 1-12.

Gajdusek DC, Gibbs CJ Jr, Alpers M (1966) Experimental transmission of a kuru-like syndrome to chimpanzees. Nature 209:794-796.

Gibbs CJ Jr, Gajdusek DC, Asher DM, Alpers MP, Beck E, Daniel PM, Mathews WB (1968) Creutzfeldt-Jakob disease (subacute spongiform encephalopathy): Transmission to the chimpanzee. Science 161:388-389.

Goudsmit J, Morrow CH, Asher DM, Yanagihara RT, Masters CL,

Gibbs CJ Jr, Gajdusek DC (1980) Evidence for and against the transmissibility of Alzheimer disease. Neurology 30:945-950.

Hadlow WJ (1959) Scrapie and Kuru. Lancet II:289-290.

Heitzman RJ, Corp CR (1968) Behaviour in emergence and open-field tests of normal and scrapie mice. Res Vet Sci 9: 600-601.

Hornabrook RW (1979) Kuru and clinical neurology. In Prusiner SB, Hadlow WJ (eds): "Slow Transmissible Diseases of the Nervous System," New York: Academic Press, Vol. 1, pp 37-66.

Kimberlin RH, Walker CA (1978) Evidence that the transmission of one source of scrapie agent to hamsters involves separation of agent strains from a mixture. J Gen Virol 39:487-496.

Koldovsky U, Koldovsky P, Henle G, Henle W, Ackermann R, Haase G (1975) Studies on a multiple sclerosis-associated agent: Transmission to animals and some properties of the agent. Infect Immunol 12:1356-1366.

Licursi PC, Merz PA, Merz GS, Carp RI (1972) Scrapie-induced changes in the percentage of polymorphonuclear neutrophils in mouse peripheral blood. Infect Immunol 6:370-376.

Madden DL, Krezlewicz AG, Gravell M, Sever JL, Tourtellotte WW (1977) Multiple-sclerosis-associated agent. Lancet II:976.

Manuelidis EE (1975) Transmission of Creutzfeldt-Jakob disease from man to the guinea pig. Science 190:571-572.

Marsh RF (1976) The subacute spongiform encephalopathies. In Kimberlin RH (ed): "Slow Virus Diseases of Animals and Man," Amsterdam: Holland Publishing Co, pp 359-380.

Marsh RF, Sipe JC, Morse SS, Hanson RP (1976) Transmissible mink encephalopathy: Reduced spongiform degeneration in aged mink of Chediak-Higashi genotype. Lab Invest 34: 381-386.

Masters CL, Gajdusek DC, Gibbs CJ Jr (1981) Creutzfeldt-Jakob disease virus isolations from the Gerstmann-Straussler syndrome: With an analysis of the various forms of amyloid plaque deposition in the virus-induced spongiform encephalopathies. Brain 104:559-588.

McDermott JR, Fraser H, Dickinson AG (1973) Reduced choline-acetyltransferase activity in scrapie mouse brain. Lancet II:318-319.

McFarland DJ, Baker FD, Hotchin J (1980) Host and viral genetic determinants of the behavioral effects of scrapie encephalopathy. Physiol and Behav 24:911-914.

Merz PA, Somerville RA, Wisniewski HM, Iqbal K (1981) Abnormal fibrils from scrapie-infected brain. Acta Neuropathol (Berl) 54:63-74.

Palsson PA, Pattison IH, Field EJ (1965) Transmission experiments with multiple sclerosis. In Gajdusek DC, Gibbs CJ Jr, Alpers MP (eds): "Slow, Latent and Temperate Virus Infection," Washington: NINDB Monograph No. 2, Publication No. 1378, Public Health Service, pp 49-54.

Sigurdsson B (1954) Rida, a chronic encephalitis of sheep: With general remarks on infections which develop slowly and some of their special characteristics. Br Vet J 110:341-354.

Sorbi S, Amaducci L, Blass JP (1981) Pyruvate dehydrogenase complex and choline acetyl transferase in aging and dementia. In Cellular and Molecular Mechanisms of Aging in the Nervous System, Int Soc for Neurochemistry Satellite Symposium, Saint-Vincent, Italy, Abstract.

Stamp JT (1962) Scrapie: A transmissible disease of sheep. Vet Record 74:357-362.

Suckling AJ, Bateman S, Waldron CB, Webb HE, Kimberlin RH (1976) Motor activity changes in scrapie-affected mice. Br J Exp Path 57:742-746.

Tateishi J, Doi S, Sato Y, Suetsugu M, Ishii K, Kuroiwa Y (1981a) Experimental transmission of human subacute spongiform encephalopathy to small rodents. Acta Neuropathol (Berl) 53:161-163.

Tateishi J, Koga M, Mori R (1981b) Experimental transmission of Creutzfeldt-Jakob disease. Acta Pathol Jpn 31: 943-951.

Wisniewski HM, Kozlowski PB (1982) Evidence of blood-brain barrier changes in senile dementia of the Alzheimer type (SDAT). Ann NY Acad Sci 396:119-129.

Wisniewski HM, Lossinsky AS, Moretz RC, Vorbrodt AW, Lassmann H, Carp, RI (1983) Increased blood-brain barrier permeability in scrapie infected mice. J. Neuropath Exp Neurol, in press.

Wisniewski HM, Moretz RC, Lossinsky AS (1981) Evidence for induction of localized amyloid deposits and neuritic plaques by an infectious agent. Ann Neurol 10:517-522.

Wisniewski HM, Terry RD (1976) Neuropathology of the aging brain. In Terry RD, Gershon S (eds): "Neurobiology of Aging," New York: Raven Press, pp 265-280.

Senile Dementia: Outlook for the Future, pages 55–68

ACETYLCHOLINE, GLUTAMATE, GABA AND NEUROPEPTIDES IN SENILE DEMENTIA OF ALZHEIMER TYPE

Professor J. Constantinidis

Medical School of Geneva, University
Department of Psychiatry. Division of
Morphological Psyhopathology
Bel-Air Clinic, 1225 Geneva, Switzerland

Abstract

In our present state of knowledge we cannot assert that Senile Dementia of Alzheimer type (SDAT) is linked to an acceleration of the natural aging process, even though the natural physiological changes play some part in the evolution of the disease. Moreover, just as it seems more appropriate to consider natural aging and SDAT as two distinct entities, it is equally difficult to assess the role of the aging process in the neurotransmitter changes observed in SDAT. Nor can we exclude that some neurotransmitter alterations proper to SDAT may be falsely attributed to the aging process.

Concerning ACH in aging, a decrease in CHAT (the synthetizing enzyme) is observed. However in SDAT, CHAT is even more decreased and ACHE (the catabolizing enzyme) is also reduced. This presynaptic impairment of the cholinergic neuron in SDAT corresponds to a relatively normal level in the ACH post-synaptic receptors.

Concerning GABA, there is a decrease in GAD (the synthetizing enzyme) in aging and an even greater decrease in SDAT, while a drop in GABA itself and in the GABA receptors is also noted in some brain areas.

Some neuropeptides (SOM, VP, ACTH, END, Subst. P, NRT, DSIP) are or may be involved in SDAT also.

The possible correlations between the brain lesions of SDAT, i.e. Senile Plaques and Neurofibrillary Tangles on one hand, and the neurotransmitters alterations on the other hand, are discussed.

The ACH, GABA, and neuropeptide alterations that seem to be implicated in the pathogenesis of SDAT led to drug treatments of SDAT with activators of ACH (Choline, Lecithine, Arecholine, Physostigmine, Deanol), of GABA (SL-76002: Progabide), and of neuropeptides (ACTH-, VP-, Naloxon-analogs), but the therapeutic results are not yet convincing.

Better knowledge of the disturbances of neurotransmitter activity in aging and SDAT would be helpful in order to obtain efficacious multifactorial therapeutics.

Introduction

Presenile and senile dementias of the Alzheimer type are forms of the same degenerative encephalopathy which occurs in advanced age. The generic name is Senile Dementia of Alzheimer type (SDAT). SDAT is clinically characterized by amnesia and aphasic-apraxic-agnosic disorders, and neuropathologically characterized by the presence of dense senile plaques (SP) and neurofibrillary tangles (NFT) in the brain (Constantinidis et al. 1978, Constantinidis, Tissot, 1979).

But these same lesions are also found in small quantities in many brains of aged subjects who did not present clinical symptoms of SDAT. These brains may be considered: 1) as normal, in which case SDAT would be an accentuation of normal aging, or 2) as pathological, constituting a subclinical state (Constantinidis 1978). Many authors refer to the process of aging, sometimes even in the case of dementia, as if dementia were an exaggeration or an acceleration of the natural aging process of the brain. But there is no proof that aging is an illness or that SDAT is the expected outcome of natural aging (Richard 1982). Perhaps some of the changes observed in the brains of elderly people, such as the increase of lipofuscine, may be considered changes of normal aging. Yet the degenerative alterations (SP and NFT) found in these brains, with or without clinical dementia, must be considered as a result of a disease rather than as a preprogrammed ineluctable consequence of advancing chronological age (De Boni et al. 1980). Clinical symptoms of dementia appear when the density of these alterations reach a threshold (Constantinidis 1978; Constantinidis et al. 1978).

These considerations point out some of difficulties involved in the comparative study between normal aging and SDAT.

In recent years, there has been much research which shows some disturbances concerning cerebral neurotransmitters (NT) in aging and SDAT. Several methods have been used for the study of the NT activity in the brain:
a) Measuring the levels of the NT and of its metabolites in various areas of the brain, post-mortem or by biopsies. The results are difficult to interpret, since the NT continues its catabolism and diffusion post-mortem and its level as well as the level of its metabolites may be influenced by drugs administered to the patient; thus, the evaluated level is not always an exact indicator of the NT activity.
b) Visualizing the NT itself and studying it microscopically in neuronal bodies and presynaptic terminals by histochemical and immunohistological methods. These extremely delicate techniques require a rapid post-mortem human brain sampling and are difficult to realize.
c) Chemically measuring or immunohistologically visualizing enzymes which synthesize or catabolize the NT in the brain. Such measures are helpful; the enzymes undergo less degradation and diffusion post-mortem.
d) Measuring the level of NT metabolites in the cerebrospinal fluid (CSF) and the urines.
e) Evaluating the density of the post-synaptic receptors by binding methods also gives results to be understood in correlation with the level of the presynaptic NT for the evaluation of the synapse activity.

Despite some differences of opinion, there is evidence from several laboratories that the activity of a number of NT and of NT synthetizing enzymes declines with age in specific areas of the brain, whereas the activity of other enzymes increases. The activity of a specific enzyme may decline significantly in one brain area, though may not be significantly affected in other areas.

ACETYLCHOLINE (ACH)

Several areas of the brain show a significant correlation between age and a decrease in the synthetizing enzyme Choline-Acetyl-Transferase (CHAT) activity (McGeer, 1978) Reductions in CHAT activity with age are particularly important in cortical areas and relatively slight in extrapyramidal and rhinencephalic structures (Bird, Iversen 1974). Others do not observe a decrease in CHAT with age in many brain areas, with the exception of a small decrease in the hippocampus (Davies 1978). Moreover, in none of the brain areas studied is there evidence of the effects of aging on either the catabolizing enzyme Acetylcholine-Esterase (ACHE) activity or the amount of the muscarinic receptors (Davies 1978; Perry, Perry 1980).

In SDAT, the CHAT and ACHE activities are reduced in the cerebral cortex and particularly in the hippocampus as compared to normal elderly subjects (Bowen et al. 1976; Davies, Maloney 1976; Davies 1978, 1979a, 1981; Davies, Werth, 1978; Perry et al. 1977; Perry, Perry 1980, 1981; White et al. 1977).

The most marked reductions in CHAT activity have been found in the temporal neocortex, hippocampus and amygdala, where reductions of 40 to 70% have been evaluated (Bowen et al. 1979; Perry, Perry 1980; Rossor et al. 1982); reductions of up to 95% from control values have also been reported (Davies 1979b); Davies' study concerned brains of relatively young cases of SDAT and generally these younger brains presented more severe cholinergic deficiency (Bowen et al. 1979; Rossor et al 1982). This study agrees with the well established fact that SDAT is more severe and of quicker evolution when it starts in the presenile period than when it starts in the senile period of life (Constantinidis 1978).

The ACH levels of the temporal lobe are lower in cases of SDAT than in that of controls, but this is not so with the choline levels (Richter et al., 1980).

The metabolism of glucose (14C) and its incorporation in ACH are reduced in the cerebral cortex in SDAT (SIMS et al., 1980).

The muscarinic cholinergic receptors do not decrease in the cerebral cortex in SDAT (Davies, Werth 1978; Bowen et al. 1979; Perry, Perry 1980). In the hippocampus, they have been found reduced (Reisine et al. 1978), or not reduced (Davies 1978).

The concept of a decrease in presynaptic ACH activity in SDAT with a relative sparing of muscarinic receptors led to therapeutic trials with ACH precursors (choline, lecithine) and cholinergic activators (physostigmine, arecholine, deanol). According to numerous reports at the Edinburgh Colloquium (Glen, Whalley 1979), in spite of the diversity of the results, it was generally agreed that these treatments provide some benefit if they are applied at the onset of the disease, when dementia is not too advanced.

GLUTAMATE (GLU)

It is known that the histological lesions of the neuronal bodies in SDAT (NFT) occur at the beginning in the hippocampus, and that the hippocampus intrinsic neurotransmitter is GLU and that zinc has a possible role in the metabolism of this NT (the GLU-Dehydrogenase is a zinc metallo-enzyme). Based on this knowledge, we hypothesised that the GLU neurotransmitter would be disturbed in SDAT through the instrumentality of zinc (Constantinidis 1979; Constantinidis, Tissot, 1982). Yet it has been found (Tarbit et al., 1980) that the hippocampal GLU level in SDAT does not differ statistically from the controls. In spite of these findings, it must be mentioned that it is difficult to distinguish metabolic GLU from neurotransmitter GLU.

GABA

The GABA synthetizing enzyme GAD (Glutamate decarboxylase) has been found to decrease with age in the nucleus caudatus and putamen (Cote, Kremzner 1974), to be unchanged in the putamen (Bird, Iversen 1974), to decrease in a widespread manner even though to a small degree, this decrease being somewhat more important in the thalamic rhinencephalic and cortical areas (McGeer, McGeer 1976, 1980; McGeer 1978, 1981).

In SDAT a 70% decrease of GABA has been found in the temporal lobe (Rossor et al 1982). The GAD activity presents a significant decrease in the thalamus, the hippocampus and the calcarinian cortex (Davies 1979a, b). The cerebral GAD decrease in SDAT correlates with the presence of NFT in numerous neuronal bodies in the calcarinian cortex and the hippocampus, of which several are GABAergic neurons (basket cells of Cajal). The epileptic seizures observed frequently at the end of SDAT evolution may be correlated to the destruction of the GABA hippocampal neurons by NFT.

A decrease in GABA receptors is found in the nucleus caudatus and the frontal cortex of patients with SDAT (Reisine et al. 1978).

On the whole, we acknowledge that GABA activity is

reduced in some brain areas in SDAT.

We administered the GABAergic SL-76002 (Progabide), which can cross the blood-brain barrier (Bartholini et al., 1979), to a patient presenting the very typical clinical symptoms of the presenile Alzheimer's disease and we observed a clear and lasting improvement in all his symptoms; in particular the archaic reflexes, oral and grasping had disappeared completely (Constantinidis 1982, 1983). At the present we are elaborating a clinical trial with this GABAergic in several SDAT patients.

It would also be interesting to treat SDAT patients with L-Cycloserine which inhibits the GABA transaminase, thus increasing the endogenous GABA in the brain (Burkard, Pieri 1982).

NEUROPEPTIDES

The limbic system is very rich in neuropeptides: 25 peptides have been identified by radioimmunoassay (RIA) in the limbic system (Stinus 1982). Some of these peptides have been observed morphologically by immunocytochemistry in the hippocampal areas and cerebral cortex in the rat brain (Roberts et al. 1982b) and in the human brain (Roberts et al., 1982a). Substance P and Enkephalins found in the limbic areas seem to be extrinsic. The intrinsic peptides of the hippocampal areas subiculum and CA1-4 are somatostatin (SOM), vasoactive intestinal peptide (VIP), cholecystokinin (CCK) and neurotensin (NRT).

These hippocampal areas are the first to present NFT in SDAT. Some of these peptides may be involved in this pathology. By RIA, SOM has been found to decrease up to 30% of control values in the cerebral cortex in SDAT (Davies et al. 1980; Rossor et al. 1980), but VIP and CCK have been found not to decrease (Rossor et al. 1980b, Rossor et al. 1981). Endorphins (END), ACTH, vasopressin (VP) are presumed to be involved in SDAT, and drug treatments have been tried with some analogs of these peptides; the naloxone analog MIF_1 (Kastin et al. 1981), the ACTH analog, Organon 2766, and the VP analog, DDAVP (Berger, Tinklenberg 1981).

Subst. P is abundant in the rat amygdaloid nucleus (Ljungdahl et al. 1978); in our immunohistological study of the human brain (Constantinidis et al., 1980) we observed that in the brain of elderly subjects with SP and NFT, subst. P density is weak in the amygdaloid nucleus.

In our immunohistological study on Delta Sleep Inducing Peptide (DSIP) (Constantinidis et al. 1983), we observed that in the rat brain the areas which are the richest in DSIP are also the limbic structures and especially hippocampus; therefore, we are wondering whether DSIP would be involved in these areas in SDAT.

Possible correlations between Senile Plaques, Neurofibrillary Tangles and some neurotransmitter alterations.

It can be said that in SDAT, in the hippocampus and the neocortex, there is a decrease of ACH activity in relation to a decrease of presynpatic ACH and a relative preservation of post-synaptic receptors.

It is agreed that the most important part of the ACH innervation of the hippocampus is provided by the ACH neuronal bodies of nucleus septi medialis (Storm-Mathisen 1978), and that an important part of ACH innervation of the neocortex is provided by the ACH neuronal bodies of the nucleus basalis of Meynert in the substantia innominata by the ascending ACH pathway (Mesulam, Van Hoessen, 1976).

In SDAT there is, in the nucleus basalis, a decrease in the number of neuronal bodies (Whitehouse et al. 1982) and in the nucleus basalis and the nucleus septi medialis a decrease of CHAT activity (Rossor et al 1982), but we observed scarce NFT in the neuronal bodies of these nuclei. In SDAT, NFT seem to involve more the GLU, GABA, and perhaps also neuropeptide neuronal bodies, for example the neuronal bodies of the pyramidal layer of the subiculum and the areas CA1-3 of the hippocampus where there are no ACH neuronal bodies.

The question arises what kind of correlations may exist between SP and NFT on one hand, and the neurotransmitters alterations on the other hand.

The following hypothesis may be formulated for discussion:
- The primum movens should be the amyloid formation and neighbouring neuritic reaction producing SP (Constantinidis, Tissot, 1979). In SP cholinergic axons are involved. In the beginning, they are not disturbed, there is neither ACH hypo-

activity nor dementia. Afterwards, the ACH axons in the SP are affected, resulting in ACH hypoactivity and clinical symptoms of dementia. It has been reported (Perry, Perry 1980) that, in the hippocampus of non-dement elderly individuals, SP and the neighbouring neuritic fibres stained positively for ACHE; in the hippocampus of elderly individuals with SDAT, there was a reduced ACHE staining in SP and neighbouring neuritic fibres. According to their hypothesis, the positive ACHE staining of nerve processes in SP suggests that these SP are partially derived from cholinergic axonal fibres and thus the decrease of ACHE staining of nerve processes may indicate a decrease in cholinergic afferent input axons in the hippocampus in SDAT.

The ACH neuronal bodies of the nucleus septi medialis and of the nucleus basalis whose ACH axons are affected by SP would present a retrograde suffering and undergo a progressive decrease. The GLU, GABA, and neuropeptide neuronal bodies of the hippocampus and of the neocortex whose dendritic neurites are implicated in SP and do not receive sufficient synaptic ACH axons, may present an anterograde hypothrophic suffering. In these neuronal bodies abundant NFT are observed in the hippocampus. NFT are constituted by abnormal proteins forming helical paired filaments of 100 Å. These alterations are observed in a great number of the pericarya of the pyramidal layers of the hippocampus, which are GLU, GABA and neuropeptide neuronal bodies, but also in the dendritic terminals of these neurons around the SP. So the problem may be discussed in the opposite way: the primum movens should be the NFT formation (helical paired filaments of 100 Å) in the neuron, particularly in the neuritic terminals. This primary degeneration of neuritic terminals should produce amyloid SP. This theory has been supported by Terry (1970). One would deduce that GLU, GABA, and perhaps also neuropeptide neurons presenting pericaryonic NFT should be affected and responsible for the amyloid SP formation, because of their terminal neuritic NFT. ACH neurons should be affected also by the involvement of their axons in the SP.

It is not our purpose here to resolve this problem, but at this point let us repeat some facts:
- SDAT is histologically characterized by the presence of SP and NFT in the brain.
- The NFT would be formed in GLU, GABA and perhaps also neuropeptide neurons, resulting in a decrease of GABA activity

(decrease of GAD), a decrease of some neuropeptides, for example SOM, and perhaps also a disturbance of GLU neurotransmitter.
- The loss of some GLU, GABA and neuropeptide NFT-containing neurons may explain the observed slight reduction of ACH and GABA postsynaptic receptors localized in these neuronal bodies and their dendrites.
- The ACH axons would be implicated in SP and affected, and this should explain the well documented ACH hypoactivity in SDAT.

We may conclude that it is impossible to limit the neurotransmitter pathology of SDAT only in an ACH hypoactivity; a GABA hypoactivity seems also well established, as a decrease of some neuropeptides, and perhaps the GLU neurotransmitter may be also involved. To these troubles we must add the well known disturbances concerning monoamines. The complexity of the alterations of many neurotransmitters in SDAT explains the poor clinical results of many drug therapeutic trials aiming to regulate the activity of only one of the disturbed neurotransmitters (see Table).

We hope that better knowledge and understanding of the disturbances in neurotransmitters and of their articulations in SDAT will unable us to try multifactorial therapeutics which would be useful in the treatment or prevention of SDAT.

Table: Some neurotransmitter disturbances in Aging and Senile Dementia of Alzheimer type and corresponding drug therapeutic trials.

↓ Slow Decrease, ↓↓ High Decrease, = Unchanged

	Aging	SDAT	Drug therapeutic trials in SDAT
Cholinergic systems			
ACH		↓	
CHAT	↓ =	↓↓	Choline, Lecithine, Physostigmine, Deanol (Coll. of Edinburgh, Glen, Whalley 1979)
ACHE	=	↓	
Muscarinic receptors	=	↓ =	
Gabaergic systems			
GAD	↓	↓↓	SL 76002 = Progabide (Constantinidis 1982, 1983)
GABA receptors		↓	
Neuropeptides			
Subst. P	↓ ?	↓	
SOM, VP, ACTH, END		↓	ACTH analog: Organon 2766 Vasopressin analog: DDAVP (Berger, Tinklenberg 1981) Naloxon analog: Propyl-leucyl-glycinamide (Kastin et al. 1981)
CCK, VIP		=	
NRT, DSIP		?	

References

Bartholini G, Lloyd KG, Worms J, Constantinidis J, Tissot R (1979). GABA and GABAergic medication: relation to striatal dopamine function and Parkinsonism. In Poirier LJ et coll. eds. " Advances in Neurology", Vol. 24, New York, Raven Press, p. 253.

Berger PA, Tinklenberg JR (1981) Neuropeptides and senile dementia. In Th Crook, S Gershon eds "Strategies for the development of an effective treatment in senile dementia", Connecticut, p. 155.

Bird ED, Iversen LL (1974). Huntington's chorea: post-mortem measurement of glutamic acid decarboxylase, choline acetyltransferase and dopamine in basal ganglia. Brain 97: 457.

Bowen DM, Smith C.B., White P, Davison A.N. (1976). Neurotransmitter related enzymes and indices of hypoxia in senile dementia and other abiotrophies. Brain 99: 459.

Bowen DM, White P, Flack RHA, Smith CB, Davison AN (1979) Brain decarboxylase activities as indices of pathological change in Senile Dementia. Lancet 1: 1247.

Burkard WP, Pieri L (1982). Different mode of action of diazepam and the GABA-transminase inhibitor L-Cycloserine on convulsions and cerebellar cyclic GMP levels. Colleg. Intern. Psychopharm., 13e Congr. Jerusalem.

Constantinidis J (1978). Is Alzheimer's disease a major form of senile dementia? Clinical, anatomical and genetic data In Katzman RD ed "Alzheimer's disease, senile dementia and related disorders", Aging Vol.7, Raven Press, NY, p.15.

Constantinidis J (1979). Zinc metabolism in presenile dementias. In Glen AIM, Whalley LJ eds " Alzheimer's disease". Early recognition of potentially reversible deficits, Churchill, Livingstone, Edinburgh, p. 48.

Constantinidis J (1982). Neurotransmitters alterations in degenerative aging brain. In "Third International meeting of the International Society for Developmental Neuroscience" Patra (Greece), Program and Abstracts p.72.

Constantinidis J (1983). Neuromédiateurs et démences de l'âge avancé. Confront. psychiat. (in press).

Constantinidis J, Bouras C, Guntern R, Taban CH, Tissot R (1983). Delta Sleep Inducing peptide (DSIP) in the rat brain: An immunohistological microscopic study. Neuropsychobiology, (in press).

Constantinidis J, Richard J, Ajuriaguerra J. de (1978). Dementias with senile plaques and neurofibrillary tangles. In Isaaks AD, Post F eds "Studies in geriatric psychiatry", John Wiley, London - New York, p.119.

Constantinidis J, Taban CH, Guntern R, Tissot R (1980). Etude morphologique de la substance P dans le cerveau humain par immunohistofluorescence. Schweiz Arch Neurol Neurochir Psychol 127: 323.

Constantinidis J, Tissot R (1979). Plaques séniles, dégénérescences neurofibrillaires et autres lésions cérébrales associées (Morphologie et théories pathogéniques). Schweiz Arch Neurol Neurochir Psychiat 124 (2): 317.

Constantinidis J, Tissot R (1982). Degenerative encephalopathies in old age, neurotransmitters and zinc metabolism. In Terry RD et al eds "Neuronal aging and its implications in human neurological pathology", Raven Press, New York, p. 53.

Cote LJ, Kremzner LT (1974). Changes in neurotransmitter systems with increasing age in human brain. Trans. Am. Soc. Neurochem. 5: p.83.

Davies P (1978). Studies on the neurochemistry of central cholinergic systems in Alzheimer's disease. In Katzman R, Terry RD, Bick KL eds ""Alzheimer's disease, senile dementia and related disorders", Aging vol. 7, Raven Press, New York, p. 453.

Davies P (1979a). Biochemical changes in Alzheimer's disease senile dementia: neurotransmitters in senile dementia of the Alzheimer type. In Katzman R ed "Congenital and acquired cognitive disorders", Raven Press, New York.

Davies P (1981). Theoretical treatment possibilities for dementia of the Alzheimer type: the cholinergic hypothesis. In Crook T, Gershon S eds "Strategies for the development of an effective treatment for senile dementia", Mark Powley, Connecticut, p. 19.

Davies P, Katzman R, Terry RD (1980). Reduced somatostatin-like immunoreactivity in cerebral cortex from cases of Alzheimer's disease and Alzheimer senile dementia. Nature 288: 279.

Davies P, Maloney AJF(1976). Selective loss of central cholinergic neurons in Alzheimer's disease. Lancet 2: 1403.

Davies P, Verth A (1978). Regional distribution of muscarinic acetylcholine receptor in normal and Alzheimer-type dementia brains. Brain Res 138: 385.

DeBoni V, Crapper-McLachlan DR (1980). Senile Dementia and Alzheimer's Disease. A current view. Life Sci 27: 1-14.

Glen AM., Whalley LJ (1979)." Alzheimer's disease. Early recognition of potentially reversible deficits". Churchill Livingstone, Edinburgh.

Kastin AJ, Olson GA, Sandman CA, Ehresing RH (1981).Possible role of peptides in senile dementia. In Crook Th, Gershon S eds "Strategies for the development of an effective treatment

for senile de mentia", Mark Powley, Connecticut, p. 139.
Ljungdahl A, Hökfelt T., Nilsson G (1978). Distribution of substance P-like immunoreactivity in the central nervous system of the rat. Neuroscience, 3: 861.
McGeer EG (1978) Aging and neurotransmitter metabolism in the human brain. In Terry RD, Bick KL eds ""Alzheimer's disease, senile dementia and related disorders", Aging vol. 7, Raven Press, New York, p. 427.
McGeer EG (1981). Neurotransmitter systems in aging and senile dementia. Prog. Neuro-Psychopharmacol. 5: 435.
McGeer EG, McGeer PL (1976). Neurotransmitter metabolism in the aging brain. In Terry RD, Gershon S eds "Neurobiology and aging" (Aging Vol 3), Raven Press, NY, p. 389.
McGeer EG, McGeer PL (1980). Aging and neurotransmitter systems. In Goldstein et al. eds " Ergot compounds and brain function neuroendocrine and neuropsychiatric aspects", Raven Press, New York.
Mesulam MM, Van Hoessen GW (1976). Acetylcholinesterase-rich projections from the basal forebrain of the rhesus monkey to neocortex. Brain Res 109: 152.
Perry RH, Perry EK (1980). Histochemistry of brain cholinesterase in normal old age and Alzheimer's disease. In Amaducci et al. eds " Aging of the brain and dementia", Aging vol. 13, Raven Press, New York, p. 167.
Perry EK, Perry RH (1981). Cerebral neurotransmitter and neuropeptide activities in Alzheimer's disease. 3rd World Congr. Biological Psychiatry, Stockholm, Abs. vol.1, S 294.
Perry EK, Perry RH, Blessed G, Tomlinson BE (1977). Necropsy evidence of central cholinergic deficits in senile dementia. Lancet I: 189.
Reisine TD, Yamamura HI, Bird ED, Spokes E, Enna SJ (1978). Pre- and post-synaptic neurochemical alterations in Alzheimer's disease. Brain Res 159: 477.
Richard J (1982). Neurotransmitter metabolism in aging and Alzheimer's disease. Medicographia (Servier, Paris), vol. 4, No. 1, p. 19.
Richter JA, Perry EK, Tomlinson BE (1980). Acetylcholine levels in post-mortem human brain tissue. Preliminary observations in Alzheimer's disease. Life Sci. 26: 1683.
Roberts GW, Crow TJ, Polak JM (1982 a). Immunocytochemical localization of peptides in the human limbic system. Poster at the "Réunion conjointe de l'Association française de Psychiatrie Biologique et de la British Association for Psychopharmacology", Paris 1982, Oct. 25-27.
Roberts GW, Woodhaus PL, Polak JM, Crow TJ (1982 b). Peptidergic circuitry of the rat hippocampus. Poster at

the "Réunion conjointe de l'Association française de Psychiatrie Biologique et de la British Association for Psychopharmacology", Paris 1982, Oct. 25-27.
Rossor MN (1982). Neurotransmitters and central nervous system disease. Dementia. Lancet II: 1200.
Rossor MN, Emson PC, Mountjoy CQ, Roth M, Iversen LL (1980a). Reduced amounts of immunoreactive somatostatin in the temporal cortex in Senile Dementia of Alzheimer's type. Neurosci Lett 20: 273.
Rossor MN, Fahrenkrug J, Emson P, Mountjoy CQ, Iversen LL, Roth M (1980b). Reduced cortical choline acetyltransferase in Senile Dementia of Alzheimer's type is not accompanied by changes in vasoactive intestinal peptide. Brain Res 209: 249.
Rossor MN, Iversen LL, Mountjoy CQ, Roth M (1982). Reduced acetylcholinesterase activity in the substantia innominata in Alzheimer's disease. Neuroscience, suppl Vol 7: 5181.
Rossor MN, Rehfeld JF, Emson PC, Mountjoy CQ, Roth M, Iversen LL (1981). Normal cortical concentration of cholecystokinin with reduced choline acetyltransferase activity in Senile dementia of Alzheimer's type. Life Sci 29: 405.
Rossor MN, Svendsen C, Hunt SP, Mountjoy CQ, Roth M, Iversen LL (1982). The substantia innominata in Alzheimer's disease: An histochemical and biochemical study of cholinergic marker enzymes. Neurosci Lett 28: 217.
Sims NR, Smith CCT, Davison AN, Bowen DM, Flack RHA, Snowden JS (1980). Glucose metabolism and acetylcholine synthesis in relation to neuronal activity in Alzheimer's disease. Lancet, 16 fév. 1980: 333.
Stinus L (1982). Neuropeptides et système limbique. Rapport à la "Réunion conjointe de l'Association française de Psychiatrie Biologique et de la British Association for Psychopharmacology", Paris 1982, 25-27 octobre.
Storm-Mathisen J (1978). Localization of putative transmitters in the hippocampal formation. In "Functions of the septo-hippocampal system", Ciba Foundation Symposium, 58: 49.
Tarbit I, Perry EK, Perry PH, Blessed G, Tomlinson BE (1980) Hippocampal free aminoacids in Alzheimer's disease. J. Neurochem. 35: 1246.
Terry RD (1970). Discussion. In "Alzheimer's Disease", Churchill, London, p. 165.
White P, Hilley CR, Goodhardt MJ, Carasco LH (1977) Neocortical cholinergic neurons in elderly people. Lancet 1: 668.
Whitehouse PS, Price DL, Strubler RG, Clark AW, Coyle JT, De Long MR (1982). Alzheimer's disease and Senile Dementia. Loss of neurons in the basal forebrain. Science 215: 1237.

Senile Dementia: Outlook for the Future, pages 69–80

THE METABOLISM OF MONOAMINES AND THEIR ETIOLOGICAL IMPORTANCE IN AGING AND IN PATIENTS WITH DEMENTIA OF ALZHEIMER TYPE

C.G. Gottfries, D.M., Ph.D.

Head of Department of Psychiatry and Neurochemistry
St. Jörgen's Hospital
S-422 03 Hisings Backa, Sweden

In high age impairment of psychic functions can be due to normal aging or dementia disorders. Usually normal aging will induce no severe mental impairment. The reserve capacity of the brain may be reduced but the old aged can still cope with social life if not too much stressed.

It is, however, not known whether there is a continuity between normal aging and dementia syndromes. In epidemiological investigations in Sweden (Adolfsson et al. 1981; Gottfries 1983a) it is shown that their is a strong correlation between age and the frequencies of dementia syndromes. In the ages between 65-74 0.8-1.6% of the population was demented. From 75-84 years the figure rose to 18.5% and above 90 years of age the per cent of dementias in the population was 43.3. The strong correlation to age may indicate that the normal aging process has etiological importance for dementia syndromes.

Dementia means a more severe impairment of mental functions. There are two main groups of dementia disorders: the ones caused by cerebral vascular diseases and the ones due to primary degenerative disorders. The non-vascular diseases are senile dementia and the presenile dementias.

In the beginning of this century Alzheimer associated two characteristic pathological changes, senile plaques and intraneuronal neurofibrillary tangles with the dementia disease with onset in the presenile age and with a progressive course. Later this presenile dementia has been given the name Alzheimer's disease (AD). Neuropathologists have, however, found that also dementia disorders with a later onset (above the age of 65) have the same neuropathological changes. These patients have been given the name senile dementia of Alzheimer type (SDAT). Usually all non cerebrovascular dementias in high age are named senile dementia (SD). As the diagnosis of AD or SDAT not can be made until the neuropathological examination is made it is at present difficult to say to what extent the patients who clinically are diagnosed as SD in fact are SDAT. It must be assumed that the group SD is very heterogenous. Above the subgroup of SDAT the senile dementia group includes dementia syndromes with other etiology as abuse and somatic illness. Also pseudodementias may be included.

In this paper disturbances of the metabolism of monoamines and their etiological importance in aging and in patients with AD and SDAT will be discussed.

There are similarities between the biochemical changes found in normal aging and in AD/SDAT. Several investigations have shown that catecholamine activity in the aged rat brain is reduced (Finch 1973, 1976; Algeri et al. 1978). The activities of tyrosine hydroxylase (TH) as well as dopadecarboxylase (DOD) have been examined post mortem in humans and highly significant agerelated decreases have been recorded (Cote and Kremzner 1974; McGeer et al. 1971; Lloyd an Hornykiewicz 1970). Postmortem studies in humans have shown reduced levels of dopamine (DA) and noradrenaline (NA) related to age (Nies et al. 1973; Carlsson and Winblad 1976; Gottfries et al. 1979). The findings indicate that at least after the age of 65 there is a slow decrease of the concentrations of catecholamines in the normally aged brain.

In AD/SDAT it was shown already in 1969 (Gottfries et al.) that the end metabolite from DA metabolism, homovanillic acid (HVA), was decreased in CSF in patients still alive. At present their are several investigations in which the reduced HVA-levels in CSF in patients with AD/SDAT has been confirmed (Mölsä 1980; Soininen et al. 1981; Shimuzu and Fujita 1981). Also in postmortem brain studies (Gottfries et al. 1969) the concentration of HVA was reduced in the caudate nucleus, the putamen and the globus pallidus in patients with AD/SDAT.

In a joint Swedish investigation (Gottfries et al. 1983) 14 brains from patients with AD/SDAT were compared with 16 brains from normally aged individuals. The hypothalamus, the caudate nucleus, the hippocampus and the cortex gyrus cinguli were dissected and analyzed for their content of monoamines, their metabolites and enzyme activities involved in the metabolism of the monoamines. It could be shown that DA was significantly reduced in the caudate nucleus in the demented group (73% of controls). HVA was significantly reduced in the nucleus caudatus but significantly increased in the gyrus cinguli(Fig. 1). NA was reduced to 57-74% of the controls and the reduction was significant in all areas investigated. 3-methoxy-4-hydroxyphenylglycol (MHPG), the end metabolite of the NA-metabolism, was, however, significantly increased in three areas investigated and the increase was in the caudate nucleus 194% of controls (Fig. 2).

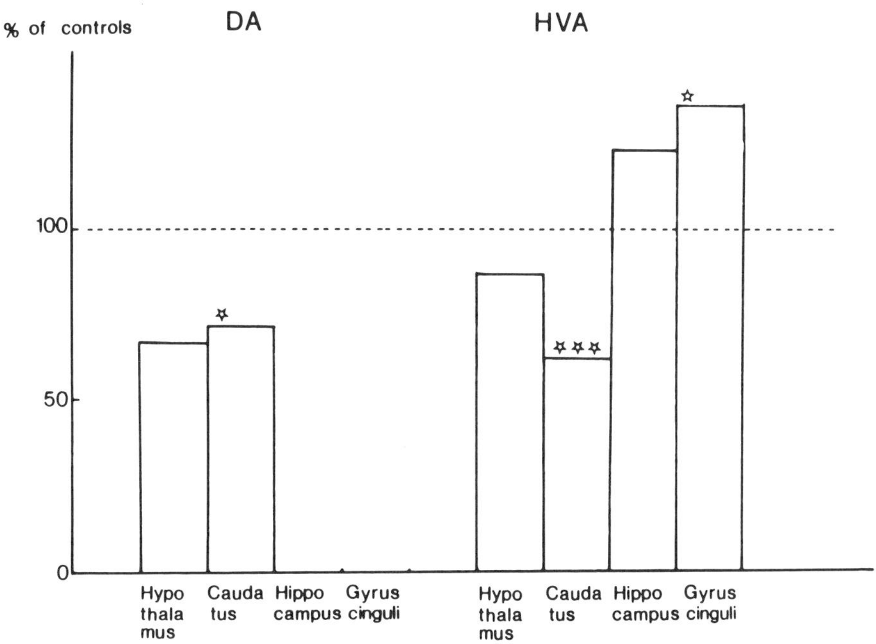

Fig. 1. The mean levels of dopamine (DA) and homovanillic acid (HVA) in a group of patients with dementia of Alzheimer type (n=14) expressed as per cent of the mean of a control group (n=16).

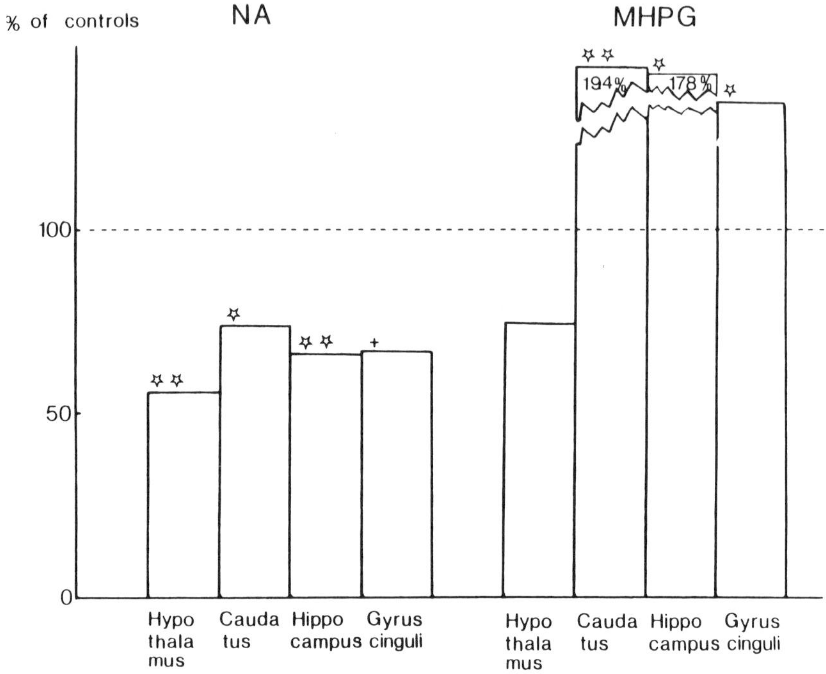

Fig. 2. The mean levels of noradrenaline (NA) and 3-methoxy-4-hydroxyphenylglycol (MHPG) in a group of patients with dementia of Alzheimer type (n=14) expressed as per cent of the mean of a control group (n=16).

In AD/SDAT it seems as if there is a severe disturbance of the metabolism of the catecholamines. The concentration of the active amines DA and NA, may reflect a decreased number of neurones. As well in normal aging as in AD/SDAT a reduced number of cells in the locus coeruleus has been reported (Brody 1976; Bondareff et al. 1981). In some areas the end metabolites, HVA and MHPG, were either normal or even increased. This may indicate that the remaining neurones have an increased release of neurotransmitters.

Studies of the metabolism of the 5-hydroxy-tryptamine

(5-HT) are more contradictory. As well increased levels of 5-HT as decreased levels in relation to age are reported in animal experiments (Samorajski and Rolsten 1973; Himwich and Himwich 1959). Relatively small but statistically significant decreases in 5-HT with age have been reported in postmortem investigations from man (Robinson et al. 1972). In other investigations (Gottfries et al. 1979) there were positive correlations between 5-HT-levels and age in some areas (brainstem areas) while there were negative correlations in cortical areas. These data are in line with data presented by MacLean et al. (1965) and Pare et al. (1969).

5-hydroxyindolacetic acid (5-HIAA), the end metabolite of 5-HT, was shown to be reduced in CSF in patients with AD/SDAT already in 1969 (Gottfries et al.). In the Swedish joint investigation (Gottfries et al. 1983) also 5-HT and 5-HIAA were studied. In AD/SDAT patients the 5-HT-levels were reduced to 21-64% of the control material. 5-HIAA was, however, not reduced (Fig. 3).

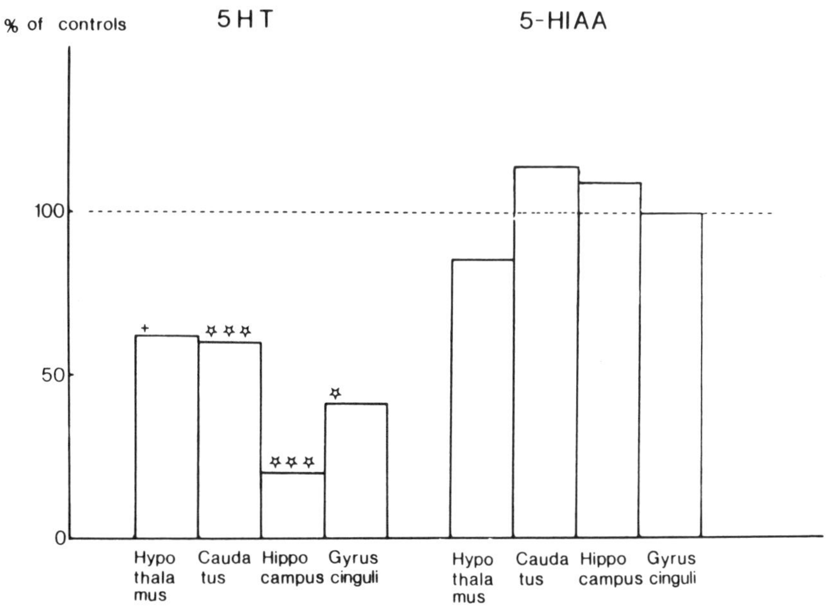

Fig. 3. The mean levels of 5-hydroxytryptamin (5-HT) and 5-hydroxyindolacetic acid (5-HIAA) in a group of patients with dementia of Alzheimer type (n=14) expressed as per cent of the mean of a control group (n=16).

Monoamine oxidase (MAO) is a key enzyme in the degradation of monoamines. The enzyme exists in two forms: MAO-A and MAO-B which have different substrate inhibitor specificites (see Fowler et al. 1980a). An increase in MAO activity with age was demonstrated by Robinson et al. (1972). This increase was found to be selective for the B-form of the enzyme (Adolfsson et al. 1980) and in later detailed analyzes the increase in activity was found to be due entirely to a variation in the enzyme concentration (Fowler et al. 1980b). A still further increase of MAO-B was recorded in patients with AD/SDAT (Fig. 4) (Gottfries et al. 1983). The increased activity of MAO-B may reflect a proliferation of extra neuronal cells.

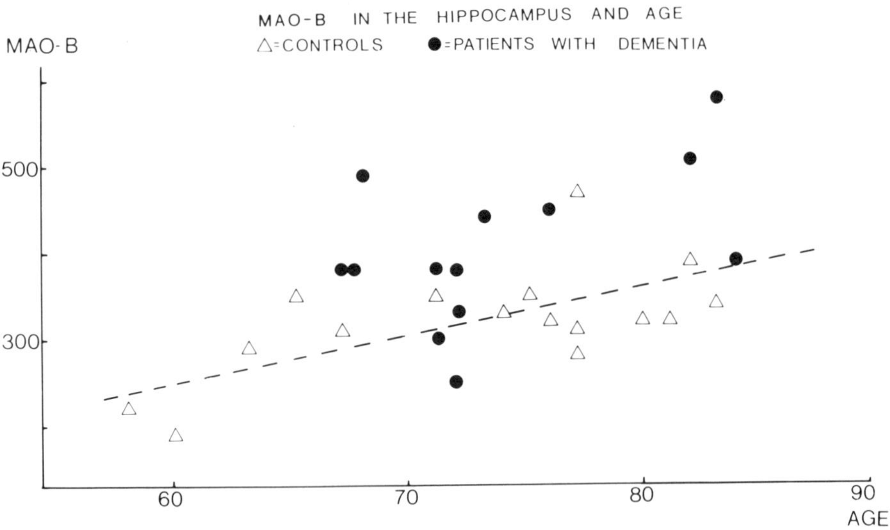

Fig. 4. The activity of MAO-B in the hippocampus (nkat/g w w) plotted against age. The dotted line is the linear regression for 16 controls (△). The circles (●) are 13 patients with dementia of Alzheimer type (AD/SDAT).

As is well known also the metabolism of acetylcholine is reported to be reduced as well in normal aging as in AD/SDAT. In the Swedish joint investigation also the activity of choline-acetyl transferase (CAT) was recorded. It could be shown that the CAT-activity was reduced in all the four areas of the brain investigated to 56-81% of the control material. This finding indicates that the same type of patients are investigated in Sweden as are investigated in the U.K. where the CAT findings are reported from.

The disturbed acetylcholine system in AD/SDAT has been given etiological importance. It seems, however, unlikely that a disease with such general disturbances of mental functions could be explained by a disturbance only in one neurotransmitter system. As is evident from the Swedish joint investigation in one and the same brain it can be shown that not only are the CAT-activity reduced but also the concentrations of the monoamines DA, NA and 5-HT. Thus one must assume that the etiology of AD/SDAT may be found beyond the neurotransmitter level. Still a disturbed neurotransmitter functioning can have pathogenetic importance. In AD/SDAT there are as well intellectual, emotional as motor impairment. Theoretically it can well be assumed that a disturbed acetylcholine system is of importance for the intellectual impairment.

From a clinical point of view it is obvious that there is an overlap between AD/SDAT and Parkinsonism. AD/SDAT-patients show parkinsonistic symptoms in 50% (Pearce 1974) and in patients with Parkinsonism dementia symptoms are reported in between 11-53% (see Gottfries et al. 1980). It is attractive to assume that a disturbed DA-metabolism is a pathogenetic base for the motor deficits found in AD/SDAT-patients. A question can, however, also be raised if there are dopaminergic systems in the brain of importance for intellectual functions, as in previous investigations a significant negative correlation between the concentration of HVA and intellectual impairment has been demonstrated (Gottfries 1981).

The reduced NA-concentration is interpreted as indicating a reduced number of neurones in the locus coeruleus. The increased levels of MHPG, even to supernormal levels, indicate a higher spead of turnover in the remaining NA-neurones. This may be due to either compensatory mechanisms or a disinhibited NA-synthesis. The NA-system is a stress system in the brain and a common clinical feature in the patients with AD/SDAT is a stress intolerance. Perhaps the high speed of turnover in the NA system explains the stress intolerance. To further study the stress situation of patients with AD/SDAT a dexamethasone suppression test has been performed in 21 patients with AD/SDAT still alive. In 57% of these patients there was a pathological dexamethasone suppression (Balldin et al. 1983).

In high age and in patients with dementia there is an increased frequency of depressive disorders. As an altered activity of serotoninergic systems is assumed to be of importance for affective disorders the reduced 5-HT metabolism in high age and in AD/SDAT patients may be associated with an increased vulnerability to depression.

Whether the increased activity of MAO is of importance for the psychiatric symptoms seen in the aged or in patients with AD/SDAT is difficult to say.

As is well known the disturbed neurotransmitter function has given clues for treatment trials. Drugs can effect a neurotransmitter system on principle on three levels: the presynaptic, the synaptic and the postsynaptic level. Several trials have been performed in which one has tried to activate the acetylcholinergic system. Some effect has been recorded but the effect is far from impressive.

Also treatment trials in which one tries to substitute or influence monoaminergic functions in CNS have been done in patients with AD/SDAT. L-dopa which activates the DA-system has been given to patients and especially the influence of this treatment on motor functional disturbances has been studied. Marginal improvement of as well intellectual as motor functioning has been reported in some investigations. There are, however, also investigations which are negative. The DA-receptor agonists bromocriptine and lisuride have also been tried. These drugs seem to cause confusion in patients with AD/SDAT (see Gottfries 1983b).

As also the concentration of 5-HT is reduced in brains from patients with AD/SDAT the precursor tryptophan has been given in treatment trials. Some positive effect has been reported but the investigations are too few and including too small patient groups to make conclusions valid (see Gottfries 1983b).

During the last years a new type of antidepressants has been introduced. Trazodone and alaproclate are drugs, which selectively block the reuptake of 5-HT in the nerve terminals. In preliminary investigations alaproclate (Bergman et al. 1983) has been studied for its effect on patients with AD/SDAT and a positive effect was recorded. Also trazodone has been reported to be of benefit in treatment of organic brain syndromes (Nair et al. 1973). Although these trials are very preliminary they may indicate a new treatment model for patients with AD/SDAT.

MAO-inhibitors have been used in the treatment of affective disorders. As these drugs have toxic effects their use has been limited. At present pharmaceutical industries have synthesisized MAO-inhibitors with a selective effect on either MAO-A and MAO-B. It can be assumed that these drugs are less toxic. Whether these drugs have effects on dementia conditions remains to be seen.

Summarizing the results of the treatment trials it seems that neither by activating the acetylcholinergic or the monoaminergic systems in patients with AD/SDAT any valuable effects on dementia symptoms can be achieved. Does this mean that the treatment model used in Parkinson's disease not can be applied in the treatment of AD/SDAT? It must be realized that in Parkinson's disease there is a selective disturbance of the DA-metabolism, while in AD/SDAT there are more general disturbances of the neurotransmitters. Perhaps it is not sufficient to substitute only one of these systems to get positive effect. Combined treatment models may be necessary. Certainly we still are on a very naive level in the treatment of patients with AD/SDAT but the biochemical findings achieved may guide us toward an effective treatment in this, for coming decades so important disease. It must also be kept in mind that although we speak of a "normal aging process" this does not exclude pharmacological treatment. It may very well be possible to alleviate symptoms which old people suffer from by substituting their failing neurotransmitter systems.

REFERENCES

Adolfsson R, Gottfries CG, Oreland L, Wiberg Å, Winblad B (1980). Increased activity of brain and platelet monoamine oxidase in dementia of Alzheimer type. Life Sci 27: 1029.

Adolfsson R, Gottfries CG, Nyström L, Winblad B (1981). Prevalence of dementia disorders in institutionalized Swedish old people. Acta Psychiat Scand 63:225.

Algeri S, Bonati M, Brunello N, Ponzio F, Stramentinoli G, Gualano M (1978). Biochemical changes in central catecholaminergic neurons of the senescent rats. In Deniker P, Radouco-Thomas C, Villeneuve A (eds): "Proceedings of the Tenth Congress of the Collegium International Neuro-Psychopharmacologicum, Quebec, July 1976", Vol. 2, Oxford: Pergamon Press, p 1647.

Balldin J, Gottfries CG, Karlsson I, Lindstedt G, Långström G, Wålinder J (1983). Dexamethasone suppression test and serum prolactin in dementia disorders. Accepted for publication in Br J Psychiatry.

Bergman I, Bråne G, Gottfries CG, Jostell KG, Karlsson I, Svennerholm L (1983). Alaproclate: A pharmacokinetic and biochemical study in patients with dementia of Alzheimer type. Accepted for publication in Psychopharmacology.

Bondareff W, Mountjoy CQ, Roth M (1981). Selective loss of neurones of origin of adrenergic projection to cerebral cortex (nucleus locus coeruleus) in senile dementia. Lancet i:783.

Brody H (1976). An examination of cerebral cortex and brainstem aging. In Gershon S, Terry RD (eds): "Neurobiology of aging", New York: Raven Press, p 177.

Carlsson A, Winblad B (1976). Influence of age and time interval between death and autopsy on dopamine and 3-methosytyramine levels in human basal ganglia. J Neural Transm 38:271.

Cote LJ, Kremzner LT (1974). Changes in neurotransmitter systems with increasing age in human brain. Abstr Am Soc Neurochem, p 83.

Finch CE (1973). Catecholamine metabolism in the brains of ageing male mice. Brain Res 52:261.

Finch CE (1976). The regulation of physiological changes during mammalian aging. Q Rev Biol 51:49.

Fowler CJ, Oreland L, Magnusson T, Winblad B (1980a). Titration of human brain monoamine oxidase -A and -B by clorgyline and l-deprenil. Naunyn-Schmiedeberg's Arch Pharmacol 311:263.

Fowler CJ, Wiberg Å, Oreland L, Marcusson J, Winblad B (1980b). The effect of age on the activity and molecular properties of human brain monoamine oxidase. J Neural Transmiss 49:1.

Gottfries CG (1981). Levels of monoamines, monoamine metabolites, and activity in related enzyme systems correlated to normal aging and in patients with dementia of Alzheimer type. In Corsini GU, Gessa GL (eds): "Apomorphine and other dopaminomimetics", Vol. 2: Clinical Pharmacology, New York: Raven Press, p 243.

Gottfries CG (1983a). Åldrandet och åldersdemenser - epidemiologiska och etiologiska aspekter. Läkartidningen 80:665.

Gottfries CG (1983b). Dementia. In Hippius H, Winokur G (eds): "Psychopharmacology 1", Part 2: Clinical psychopharmacology, Amsterdam: Elsevier Science Publishing Co, p 271.

Gottfries CG, Gottfries I, Roos BE (1969). Homovanillic acid and 5-hydroxyindoleacetic acid in the cerebrospinal fluid of patients with senile dementia, presenile dementia and Parkinsonism. J Neurochem 16:1341.

Gottfries CG, Adolfsson R, Oreland L, Roos BE, Winblad B (1979). Monoamines and their metabolites and monoamine oxidase activity related to age and to some dementia disorders.In Crooks J, Stevenson IH (eds): "Drugs and the elderly. Perspectives in geriatric clinical pharmacology. Proceedings of a symposium held in Ninewells Hospital, University of Dundee, on 13 and 14 September 1977", London: Mac Millan, p 189.

Gottfries CG, Adolfsson R, Aquilonius SM, Carlsson A, Oreland L, Svennerholm L, Winblad B (1980). Parkinsonism and dementia disorders of Alzheimer type: Similarities and differences. In Rinne UK, Klinger M, Stamm G (eds): "Parkinson's disease - current progress, problems and management", Amsterdam: Elsevier/North-Holland Biomedical Press, p 197.

Gottfries CG, Adolfsson R, Aquilonius SM, Carlsson A, Eckernäs SÅ, Nordberg A, Oreland L, Svennerholm L, Wiberg Å, Winblad B (1983). Biochemical changes in dementia disorders of Alzheimer type (AD/SDAT). Submitted for publication in Neurobiol Aging.

Himwich WA, Himwich HE (1959). Neurochemistry of aging. In Birren JE (ed): "Handbook of aging and the individual", Chicago: The University of Chicago Press, p 187.

Lloyd K, Hornykiewicz O (1970). Occurrence and distribution of L-dopa decarboxylase in the human brain. Brain Res 22:426.

MacLean R, Nicholson WJ, Pare CMB, Stacey RS (1965). Effect of monoamineoxidase inhibitors on the concentrations of 5-hydroxytryptamine in the human brain. Lancet ii:205.

McGeer EG, McGeer PL, Wada SA (1971). Distribution of tyrosine hydroxylase in human and animal brain. J Neurochem 18:1647.

Mölsä P (1980). "Dementia. A clinical study in the Finnish population". Research reports from the department of neurology, University of Turku, Finland.

Nair NPV, Ban TA, Hontela S, Clarke R (1973). Trazodone in the treatment of organic brain syndromes, with special reference to psychogeriatrics. Curr Ther Res 15:769.

Nies A, Robinson DS, Davis JM, Ravaris CL (1973). Changes in monoamine oxidase with ageing and depression in man. In Eisdorfer C, Fann WE (eds): "Psychopharmacology and aging: Advances in behavioral biology", New York: Plenum Press, p 41.

Pare CMB, Young DPH, Price K, Stacey RS (1969). 5-hydroxytryptamine, noradrenaline, and dopamine in brainstem, hypothalamus and caudate nucleus of controls and patients committing suicide by coalgas poisoning. Lancet ii:133.

Pearce J (1974). Mental changes in Parkinsonism. Brit Med J Letter 1:445.

Robinson DS, Davis JM, Nies A, Colburn RW, Davis JN, Bourne HR, Bunney WE, Shaw DM, Coppen AJ (1972). Ageing, monoamines, and monoamine oxidase levels. Lancet i:290.

Samorajski T, Rolsten C (1973). Age and regional differences in the chemical composition of brains of mice, monkeys and humans. In Ford DH (ed): "Progress in brain research". Vol. 40: Neurobiological Aspects of Maturation and Aging, Amsterdam: Elsevier Scientific Publishing Co, p 253.

Shimizu T, Fujita M (1981). Monoamine metabolite levels in the cerebrospinal fluid of patients with dementias. Paper presented at the 12th World Congress of Neurology, Kyoto, Japan, September 20-25, 1981.

Soininen H, MacDonald E, Rekonen M, Riekkinen PJ (1981). Homovanillic acid and 5-hydroxyindoleacetic acid levels in cerebrospinal fluid of patients with senile dementia of Alzheimer type. Acta Neurol Scand 64:101.

III. CRITICAL EVALUATION OF SENILE DEMENTIA RESEARCH

Presided by D. Danon (Rehovot, Israel)

Senile Dementia: Outlook for the Future, pages 83–92

CRITICAL EXAMINATION OF CONTEMPORARY PROGRESS IN DEMENTIA RESEARCH

Robert N. Butler, M.D.

Brookdale Professor of
Geriatrics and Adult Development

We are in the midst of a wave of enthusiasm related to senile dementia of the Alzheimer's type. Alzheimer's disease: is becoming a household word, and overdiagnosis is occurring. New "treatments" — from physostigmine to naloxone to blue-green algae! — are enthusiastically endorsed by the press, and families despair when these "treatments" fail. It is time to take stock critically. How far has dementia research come? What is our present knowledge of causes and treatments? Where must we go?

Where Have We Been

Twenty-five years ago there was very little research or activity concerning senility in any of its forms. There were no significant biochemical or neurotransmitter leads; indeed, until recently little knowledge of neurotransmitters or of neurotransmitter chemical activity existed. We had available the Kety-Schmidt method for measuring total cerebral blood flow, glucose and oxygen consumption, but we did not have techniques for precise, quantitative, regional measurements of cerebral metabolism.

Our diagnostic formulations were extremely weak, even downright misleading. Until 1965, in what was then the most widely used psychiatric textbook in the United States, Modern Clinical Psychiatry, authors Noyes and Kolb urged us that when there was a doubt between psychosis with cerebral arteriosclerosis and senile psychosis, to favor cerebral arteriosclerosis in making a diagnosis. This statement apparently derived from the New York State book on nomenclature. I am certain that many hospital records, particularly in New York, for years carried a heavier emphasis upon cerebral arteriosclerosis than was justified by clinical examination.

A quarter of a century ago cerebral arteriosclerosis was the predominant diagnosis for brain disease in old age in the United States, and medical practitioners were telling family members that the parent or spouse who was suffering from "hardening of the arteries" was nonetheless senile. Senility was popularly viewed as inevitable with chronological aging and irreversible. (The legitimation of diseases subsumed under the category of "senility" has taken time indeed.)

Twenty-five years ago Alzheimer's disease was considered a very rare neurological disease of the middle years. Until the introduction of Medicaid and Medicare in 1965, older patients were largely in public mental hospitals. They received minimal, custodial treatment. Very little research activity was devoted to organic brain diseases of old age. As recently as 1976, when the National Institute on Aging was founded, only twelve grants related to organic brain diseases in old age were supported by the Mental Health, and the Neurology and Aging institutes within the National Institutes of Health.

Where Are We Now

Today in the United States most of the older patients with significant brain disease are in the 18,000 nursing homes throughout the country.[1] In part because of the failure of American general hospitals, academic hospitals, and public mental hospitals to show sufficient interest in this very common disease, nursing homes are beginning to move directly into the care of patients with senile dementia of the Alzheimer's type (SDAT); for example, in Phoenix, Arizona, a proprietary nursing home corporation is working directly

[1]The nursing home industry is beginning to experience a kind of "McDonalization"; some 20 to 25 individuals now manage approximately 40% (about 400,000) of the nursing home beds in the United States. (The National Council of Health Centers represents the chain corporations).

with the Alzheimer's Disease and Related Disorders Association chapter to develop settings for the care and treatment of people suffering from SDAT.

Of the older patients who have remained in public mental hospitals, many, particularly in areas of Washington, D.C., New York City, and Chicago, are wandering confused in the streets as a consequence of what had appeared to be an enlightened public policy, called "deinstitutionalization."

We have seen some improvement in diagnosis. Distinctions between multi-infarct dementia and senile dementia of the Alzheimer's type have been clarified. However, SDAT is still a diagnosis by exclusion, for--despite exciting developments in the technology of scanning, Sokoloff's 2-D deoxyglucose method which is the intellectual basis for PET scanning, and the prospect of nuclear magnetic resonance (NMR)—we do not have clear biochemical, neurotransmitter, or other forms of direct indications. In addition, although recent emphasis on the potential reversibility of some forms of mental confusion is well placed, it is likely that we are more enthusiastic than is warranted by the facts. We do not have the epidemiological data necessary to support the oft-stated claim that 30% of cases of "senility" can be reversed. (I personally believe that we overestimate the reversibility of dementias compared to deliria.)

The Lack of Data

Indeed, we do not have the data, epidemiological or otherwise, to support most of our presently held notions, including how many persons are suffering from senile dementia of the Alzheimer's type and the degree to which the disease curbs life. While we call it the number four or five cause of death and are increasingly convinced of its commonness, the epidemiological data base remain too poor to provide an accurate portrait of the incidence and prevalence of psychopathology in late life. Screening methods are uncertain and tend to vary from study to study.[2] Post

[2]Soon we will have some useful data from the Yale-New Haven study — a collaboration of the National Institutes on Aging, Mental

mortems are rarely performed are rarely performed in nursing homes, where death certificates are woefully inadequate. We lack the final peer review. We have no neuro-pathological data on deceased subjects of the few longitudinal studies in which extensive psychometric testing was done. We do not have reliable genetic information with which to compare the genetic-familial form of SDAT with the sporadic type.

We cannot even be certain that senile dementia of the Alzheimer's type is one, unitary disease. At an important conference on senile dementia held by the aging, neurology, and mental health institutes, a commission was established to come to grips with the question of nomenclature. We decided that we should be very careful to use the term senile dementia of the Alzheimer's type, not "Alzheimer's disease". We did not want to foreclose the possibility that the disease could reflect more than one, quite separable conditions. If the cholinergic neuron hypothesis of SDAT is correct, why, then, did only 60% of the David Bowen brain biopsy series show reductions in choline acetyltransferase even though they were identified as clear-cut cases of senile dementia of the Alzheimer's type? Needless to say, combining different conditions is a serious matter, confusing clinical studies on dementia, especially clinical trials.

So too, the importance of neurofibrillary tangles and plaques that is, the degree to which they may be specific to senile dementia of the Alzheimer's type has possibly been over-interpreted. After all, a number of conditions present NFTs: post-encephalitic parkinsonism, dementia pugilistica, Down's syndrome and even aging itself. While NFTs may prove important — indeed, they are found only in humans, not in animals -- we may be dealing with changes associated with certain kinds of "causes" of dying cells. We know too little about the biochemistry of neurofibrillary tangles and neuritic plaques, including the chemical character of amyloid.

Health, and Neurology — in which the community population oversampled with regard to the 65+ population. In addition, we can look abroad to the work in Lund, Sweden and to the earlier work of Sir Martin Roth in the United Kingdom.

What about the currently prevalent hypotheses concerning the etiogenesis of senile dementia of the Alzheimer's type? Some are of uncertain significance. The slow virus hypothesis is exciting yet - for instance, if cholinergic deficiency is important, why is there no marked cholinergic deficiency in Creutzfeldt-Jacob disease, apparently due to a slow virus? In parkinsonism-dementia there are only mild changes in cholinergic enzymes.

The aluminum hypothesis has created a great stir -- some members of the public apparently are now afraid to use antacids, deodorants, and aluminum pots and pans — but here too we are left uncertain as to the degree to which it plays a primary or even a significant secondary role.

Even with regard to the cholinergic deficiency hypothesis, one cannot help but wonder. Could the central nervous system have been built so fragilely during the evolutionary course of human cerebral development that one neurotransmitter system would become so central and its deficiency have such an awesome repercussion? Undoubtedly, there is a multiple system deficiency in senile dementia of the Alzheimer's type.

The Research and Funding Needs

The questions we ask are challenging and our research needs are immense on all levels, from the most basic to the most practical. We require national population laboratories to study changes in biomedical, biochemical and behavioral aspects of human performance over time among diverse social, economic and ethnic groups and to have well-characterized study groups for clinical trials.

We lack a variety of animal models; SDAT is a uniquely human disease, yet because of its central nervous system location we cannot study it in human subjects as we might other diseases. At John Hopkins there is animal work on the cholinergic model. The National Institute on Aging has coordinated some colonies of characterized non-human primates. But aging pedigreed cats, essential for classic neurophysiological studies for example, are largely unavailable.

We must also develop the neuropsychology of old age in general and of the differential diagnoses of the various dementias, depressions, and paranoia states. If we are correct in thinking that there are more rapid, fugitive, and subtle neurochemical events in senile dementia, then the type of neuropsychology needed would involve rapid appraisal, essential for the examination of outcomes when any type of intervention is introduced. Interactive computers ("videogames") might be useful for more rapid appraisal involving stimuli and responses.

While simple mental status tests are useful for screening, we need to develop validated and reliable comprehensive methods of assessment encompassing medical, sociological, and psychological factors.

And need we remind ourselves how little we know about basic memory and the develomental phase of late life itself? How little, in terms of the chemistry of memory, we know of the role of pituitary hormones (ACHTH, vasopressin, etc.) alone.

Research needs require research funding. The level of dementia research funding may be remarkable relative to what it was a few years ago, but it is still just a drop in the bucket. Among the three pertinent institutes of the NIH, the combined total comes to about $20 million per year. Dementia research has some good friends now in Congress, in both Senate and House appropriations committees, and the generous support of the Commonwealth Fund, which supports three Commonwealth Fund Fellowships. But what is $20 million compared to the billion dollars a year available for research in cancer from the U.S. National Cancer Institute alone? (I do not question the justification of extensive support for cancer research, of course). Given the extent, costs, impact upon families, personal anguish, etc., caused by dementia, $20 million is a minimal investment in research that is, investment in the future.

Care and Treatment of SDAT Patients

The impact of senile dementia of the Alzheimer's type on the American family is made all the worse by reimbursement limitations which dramatically affect the care of the patient at home and in nursing homes. The private insurance industry has made only a minimal contribution to coverage of people suffering from senile dementia of the Alzheimer's type. Unquestionably, the behavior of doctors is influenced by reimbursement schemes, and there is not the level of reimbursement for the care and treatment necessary for of people who suffer from SDAT.

Neither does the insurance industry contribute vastly to nursing home care as a whole. From all sources, $24 billon was spent on nursing homes in 1981 in the Unites States. Only $200 million of that came from private, third-party insurance coverage. "Market segregation", or cream skimming, leads to nursing homes taking the patients easiest to handle and most able to pay out of their own pockets -- in short, the most manageable and the richest.

If SDAT proves as common as we now believe, patients are hardly clustered among the rich. Exhibiting progressively debilitating symptoms, neither are they easily managed. Indeed, treatment of the patient with senile dementia of the Alzheimer's type must be aggressive in its interventions.

It is important to distinguish between treatment and cure of SDAT, a distinction which isn't always clearly made, particularly in the media. The public should not be lead to think that there is a cure at hand, but they should be made aware that there are ways in which presently available treatments can be helpful. The replacement of certain significant enzymes of the cholinergic system and the development of chemicals that would help in re-establishing circuitry of healthy brain cells to make up for those that are damaged or dead are treatments that depend on future knowledge about the basic cause of SDAT. Until more is known, the goal is to preserve existing functioning and even to enhance it whenever possible. This is accomplished by:

1. Direct treatment of primary symptoms, such as disorientation and confusion, through the provision of memory aids and orientation procedures such as cues, calendars, and clocks.

2. The treatment of the common secondary symptoms, which derive from the patients' self-incapacity and their reactions to this incapacity.

Such symptoms and treatmens include:

a. Painful self-awareness, such as agitation, anxiety, depression, which are patient reactions to psychological and motor symptoms. Treatment includes counseling the patient and family to provide emotional support and teaching specific skills with which to handle the patient's hostility, anxiety, agitation, and depression. The judicious use of medications (mild to major tranquilizers, antidepressants) may be in order. Agitation and restlessness can often be lessened through exercise.

b. Self-incapacitation -- symptoms directly arising from physical and mental incapacitation, including malnutrition, falling, leaving the stove on, making mistakes in taking medications, and confused wandering. The provision of proper nutrition and a secure environment is indicated.

c. Stimulation-threshold problems -- symptoms reflecting overstimulation by the environment, that is, stimulation beyond the capacity of the patient (e.g., the Goldstein catastrophic reaction with anxiety, irritability). Here the development of simple routines and techniques for stress reduction is helpful.

Where Do We Go From Here?

Dementia is an extraordinarily exciting research topic to pursue because it draws together a variety of disciplines: neurology, immunology, genetics, molecular biology, the neurosciences, neuropsychology. One might question how truly effective we have been in this country in creating multidisciplinary, or more importantly interdisciplinary, programs, yet these are just the types of programs that we must begin to plan. The importance of planning in all manifestations of our work cannot be overstated. In the Unites States today we can no longer depend upon foundations or Congress to support biomedical research adequately or to know how to make decisions regarding allocation of those precious dollars that do exist. We must thus be more "planful" in our approach to them, helping to make their decisions for them.

The National Institute on Aging's effort, A National Plan for Reseach on Aging, subtitled "Toward an Independent Old Age," illustrates such an approach. Twenty-nine scientific advisers and 213 consultants participated in describing opportunities and needs in four important areas with regard to aging. Policy makers can consider adopting and supporting those portions of that plan which bear upon the support of fundamental neurobiology, not solely studies of senile dementia of the Alzheimer's type. This plan has been provided to the various research programs on aging around the world through the World Health Organization.

We must become much more effective in our presentations before foundations and individual philanthropists. We should consider, too, turning to corporations for assistance. Aging research can be shown to be very much in the interests of U.S. industry, for the work force will be increasingly aging. The mandatory retirement age has been moved up to 70, the age of eligibility for social security has been advanced to 67 in a long phasing-in, and starting in 1990 a shortage of skilled workers is predicted. This could lead to job opportunities for older workers in the U.S. Corporate personnel officers are going to have to look beyond their present concerns with motivation, organizational ability, and aptitudes among employees and consider the impact of aging on both behavioral and biological functioning.

The nursing home industry is itself an important resource. Having come of age, it is becoming much more receptive to the importance of both education and research in its institutions.

We must utilize resources that are available to us through the U.S. Society of Neurosciences. David Drachman has urged the development of Alzheimer's and related disorders "centers of excellence" throughout the country. Lewis Thomas has stressed the importance of ten-year stable funding arrangements to pursue possible slow virus etiology. Both the Robert Wood Johnson Foundation and the National Institute on Aging have supported the development of "teaching nursing homes". All three of these approaches could provide centers with populations, computer capability, animal resources, etc., needed to mount effective research efforts.[3] Training could provide opportunities for transfer of already established scientists.

A most significant and rewarding resource presently available to SDAT researchers is the Alzheimer's Disease and Related Disorders Association, an organization of rapidly developing support groups. It is a very important Association both for the families[4] and for its role in advocacy, including advocacy in behalf of research.

In conclusion, much has happened in dementia research and treatment over the last 25 years, and now before our eyes are tantalizing leads. Yet despite progress, we continue to search for new hypotheses and new technology, for greater diagnostic precision and certainly for new therapeutic interventions. In truth, we do not know the causes and we do not have the means for definitive diagnosis or cure. We had best invest more in research right now, for with the extraordinary increase in the size and proportion of older persons that is imminent, we will be confronted indeed with the "disease of the century".

[3]An important obstacle to SDAT research is posed by informed consent requirements. The National Institute on Aging has sponsored a conference to develop guidelines (not requirements) that would be important for institutional review boards in evaluating the acceptability of studies in patients with the disease. The disease itself can impair the very capacity necessary to give informed consent. The guidelines, and the results of the conference, will be published soon.

[4]Families of dementia patients pay a heavy toll. Pressures on the caretakers, largely women, are more than considerable. The risk is great that the caretaker will become ill or depressed and that one patient will turn into two. The Thirty-Six Hour Day, a book by N.L. Mace and P.V. Rabins, is a valuable aid for families.

Senile Dementia: Outlook for the Future, pages 93–104

ONE ROAD OR MANY TO THE CLINICAL RECOGNITION OF ALZHEIMER'S DISEASE ?

Jean Wertheimer

Professeur
Service Universitaire de Psycho-Gériatrie
1008 Prilly - Suisse

A survey of the literature relating to the identification of presenile Alzheimer's disease and senile dementia creates confusion as to the uniformity of criteria throughout the world. We find a variety of modes of clinical approach, with a choice of psychiatric, neurologic or neuro-psychiatric orientations. We also find an exclusive devotion to psychological concepts, exemplified by tests or scales of evaluation designed to assess only mnestic functions and, more rarely, instrumental functions. Confronted by this multiplicity of approaches to diagnosis of the disease, a preliminary question comes to mind : Is there such a close internal coherence among them that the recognition of any one of its signs or symptoms necessarily implies that all the others must be present and that there is no need to identify all of them ? If such is the case, no matter what angle of observation is chosen, psychological, neurologic or neuropsychological, it is logical to say that the identification of a single one of the manifestations of the condition is sufficient for diagnosis. If, on the contrary, the evidence of this inner logic is less certain, isn't there a danger that an approach limited to only one route of access may lead to a wrong diagnosis ?

Generally speaking, the identification of a disease passes through three successive phases. The first is the phase of analysis, based on the anamnesis and then the uncovering of signs and symptoms. This is followed by the phase of synthesis, which brings together an image in relief, in which we see what is observable at the moment, in the deeper context of its historic evolution. In the third phase, we arrive by deduction at the nosological entity which corresponds to this image, excluding all others. This differential diagnosis is carried out by taking into consideration how two or more diseases are related, by characteristics they have in common and above all, by what distinguishes them, the characteristics which make them different.

The process of investigation begins and then develops at some point in the evolution of the disease, which is determined by one of two typical situations. The first clinical situation is defined by the suffering of the patient and sometimes, especially in the psychiatric domain, by the observations of persons around him. The second situation is epidemiological, when the sick subject is identified through the happenstance of a survey. In the former case, the commonly long and complex investigations are more easily accepted than in the second case.

Should Alzheimer's disease therefore be approached in two different manners, one clinical and the other epidemiological, the former in a highly elaborated way while the other is limited to what is most essential? In this case, we must be sure that we have chosen well what is essential.

General Characteristics

Some of the major characteristics of this condition should be emphasized to give us a better view of the contours of the terrain which the clinician or the epidemiologist will explore. The principal one of these characteristics is the fact that we are dealing with an evolutive disease. This implies that the moment when the patient first comes into contact with the medical world very seldom corresponds to the beginning of the evolution, except in the case of an epidemiological study of the whole population in a community. In the latter case, it seems essential to be up to the minute on early diagnosis. This is not at all easy, as reported by Sir Martin Roth (1979). In a study in Newcastle, from 2 to 4 years after initial interviews with 711 subjects of 65 years or more, he found 30 dements, of whom only 6 had been identified at the outset.

It is therefore clear that another fundamental variable plays an important role, the rapidity with which the symptoms become established. In one of our studies (Brull, Wertheimer, Haller 1979), we report on the observation on a neuro-psychological basis of the 4-year evolution of a group of 41 dements. It was found that 2 groups, respectively slightly and moderately deteriorated at the outset, did not become worse during the period of study, whereas a third group, moderately affected in the beginning, became significantly worse.

Individual evolutionary variations result from interactions between five variables. The first, related to the disease itself, is composed of variations in the relative intensity of mnestic, phasic, praxic and gnostic disorders. The disease does not always begin with memory difficulties. We know of presenile cases of patients who suffer from precocious language difficulties (Wechsler 1977). In both the presenile and senile forms we may find focal signs, notably parietal (Lauter, Meyer 1968). The second variable is the rapidity of evolution, which is recognized as being more pronounced in the presenile forms. The third is the intervention of another pathology, either general or cerebral. The latter variable is exemplified by bronchopneumonia which may trigger a confusional-oneiric state in a subject hitherto suffering only from subclinical Alzheimer's disease. It is sometimes observed in the cases that recuperation is incomplete following the acute phase, as the limited function of the affected brain does not permit optimal recuperation of the capacity to cope with the environment (Wertheimer 1979). This vulnerability of mental functioning in the limit forms of this condition is also illustrated in the clinical picture of "pseudo depressive dementia". In the depression of aged people whose neuronal reserves are diminished, the slowing up of psychomotor activity and withdrawal from the outside world, related to thymic disorders, may induce alteration in memory fixation, a lowering of intellectual efficiency and poor orientation, phenomena which improve with a resumption of normal affectivity (Lishmann 1978). The fourth variable depends on the permanence or modifications in the social, relational or environmental surroundings. A changing of furniture, a move, a period of hospitalization, for example often entail a break in the life of the patient, who loses permanently some of his points of reference. In addition, studies carried out through a psychological approach suggest that such socio-economic factors as educational levels may affect the prevalence of the disease, to the detriment of disadvantaged classes (Gurland 1981). The final variable is the mode of psychological reaction to the disease, which itself depends largely upon pre-morbid character and the functional psychopathological history. This enumeration of the factors contributing to the individual clinical image of senile dementia brings to light another major characteristic of the disease, its plasticity. Each case does not only present characteristics it has in common with others but also variations which are peculiar to itself and which often call for particular therapeutic measures. This variability in the clinical picture is also observed in the same individual, from day to day, resulting from factors which are difficult to identify. Accordingly, we may observe variations in performance in the copying of a house, done by a patient at intervals of a few days, but at the same time of day (Fig. 1). Finally, the extent of this plasticity varies in terms of the degree of predominance of the disease. The variability will thus be greater at the beginning of the evolution, when the personality is still firm, and

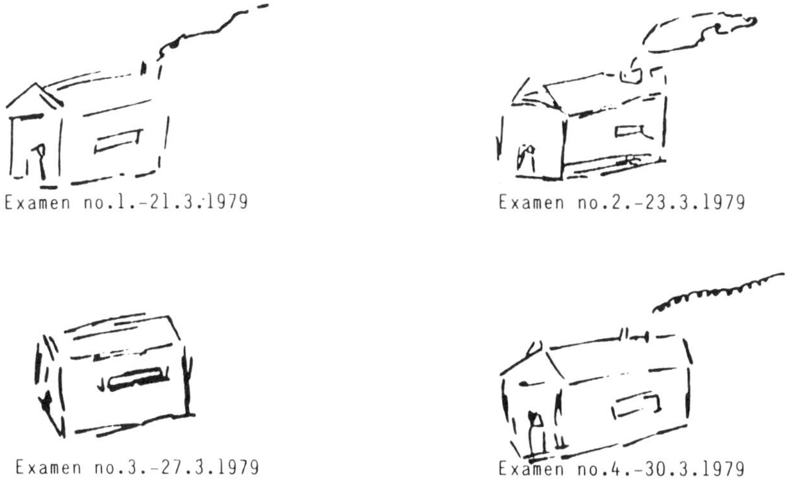

Figure 1.- 84 years old patient. Variations in performance while copying a house drawing, at the same hour, but not on the same day.

becomes lost in a general and common clinical picture at the end of the evolution, when the patient has become entirely dependent and presents a profound aphaso-aprxo-agnosic syndrome.

Also, Alzheimer's disease sweeps up in the whirlwind of its evolution mental operations, affectivity and behavior. It is accompanied as well by neurological manifestations. Thus, the clinician first becomes acquainted with his patient at a given moment in this evolution, and is confronted by a multitude of signs and symptoms, among which he must put his finger on the ones which are common to all cases and which consitute the signature of the disease at a particular phase in its development. What are these signs and symptoms ?

At the outset

Mnestic disorders can be objectified in the clinical situation by the immediate memory test of numbers in direct and reversed order and by the learning of 10 words after 5 repetitions. The repetition of numbers in direct order remains relatively good, while that in reverse order deteriorates precociously. In the learning of words, we find that the acquisition remains satisfactory for the first three (the effect of primacy) and for the last three (the effect of recency), to the detriment of words in the middle of the list. The words which are not remembered are nevertheless recognized when some hints are given, for example when they are inserted in another list of related words. It is therefore apparent that the pathogenesis resides in the capacity to rediscover the correct words. The hypothesis may be proposed of interference (Brooks, Baddeley 1976), whereby the ability to remember depends on inhibiting non-significant information for the sake of relevant information. Supplying a hint reduces the range of choice.

Attention, evaluated by the ability to follow with the eyes the course of lines interlaced with others, and when this is impossible, to do so with a finger, shows disturbances for the first modality.

Temporal orientation is altered earlier than spatial orientation. The patient, near the beginning may find it hard to locate himself with respect to the year, the season, month or day and may make mistakes in estimating the duration of events. Difficulties with regard to space often manifest themselves on the occasion of a trip, when it is necessary to learn new points of reference.

Language functions are also found to be affected quite early. In expression, this may be shown by the forgetting of such words as proper nouns and the designation of details of objects. In such cases, we often find recourse to periphrastic phrases. The disease often begins quite definitely with a predominance of aphasic signs, with disturbance of verbal fluency, a pronounced impoverishment of vocabulary and semantic, morphologic and phonemic paraphasias. The comprehension of spoken language, evaluated by the three papers test of Pierre-Marie, is also altered.

Analysis of writing shows quite early a variety of signs : the forgetting or repetition of words, syllables or letters, or the doubling of downstrokes.In mental arithmetic,automatic operations are conserved for a relatively long time. It is quite different with non-automatic calculations, in which there is an early deterioration. Written arithmetical operations provide a highly varied symptomatology specific to Alzheimer's disease, even at the beginning. We may observe disturbances of spatial arrangement, the loss of the principle of an operation, especially in division and multiplication, the shifting in the midst of one procedure to another (a mixture of subtraction and addition, for example) or the spelling out of numbers or signs. The patient may also write tens, hundreds and thousands separately (1000211 instead of 1211, for example).

The study of praxes is especially informative. Very early in the evolution of the disease, the patient imitates the simulation of a butterfly by the examiner in a reversed form: when the examiner crosses his thumbs with the palms of his hands facing inward, the patient will turn his palms outward, away from himself. When the patient is asked to mime the use of an object, such as a comb or toothbrush, he often takes his own body as the object. Damage to ideational praxes usually comes later in the evolution, but it may sometimes occur relatively early, which imposes a serious handicap upon the patient, who loses his capacity to proceed logically from his intention to the elementary gestures which constitute the action.

Constructives praxes, evaluated either graphically by a spontaneous or copied drawing of a cube a 3-dimension house and a 2-dimension bicycle, or by the reconstitution of a model presented in the form of separate pieces (Wechsler's man), are also precociously altered. The most common observation is the absence of representation of perspective by the diminishing of planes in copying a cube or the transposition of the arms and legs of Wechsler's man.

Visual agnosia is manifested relatively early in the difficulty of recognizing the entangled figures en Poppelreuter's test. In the field of corporal gnoses, we should note the difficulties encountered quite early in the naming and indication of the middle and ring fingers.

In the neurological field, signs of the onset of the condition are not pronounced, being limited sometimes to traces of archaic reflexes (oral-visual, grasping, palm-chin).

Affectivity is fairly often altered, tending toward depression, early in the evolution. Gustavson, for example (Gustavson 1975) found in a group of 57 patients suffering from presenile Alzheimer's disease that depression was the reason for the first consultation in one-third of the cases.

Advanced forms of the disease

We shall not undertake a detailed description of the neuropsychological manifestations which evolve toward a major amnesic and also aphasic, apractic and agnosic syndrome. It is appropriate however to draw attention to some of the particular characteristics of these advanced forms. The diffuse cortical alterations are not simply additive in their effects. Their simultaneous occurrence is reflected by the appearance of particular forms of behavior which represent compromises resulting from interactions between altered fundamental functions. We may for instance observe alterations in relation to the specular image. Thus, the patient will have difficulty in identifing an object and the reflection of the same object in a mirror; in accepting the identity of the reflection of the experimenter and the experimenter himself; finally, in recognizing his own reflection (Ajuriaguerra,Strejilevitch, Tissot 1963).

The Geneva school describes three types of functional disintegration:

- dissolution with a return to chronologically earlier levels of organization, corresponding, in involuted stages, to the natural articulations of development;
- dissolution with a return to primitive forms of organization, characterized by a tendency

to disappear ontogenetically and to give way to voluntary functions (archaic reflexes, for example);
- disorganization which has only a distant and doubtful relationship with stages in maturation, such as stereotypes (Richard, Constantinidis 1970).

Neurological manifestations are accentuated. Archaic reflexes are easily and regularly evoked. Walking becomes less rhythmic. We find a paratonia and sometimes disturbances in both voluntary and automatic oculomotor functions (Richard 1974).

The affective alterations in advanced forms of Alzheimer's disease have given rise to a classification into sub-groups :

- simple senile form : monotonic humour
- hypochondriac-melancholic form : anxiety about poverty, ruin, bodily degeneration
- manic-expansive form : exaggerated efforts at self-affirmation through activity
- paranoid-hallucinatory form : delirious ideas of prejudice and thefts.

Paraclinical examinations

In the diagnostic approach to Alzheimer's disease, the EEG is very useful, in showing diffuse slowing of waves. The CT scan has made possible a great step forward. It must be recognized however that correlations between the extent of atrophy and that of injury to mental operations are often uncertain (Huckmann, Fox, Topel 1975). We may for example observe the existence of atrophy in subjects with normal mental activity and an absence of atrophy in some dements. It is also apparent that neither the EEG nor the CT scan should be regarded as absolute means of diagnosis; their results must be integrated into the clinical observations as a whole. Measurement of regional cerebral blood flow is difficult to apply to large populations. Great hopes have been placed in the PET, in the belief that it may enable us to gain a better understanding of metabolic activities in the brain in Alzheimer's disease and possibly make a better assessment of the evolutionary stage.

Psychological approaches

Description of the clinical aspects of Alzheimer's disease demonstrates that we cannot limit ourselves in the diagnostic approach to the evaluation of any single modified function. The psychological approach, for example, utilizes both tests of memory and of orientation, such as the Mental Status Questionnaire (MSQ) (Kahn, Pollack, Goldfarb 1961) or the Short Portable Mental Status Questionnaire (SPMSQ) (Pfeiffer 1975). It resorts to tests of memory and learning (Inglis Paired Associate Learning Test, Synonym Learning Test, Object Learning Test, Digit Copying Test) (Miller 1981) and to tests described as diagnostic for dementia (Benton, Bender) or to scales for evaluating intelligence, such as the Wechsler-Bellevue Scale, the WAIS, Raven's Progressive Matrices and the Primary Mental Abilities Scale. Even if we grant that the majority of psycho-organic syndromes in old age consist of senile dementias of the Alzheimer type, it is unjustified to conclude from this that injury to mental operations detected by these tests is a positive identification of this condition. In the situation of an epidemiological survey, it is advisable to regard the psychological approach as a preliminary. It enables us to identify subjects suffering from psycho-organic syndromes, thus clearing the way for a subsequent rigorous clinical approach. The same principle is applicable to such neuro-psychiatric tests as the Face-Hand Test. Disturbance of perception of the two simultaneous tactile stimuli is not exclusive to Alzheimer's disease. It is also encountered in focalized parietal lesions. The disclosure of evidence of a deficit in this test is therefore the proper preliminary to a complete clinical study.

Conclusions

The clinical picture of Alzheimer's disease, whose plasticity we have emphasized, can be examined from various points of view, affective, behavioural, neuropsychological, neurological, radiological, etc. No single one of these is specific enough however to make a diagnosis. It is through a synthesis of the signs and symptoms in all these fields, taking into account not only what can be observed at a particular moment but also the evolutionary history, that the condition can be understood. Only then shall we be able not only to recognize the existence of a psycho-organic syndrome, but also to identify its nature and exclude other hypotheses. We may add that the effort to identify Alzheimer's disease in aged people serves as a central fulcrum for the differential diagnosis of psycho-organic syndromes as a whole. In response to the question presented in the title of this article, we may say that the routes of access to the diagnostic hypothesis of senile dementia are multiple, but that the effort thus undertaken is unique, entailing a synthesis of the psychiatric, neuropsychologic and neurological aspects of the disease.

References

Ajuriaguerra J., Strejilevitch M., Tissot R.(1963) A propos de quelques conduites devant le miroir de sujets atteints de syndromes démentiels du grand âge. Neuropsychologia 1 : 59.

Brooks D.N., Baddeley A.D. (1976). What can amnesic patients learn? Neuropsychologia 14 : 111.

Brull J., Wertheimer J., Haller E. (1979). Evolutive Profiles in Senile Dementia. A Psychological and Neuropsychological Longitudinal Study. Springer. Brain Function in Old Age, p. 188.

Gurland B.J. (1981). The Borderlands of Dementia : The Influence of Sociocultural Characteristics on Rates of Dementia Occuring in the Senium. Raven Press, New York. Aging 15 : 61.

Gustafson L.(1975).Psychiatric symptoms in dementia with onset in presenile period. Acta Psychiat. Scand. Suppl. 257:9.
Huckmann M.S.,Fox J.,Topel J.(1975).The validity of criteria for the evaluation of cerebral atrophy by computed tomography. Radiology 116:85.
Kahn R.L.,Pollack M.,Goldfarb A.I.(1961).Grune & Stratton New York.Psychopathology of Aging,p.104.
Lauter H.,Meyer J.E.(1968).Clinical and Nosological Concepts of Senile Dementia.Senile Dementia Clinical and Therapeutic Aspects, p. 13.
Lishmann W.A.,(1978).Senile dementia, presenile dementia and pseudo-dementia. Organic psychiatry, the psychological consequences of cerebral disorders. Blackwell Scientific Publications, Oxford Chap. 10:527.
Miller E.,(1981). The Differential Psychological Evaluation. Raven Press New York.Aging 15:121.
Müller Ch.,WertheimerJ.(1981).Abrégé de psychogériatrie. Masson Paris.
Pfeiffer E.(1975).A short portable mental status questionnaire for the assessment of organic brain deficit in elderly patients.J.Am.Geriatr.Soc.23:433
Richard J.,Constantinidis J.(1970).Les démences de la vieillesse. Confrontations psychiatriques 5:39.
Richard J.(1974).Neuropsychologie et gériatrie. Méd.& Hygiène 32:1189.
Sir Martin Roth (1979).The early diagnosis of Alzheimer's disease:an introduction. Churchill Livingstone.Alzheimer's disease p.65.
Roth M.(1959). Some diagnosis and aetiological aspects of confusional states in the elderly. Gerontologia 1:83.
Wechsler A.F.(1977) Presenile dementia presenting as aphasia. Journal of Neurology,Neurosurgery and Psychiatry 40:303.
Wertheimer J.,Lobrinus A.,Brull J.(1977). Zu einer Langzeitstudie der Senile Demenz.Janssen Symposium.Gerontopsychiatrie 6:296.
Wertheimer J.(1979) Plasticité de la démence sénile. Médecine & Hygiène 37:3824.

IV. AGING OF NERVE TISSUE AND LESIONS OF ALZHEIMER'S DISEASE

Presided by M. Yoshikawa (Tokyo)

Senile Dementia: Outlook for the Future, pages 107–112

SENILE AMYLOIDOSIS:CLINICAL AND ANATOMICAL ASPECTS

Diana D. Orlovskaya and Akim I.Oifa

All-Union Research Center of Mental Health
Academy of Medical Sciences of the USSR
Moscow

Amyloid deposits in the central nervous system are one of the main neuronal aging manifestation (Divry I932, I939,I956;Schwartz I970). They are commonly found in aged animal and people,especially in patients with senile dementia and Alzheimer disease.The brain amyloid is mostly presented in the form of senile plaques.

Although in neurohistopathology the senile amyloidosis has become fairly well defined its origin and pathogenesis is not known completely.

There are several hypotheses, that attempt to interpret the amyloid plaque formation (Terry I932;Wisniewski et al. I932,I933).

Wisniewski et al. (I933) underline the role of the microglia in the process of amyloid production. According to their electron microscopic findings microglial cells are commonly located in and around senile plaques and the amyloid-associated microglia often have a protrusion of cytoplasmic processes extending into the amyloid. They also found amyloid fibers streaming from their processes.There are not only electron microscopic evidences of microglia participation in the amyloidogenesis but also histochemical ones (Wisniewski et al. I932). The idea about the the role of the microglial cells in the brain amyloid formation coincides the suggestion of Rowers and Spicer (I977)that the amyloid may arise from local brain factors rather than circulating systemic factors.

In spite of the above-mentioned data the role of microglia in the formation of the amyloid plaques remains definitively unconfirmed. In connection with this problem it may be interesting the relationship between the senile process in the brain and schizophrenic process.

In psychiatric literature some kind of a competition between schizophrenia and senile process can be found. Besides the somatic infantilism was emphatized in schizophrenic patients. As to anatomical level many histopathological fenomena in schizophrenic brain were described including the loss of the microglial cell reactivity (areactivity) and the features of atrophy of these cells (mainly in nuclear forms of schizophrenia and in a long course of disease).

If the microglia really plays the important role in the amyloid production the frequency of senile plaques in schizophrenic brain must be much more less than in control ones.

Dusheiko (1972) determined the frequency of senile plaques in 300 patients aged 60-90 years with different mental disorders. He established rather active senile plaques formation in schizophrenic brain tissue. The proportions of cases with senile plaques were following: senile dementia - 100%, schizophrenia - 75%, vascular (atherosclerotic) psychoses - 47,3%. But in this study the schizophrenic group was too small (8 cases) for final conclusion.

This paper concerns to some results of senile amyloidosis screening in the brain and some visceral organs according to " Schwartz's triada" - brain, heart, pancreas in 3 group of aged persons - non-demented geriatric patients, schizophrenics and patients with senile dementia.

A total amount of 190 cases was examined. According to their clinical diagnoses they distribute the following way: non-demented geriatric (normal) patients -77, schizophrenics 50, senile dementia -63. The age of all patients was between 60 and 88 years; women were 127, men -70. Normal aged people came from a geriatric unit of a general hospital, schizophrenic and patients with senile dementia from the wards of mental hospital. The other words, our study was based on unselected cases from autopsy room. In all cases the leading causes of death were extracerebral diseases.

The frequency and distribution of amiloid deposits in different organs were studied by fluorecsent histochemical methods with thiozine-red (the delusions of fluorochrome were I:I0000 -I:I00000) and in polarized light after the staining with Cóngo-red.Amyloid deposits in the fluorecsent pictures gave a bright orange-red color in the green background. Eight or nine regions were taken for examination, namely frontal,temporal,parietal and ocipital brain cortex, hyppocampus,corpus striatum,hypotalamic area.

The distribution of senile amyloidosis in the group of non-demented patients is presented in table I.

Table I

The frequency of amyloidosis in internal organs and brain of non-demented geriatrics patients

Age	Number of cases	Frequency of amyloidosis (%)	
		All organs, including brain	Brain
6I-65	3	0	0
66-70	I0	60	33
7I-75	29	5I	36
76-80	I9	78	6I
8I-85	II	63	54
86-88	5	I00	I00
Total	77	58	46

A highly significant correlation was established between the frequency of amyloidosis of different organs and age.This correlation was mainly determined by the cerebral amyloid deposits.In all age groups brain amyloidosis was seen in 46% of the cases, heart amyloidosis in25% and amyloidosis of pancreas in 24%.The conclusion is maid that in senile amyloidosis there may be developed an isolated lesion of the brain tissue.The full "Schwartz's triada" was found only in 5 cases(6,5%).

The autonomous aging process in the brain may partially explain a dissociation between somatic and mental aging changes. It is well known that mental deterioration can develop without corresponding somatic alterations and vice versa.

In table 2 the results received in schizophrenic group is shown,

Table 2

The frequency of amyloidosis in internal organ and brain of schizophrenic patient group

Age	Number of cases	Frequency of amyloidosis (%)	
		All organs, including brain	Brain
6I-65	9	56	33
66-70	II	55	27
7I-75	I6	75	69
76-80	8	50	50
8I-85	6	33	83
Total	50	64	52

According to described data the conclusion can be developed that the brain amyloidosis was produced in schizophrenia rather actively and earlier comparatively to non-demented geriatric patients. Its frequency in the age groups of 6I-65 years, 7I-75 years and 8I-85 years was higher than in a control one (table I). The percentage of the cases with manifestation of brain amyloidosis in different clinical group were as follows: non-demented geriatric patients -46%, schizophrenics - 52%, senile dementia - I00%.

In the light of the microglia function in the amyloid fibers production we analyesd the histological appearance of the microglial reaction in schizophrenic brain with amyloidosis (52%) and without it (48%).

In schizophrenic brain with amyloidosis the active reaction and hyperplasia of the microglial cells were determined, especially in and around the senile plaques. In connection to these finding it is important to stress that we studied long developed schizophrenia and in these cases we could expect areactivity of the microglial cells, which had been mentioned in the literature (Aleksandrovskaya 1950; Wildi et al. 1967; Suchorukova 1972). The loss of a reactivity of the microglia was only found in schizophrenic brain tissue without senile amyloid deposits.

The correlation between the amyloid plaques formation and the microglial cells reaction supports of hypothesis about the key-role of the microglia in the production of the amyloid in the nervous system. It may be explained from the immunological theory of brain aging and amyloidogenesis. Apparently for the microglial reaction the most important is brain local immunological status and the presence of corresponding immunological stimula.

Aleksandrovskaya M (I950). Neuroglia in different psychoses Moscow:Medgiz,246 p.
Divry P(I932). Method de demonstration rapide des plaques seniles. Riv Patol Nerv Ment 40:399.
Divry P (I939). Le probleme des plaques seniles. J Belge Neurol Psych 6:444.
Divry P (I956). De la notion d'amyloidose cerebrale dans les processuse seniles. Experientia Suppl 4 p.II2.
Dusheiko SD (I972). Concerning senile plaques and Alzheimer changes of Neurofibrilles in Mental patients Deceased in Old Age. Zh Nevropat psikiat (Moscow) 72:I029.
Powers JM, Spicer SS (I978). Histochemical Similarity of senile plaque amyloid to apudamyloid. Virchows Arch A (Pathol Anat) 376:I07.
Schwartz Ph (I970). Amyloidosis.Cause and Manifestation of senile Deterioration . Springfield Ill:Ch C Thomas Publisher p.4I6.
Suchorukova LI (I972). The changes of a neuroglia in schizophrenia. In Romasenko VA (ed): "The Pathologic anatomy and certain problem of the Thanatogenesis of Schizophrenia".Moscow:Medizina 23o p.
Terry RD (I982). Brain Disease in Aging,Especially Senile dementia. In Terry RD,Bolis CL,Toffano G (ed):" Neuronal Aging ant Its Implication in Human Neurological Pathology" New York:Raven Press p.43
Wildi E, Costoulas G, Linder A (I967). Schizophrenie et involution cerebrel senile. Etude anatomo-pathologique et statistique de 75 cas. Psychiat et neurol I54:I
Wisniewski H.M.et al.(I983). Morphology and Biochemistry of Neuronal Paired Helical Filaments and Amyloid Fibers in Human and Animals. In Zimmerman HM (ed):" Progress in Neuropathology" New York:Raven Press p.I39.
Wisniewski H.M. ,Vorbrodt AM,Lossinsky AS, Grundke-Iqbal I (I982). Pathogenesis of Neuritic (Senile) and Amyloid plaque Formation. Experiment Brain Res Suppl 5:3.

Senile Dementia: Outlook for the Future, pages 113–123

MODIFICATIONS IN THE GENETIC EXPRESSION IN THE AGING BRAIN

Jorge Cervós-Navarro, M.D.

Director Institute for Neuropathology
Free University Berlin (FRG)
Hindenburgdamm 30, 1000 Berlin 45

Aging in brain is a complex process which is characterized by alterations of morphological and chemical parameters. Brain tissue consists of different cell types with distinct biochemical and functional features and the interactions among cells may be quite complex during aging. However, histological and ultrastructural information on aging brain strongly suggests that changes in the biological parameters of neurons play the primary role in the process.

In spite of the universal character of the aging process in the cellular level when studies of the molecular mechanisms of cellular aging are conducted of different times, the question arises if the cells to be investigated remain constant throughout the time. The cellular and organismal life spans are identical only for postmitotic cells. Although there is considerable neuronal plasticity possible in the mature neuron (Szekely 1979) in the postnatal life differentiated neurons are not capable of mitosis. Thus comparative examinations of neuronal populations can be carried out at different times during aging, whereas in the case of mitotic cells the cellular composition of a population at different autogenetic times is a function of the cycle of generations of the respective cells. Another advantage of postmitotic cells lies in their natural synchronization and in the lower microheterogenity of their chromosomal material.

The biological parameters varying as a function of aging reflect modifications in the expression of genetic information encoded in the genome. The fact that genetic expression and transfer of genetic information may be hampered at different cellular levels led to the development of a large number of genetic theories on aging. They did not really represent independent theories on aging but merely described different aspects of age-dependent modifications of genetic expression.

In eukaryotic cells the genetic information is contained in code in the DNA of chromatin by means of the linear arrangement of the nucleotide and is transcribed to RNA by the nuclear DNA-dependent RNA polymerase. The transcription process is composed of several highly specific steps. In the present study we investigated the age-dependent changes in several of these steps.

Material and Methods

Two groups of female Sprague-Dawley rats, 150 to 180 g, of different age (12 and over 30 months old) were used. Cerebral rat brain nuclei were isolated and purified neuronal and oligodendroglial chromatin was isolated by discontinuous sucrose gradient centrifugation corresponding morphologically to those described by Austocker et al.(1972). The isolated chromatin was fractionated by nucleolytic digestion with DNAase II into fragments of the average size of transcriptional units. The procedure permits the separation between transcriptionally active and repressed chromatin.

The total number of initiation sites on neuronal chromatin was titrated under conditions completely eliminating reinitiation and non-specific initiation using the technique described by Axel et al.(1974), which allows only one RNA molecule to be synthesized at each available RNA initiation site. Either a fixed amount of E. coli RNA polymerase (2.4 units) was incubated with increasing amounts of neuronal chromatin (0 to 12 μg DNA) or various amounts of RNA polymerase (0 to 10 units) were incubated with fixed amounts of neuronal chromatin (2 μg DNA) (Sarkander et al. 1978). The absence of CTP in the assay during the initiation period prevents extensive RNA chain elongation, and thus repeated initiation of RNA chains at the same initiation site. After formation of the initiation complex (15 min), RNA chain elongation was permitted under high ionic strength conditions, which prevents further initiation by addition of $(NH_4)_2SO_4$, $MgCl_2$ and CTP.

With increasing template-to-enzyme rations, the final (^{3}H)UMP incorporation at the end of the elongation period increased until saturation of RNA initiation sites was reached, representing the point at which all of the RNA polymerase molecules are bound to the chromatin template (saturation point). The number of RNA chains initiated under conditions preventing reinitiation and non-specific initiation is equal to the number of RNA initiation sites on the template.

The in vitro up-take of acetate in nucleosomal DNA-bound histones were measured to asses its biological significance. For the purpose neuronal and oligodendroglial DNA-bound histones were acetylated up to maximum values in the presence of saturating amounts of (^{3}H)acetyl-conenzyme A. Densitometric scans and photographs of acetylated and deacetylated histones were separated by polyacrylamide gel electrophoresis. Thereafter acetylated and non-acetylated templates were comparatively transcribed by exogenously added RNA polymerase B molecules 15 min in assays described elsewhere (Sarkander, Uthoff 1976).

Results

As summarized in tab. 1) the amount of template-active portions as compared to repressed portions is markedly different between neuronal chromatin isolated either from 12 or 30 months old rats. Assuming identical DNAase II susceptibility of chromatin, neuronal chromatin isolated from adult rats contains a higher proportion of transcribable sequences than chromatin isolated from senile rats.

Age of animals (month)	DNAase II sensitive	transcrip-tionally-active	transcrip-tionally-inactive
12	87.4 ± 5.2	20.8 ± 2.1	66.1 ± 3.7
30	89.5 ± 5.7	13.3 ± 1.9	75.6 ± 5.2

Table 1: Percent of chromosomal DNA of DNAase II fractionated chromatin isolated from 12 and over 30 months old rats.

In fig. 1 can be seen the different inflection points (arrows) of the RNA polymerase saturation curves in comparision to unfractionated neuronal chromatin. From 30 months old rats a greater

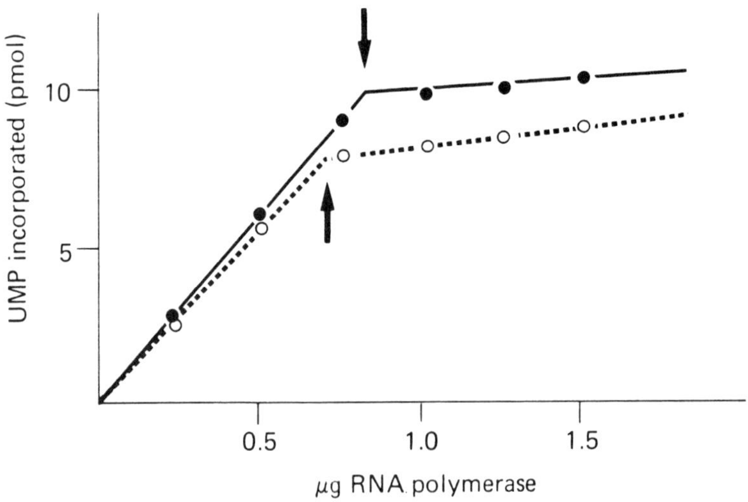

Fig. 1: Titration of the total number of RNA initiation sites on unfractionated neuronal chromatin from 12 (0—0) and over 30 months (0--0) old rats.

quantity of RNA polymerase was needed to saturate the initiation sites present on unfractionated chromatin of 12 months old rats, indicating a greater number of RNA initiation sites on chromatin in adult rats.

In template-active neuronal and oligodendroglial chromatin the differences in the number of neuronal and oligodendroglial RNA initiation sites is much smaller than the differences measured when under the same conditions unfractionated chromatin of both cells is used for the determination of the RNA initiation sites (fig. 2).

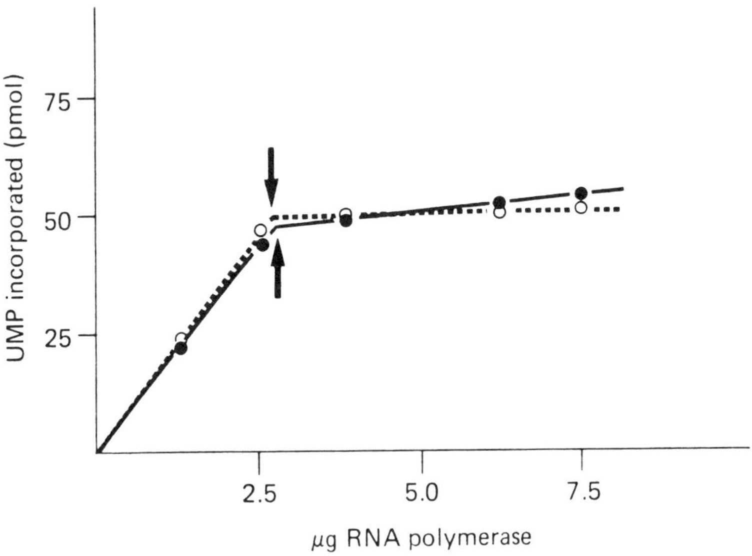

Fig. 2: Titration of the total number of RNA initiation sites on transcriptionally active neuronal chromatin from 12 (0—0) and over 30 months (0--0) old rats.

Fig. 3 shows the number of RNA initiation sites available for exogenously added RNA polymerase B molecules on acetylated and non-acetylated template-active neuronal chromatin fractions prepared from adult and senile rats. The different position of the inflection points of the titration kinetics of RNA polymerase saturation curves of "adult" neuronal chromatin signifies that the enzymatic acetylation of template-active neuronal chromatin creates an additional availability of RNA initiation sites on the acetylated chromatin. However, the position of the inflection points of the titration curves of RNA initiation sites of acetylated and non-acetylated neuronal template-active chromatin isolated from senile rats was almost identical. This indicates that the acetylation of the senile template-active neuronal chromatin causes no or only a negligible increase in the number of RNA initiation sites on the acetylated "senile" chromatin(fig. 4).

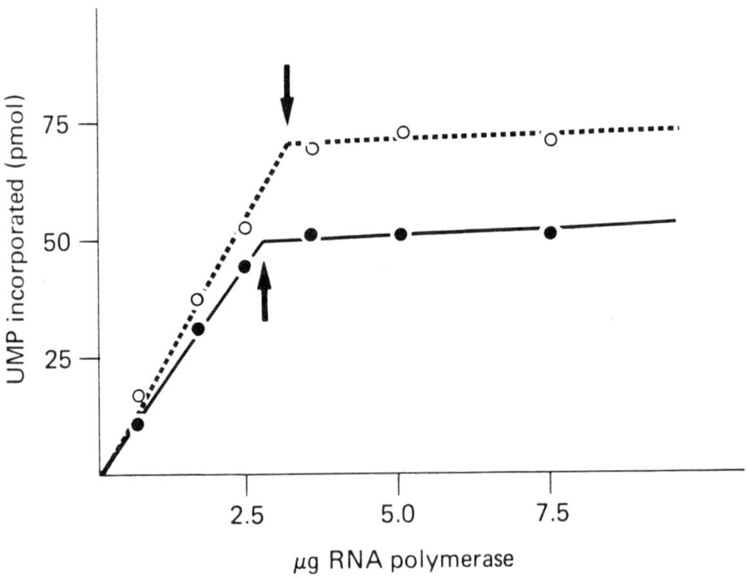

Fig. 3: Neuronal RNA polymerase B saturation curves of acetylated (0--0) and non-acetylated (0—0) transcriptionally active chromatin isolated from adult rats.

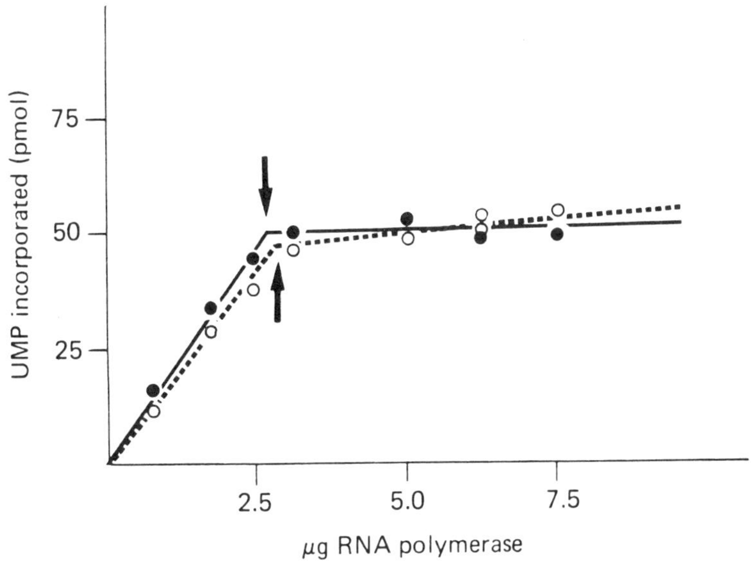

Fig. 4: Neuronal RNA polymerase B saturation curves of acetylated (0--0) and non-acetylated (0——0) transcriptionally active chromatin isolated from senile rats.

Discussion

Our results allow a comparative compositional and functional chromatin analyses of the postmitotic neuronal and of the mitotic glial cells of the brain at different points in time during the aging process. The aim of these types of molecular biological studies has been to detect the control regulation mechanisms of gene expression and their age-dependent modifications.

All experiments on age-dependent compositional changes of the chromatin-templated transcription performed to date have been carried out using total chromatin (Thompson 1973; Banks-Schlegel, Johnson 1975; Ryan 1975). Since, however, in differentiated cells only a small portion of selected DNA sequence (10 %) is transcribed in RNA, results obtained from investigations carried out on total chromatin are related to chromatin mainly in its transcriptionally inactive biologically repressed state. The amount of DNA sequences without transcriptional activity depends on the genetic restriction of the chromatin. For the purpose of recognizing regulatory mechanisms and the components involved in genetic expression, the phenomenon of genetic restriction of chromatin, and the identification of molecular mechanisms of age-specific modifications of the transcription process it becomes indispensable to separate chromatin into its transcriptionally active and inactive DNA sequences. This makes it possible to examine the compositional and functional properties of those DNA sequences that in vivo encode for the cellular RNA.

Previous results showed considerable differences in quantities and relationship between transcriptionally active and repressed neuronal and oligodendroglial fractions and the age-dependent shift of the relation within the neuronal and oligodendroglial chromatin (Cervós-Navarro et al. 1980). It is well established that oligodendrocyte rat brain nuclei display a higher restricted endogenous RNA polymerase A and B reaction and a several times lower in vivo labelling of RNA than neuronal and astrocyte nuclei. These are presumably due to the difference in the internal organization and arrangement of their nucleosomes which determine both the morphological and gross functional properties of neuronal, astrocytic, and oligodendroglial chromatin.

There is a marked difference between the portions of transcriptionally active DNA sequence in the Mg^{2+}-solube of adult and senile animals. This means that neuronal and oligodendroglial chromatin isolated from adult animals has a higher content of transcribable DNA sequences than the neuronal or oligodendroglial chromatin of senile animals. Results clearly prove that in the course of the aging process structural modifications of the neuronal and chromatin develop that age-dependently restrict the transcription of transcribable DNA sequences originally available in adult animals.

Interestingly we found an equal number of RNA initiation sites on neuronal chromatin isolated from 12 and over 30 months old rats. This brings to light that the large capacitive differences between neuronal and NAG in vivo and in vitro RNA synthesis (Thompson 1973; Fleischer-Lambropoulos et al. 1974; Sarkander, Dulce 1979) are more the consequence of the different mass ratio of transcriptionally active and repressed DNA sequences within the neuronal and NAG chromatin than of quantitative transcriptive differences between the transcriptionally active DNA fractions of both types of cells. Since the transcribable DNA sequences of senile animals is lower it has to be assumed that the transcription rate increases in the course of aging process.

Several molecular mechanistic events may be in part responsible for the realization of the neuronal transcription rate, increasing in old age as well as for the age-dependent NAG chromatin-directed transcription; (a) differences in the number of RNA initiation sites on the templates compared; (b) differences in the initiation frequencies with which the RNA polymerase molecules utilize the RNA initiation sites localized on every one of the templates; and/or (c) different velocities of the RNA chain elongation.

It has been shown that the acetylation of chromatin brings about an increase in the number of available RNA initiation sites on the acetylated template and that the amount of acetate uptake correlates positively with the degree of increase of RNA initiation sites (Oberhauser et al. 1978; Sarkander, Dulce 1978; Sarkander 1983).
Therefore the different in vitro acetylation rates of the chromatin-bound histone fractions in senile rats indicate that neuronal chromatin has a different structure at these times of development. In particular we found that the strength of histone binding to nucleosomal core particle DNA decreases with age. The greater capacity for acetylation of chromatin isolated from older rats may be the molecular basis for rendering additional RNA initiation site on chromatin available for RNA polymera-

se molecules. However, there is reason to assume that the age-related loss of stability of chromatin may lead to a decrease of the fidelity of the genetic outflow of information of chromatin. Moreover, the fact that the acetylation of the senile neuronal chromatin does not increase the number of RNA initiation sites was a surprising finding. It could be interpreted as the fact that the higher acetylation capacity of the histones localized in the template-active sequences of the "senile" chromatin by comparison with "adult" chromatin may already be a compensatory mechanism and signifies that neuronal chromatin in old age is already transcribed with a capacity that cannot be increased further by the acetylating mechanisms.

Every cellular event is characterized by its relative position with respect to the preceding step and by the temporal difference between the latter and the previous events. Since the genetic information is not expressed simultaneously but sequentially, DNA not only serves as a carrier of genetic information, i.e., as a matrix for other molecules, but also as a "biological clock". Such considerations are of special importance for the aging process.

In essence, the age-related destabilisation of neuronal chromatin may be one of the mechanisms triggering cellular and organismal aging due to faulty transcription of the genetic information as assumed in the "error theory of aging".

References

Austocker J, Cox D, Mathias AP (1972). Fractionation of nuclei from brain by zonal centrifugation and a study of the RNA polymerase activity in the various classes of nuclei. Biochem J 129:1139.

Axel R, Cedar H, Felsenfeld G (1974). Chromatin template activity and chromatin structure. Cold Spring Harbor Symp. Quant.Biol.38:773

Banks-Schlegel SP, Johnson TC (1975). RNA metabolism in isolated mouse brain nuclei during early postnatal development. J Neurochem 24:947

Cervós-Navarro J (1980). Pathologie des Nervensystems I. Gefäßerkrankungen und Durchblutungsstörungen des Gehirns, Bd 13/1, Springer Verlag Berlin Heidelberg New York

Fleischer-Lambropoulos H, Sarkander HI, Brade WP (1974). Phosphorylation of nonhistone chromatin from neuronal and glial nuclei-enriched fractions of rat brain. FEBS Lett 45:329

Oberhauser H, Csordas A, Puschendorf B, Grunicke H (1978). Increase in initiation sites for chromatin RNA synthesis by acetylation of chromosomal proteins. Biochem Biophys Res Commun 84:100

Ryan JM (1975). Alterations in chromatin functions during ageing in vitro. Adv Exp Med Biol 53:123

Sarkander HI, Uthoff CG (1976). Comparison of the number of RNA initiation sites in rat brain fractions enriched in neuronal or glial nuclei. FEBS Lett 71:53

Sarkander HI, Dulce HJ (1978). Studies on the regulation of RNA synthesis in neuronal and glial nuclei isolated from rat brain. Exp Brain Res 31:317

Sarkander HI, Knoll-Köhler E, Cervós-Navarro J (1978). Repression of glial RNA transcription during the development of 6-aminonicotinamide (6.AN)-induced acute gliopathy. J Pharmacol Exp Ther 20:503

Sarkander HI, Dulce HJ (1979). Characteristics of transcriptionally active and inactive neuronal and nonastrocytic glial rat brain chromatin fractions. Exp Brain Res 35:109

Sarkander HI (1983). Age-dependent changes in the organization and regulation of transcriptionally active neuronal and nonastrocytic glial chromatin. In Cervós-Navarro J, Sarkander HI (eds): Brain aging: Neuropathology and Neuropharmacology (Aging Vol 21) Raven Press NY, p 301

Szekely G (1979). Platicity of neurons. Trends in Neurosci 2:245

Thompson RJ (1973). Studies on RNA synthesis in two populations of nuclei from the mammalian cerebral cortex. J Neurochem 21:19

Senile Dementia: Outlook for the Future, pages 125–135

STEREOLOGIC FINDINGS IN NORMAL BRAIN AGING AND ALZHEIMER'S DISEASE

W.Meier-Ruge, M.D.[1], J.Ulrich, M.D.[2],
S.Abdel-Al, B.Sc.[1]
[1]Gerontol. Brain Res., Sandoz Ltd.,CH-4002 Basel
[2]Inst. Pathol., University, CH-4003 Basel

In the past the decrease in brain weight and brain volume in old age was considered to be the result of a progressive nerve cell loss (Brody and Vijayashankar 1977). Morphometric investigations of brain stem nuclei in aging individuals, however, showed only a few brain structures with an age-dependent decrease in nerve cells (Konigsmark and Murphy 1970, 1972; Vijayashankar and Brody 1979; Monagle and Brody 1974; Sandoz and Meier-Ruge 1977; Meier-Ruge et al. 1978). Nerve cell loss in old age seemed not to be a universal phenomenon in the brain.

Recent investigations by Miller et al. (1980) established the fact that hemisphere volume decreases by 3.5 % per decade in males and 1.9 % per decade in females. A subsequent increase in the ratio of grey matter to white matter volume, however, could not be explained unambiguously.

In order to obtain better insights into shrinkage phenomena of the brain we investigated the three-dimensional network of the brain capillaries, which promised to give through expansion or drawing together of the capillary net - the most relevant information about volume changes in selected brain structures. We were able to show that post-mortem changes in the stereologic parameters of the brain capillaries are of minor importance (Hunziker and Schweizer 1977). The use of native brain slices which allowed an elective staining of the capillaries with an alkaline phosphatase reaction avoided the introduction into the stereologic calculations of a correcting factor as compensation for shrinkage artefacts due to any fixation procedure (Haug,1967, 1972). All stereologic investigations were made (Fig. 1) with an optic electronic image analysis system (Texture Analyzer TAS Leitz).

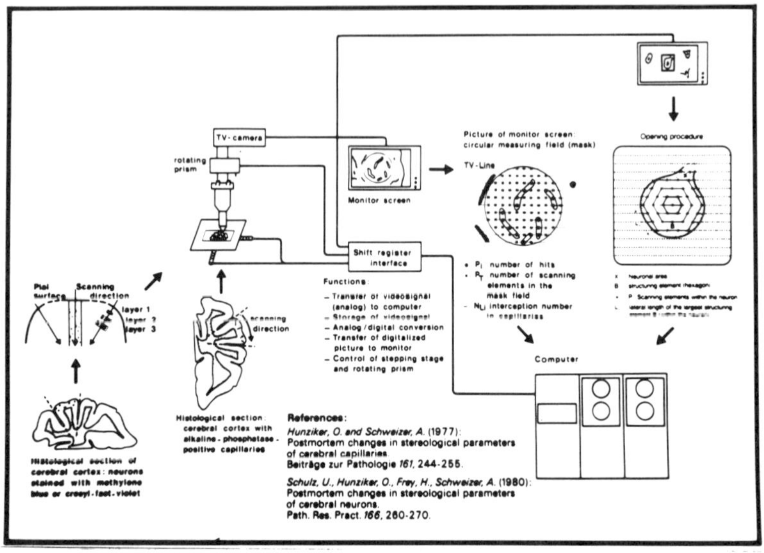

Fig. 1. Schematic representation of the morphometric procedure.

The investigation of normal aging brains (Hunziker et al. 1978; Meier-Ruge et al. 1980) demonstrated that the capillary parameters of the cortex of the medial frontal gyrus did not show any trend with increasing age towards changes in the capillary length, the capillary volume or the intercapillary distances (Meier-Ruge et al. 1980). All values merely oscillated around the mean value measured in the group of young brains between 19 and 54 years of age (Fig. 2). In contrast to the brain cortex, an age-dependent increase in capillary length and capillary volume, and a decrease in intercapillary distances could be measured in the putamen (Fig. 2).

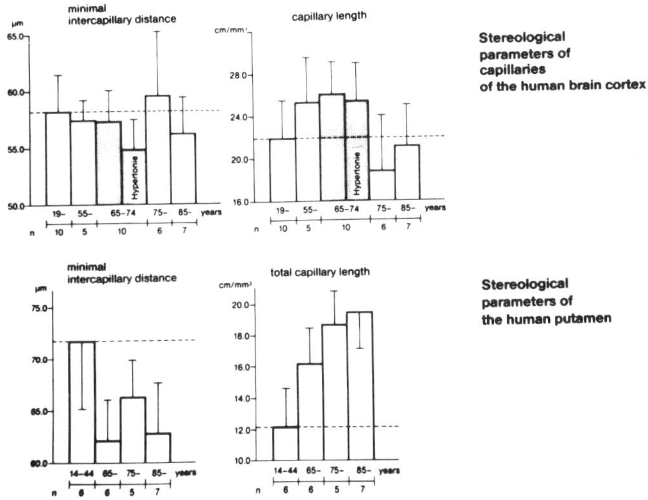

Fig. 2. Stereologic results from the cortical capillaries (precentral gyrus, top) in comparison with the results from the putamen (bottom). Shrinkage phenomena in the putamen are characterised by an age-dependent increase in the capillary length and a decrease in the intercapillary distances. The values of the cortex merely oscillate around the level of values in the youngest brain group.

This surprising observation stimulated us to study the subcortical white matter in the same cortical areas. In fact, we observed also in the white matter of normal aging brains an age-dependent increase of the capillary volume and the capillary length similar to that seen in the putamen.

Consequently the intercapillary distances decrease (Fig. 3).

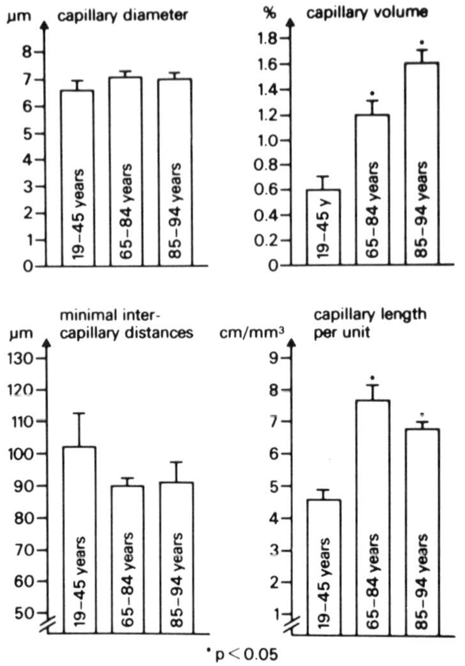

Stereological parameters of capillaries in the subcortical white matter of the human brain. Comparison of mean values (± S.D.) between young (19–45 years; n = 6) and aged (65–84 years; n = 12; 85–94 years; n = 6) individuals.

Fig. 3. The capillary lengths in the white matter (mean values for the medial frontal gyrus, the medial temporal gyrus and the precentral gyrus) increase significantly by ∿ 50 % in the age group 65-74 years in comparison with the group aged 19-45. After 75 years of age only gradual changes could be observed.

If we draw a conclusion from these findings, we may say that the loss in volume of normal aging brains is mainly the result of a shrinkage of the white matter and not of the brain cortex (Miller et al. 1980). Therefore the increase in the liquor space and the ventricular system seems to be a normal aging phenomenon. The comparison of the capillary net in the putamen of age-matched controls with that of cases of Alzheimer's disease demonstrates that

Alzheimer's disease is not accompanied by an additional shrinkage of white matter containing brain structures (Fig. 4).

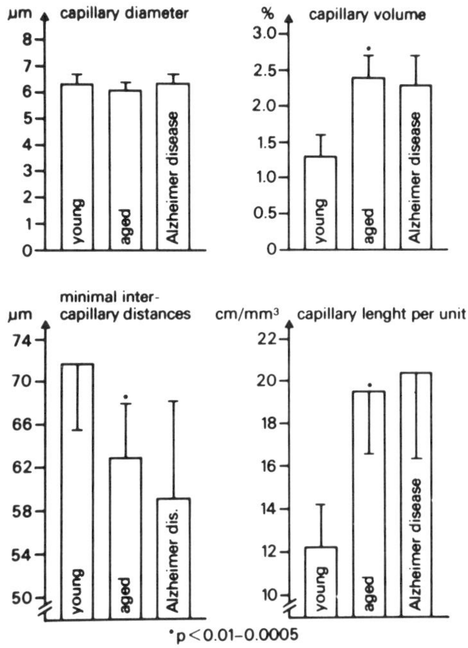

Stereological parameters of capillaries in the putamen of the human brain. Comparisons of mean values (± S.D.) between young (19–45 years; n = 6), aged (85–95 years; n = 7) and Alzheimer patients (85–95 years; n = 3).

Fig. 4. Comparison of stereologic parameters of the capillaries in the putamen in old age and Alzheimer's disease shows that the latter is not accompanied by an additional significant shrinkage of the putamen.

Bearing these findings in mind, it seems questionable to diagnose a dementing brain disease from a CT-scan finding of an enlarged ventricular system.

The observation that normal brain aging is not attended by a volume loss of brain cortex again raised the old question of a progressive nerve cell loss due to aging

(Brody 1955). We therefore started nerve cell measurements which were made, like the morphometric studies of the capillaries, in native cryostat slices with an optic electronic image analysis system. The nerve cell perikarya were stained with cresyl fast violet. The basic stereologic parameters measured were the area per nerve cell in μm^2 and the circumference in µm (Hunziker et al. 1976; Schulz et al. 1976). The post-mortem influence on the stereologic parameters of the brain nerve cells had been investigated in a preceding experiment (Schulz et al. 1980).

In view of the fact that the absolute number of nerve cells in the brain cortex cannot be quantified exactly because of the non-defined extension of the brain cortex and the variation of the nerve cell layers in the different brain cortex regions, we investigated only the nerve cell size in defined cortex areas. It is known from investigations by Scheibel et al. (1975), Buell and Coleman (1981) and others that a loss of dendrites is always accompanied by a deterioration in shape and decrease in size of the nerve cells. Before the nerve cells die a decrease in the number of dendrites and a shrinkage of the perikaryon can be shown (Scheibel and Scheibel 1977). It therefore seemed reasonable to us to use the nerve cell size as an indirect parameter of a nerve cell atrophy.

Our stereologic measurements of the nerve cell areas and perimeters in the brain cortex of normal aging individuals demonstrated that the size and shape of neuronal perikarya do not change significantly up to an age of about 75 years. The observations, which are consistent with previous reports by Treff (1974), Hall et al. (1975) and Haug (1983), are remarkable because age-dependent changes in perikaryal size and shape do not become obvious until an age of 85 to 94 years (Fig. 5). The most pronounced decrease in perikaryal area was observed in the pyramidal layers, particularly in the external pyramidal layer II and pyramidal layer III, which in normal life have the greatest glucose turnover in the brain cortex. The surprising observation that, under normal aging conditions, a significant decrease in nerve cell size cannot be observed until a late period of life is to a certain extent in accordance with the findings of Sokoloff (1975), who observed in normal elderly with a mean age of 71 years rates of cerebral blood flow and oxigen consumption which were identical with those in normal young adults (mean age 50 years). Nerve cell measurements in the putamen gave similar results.

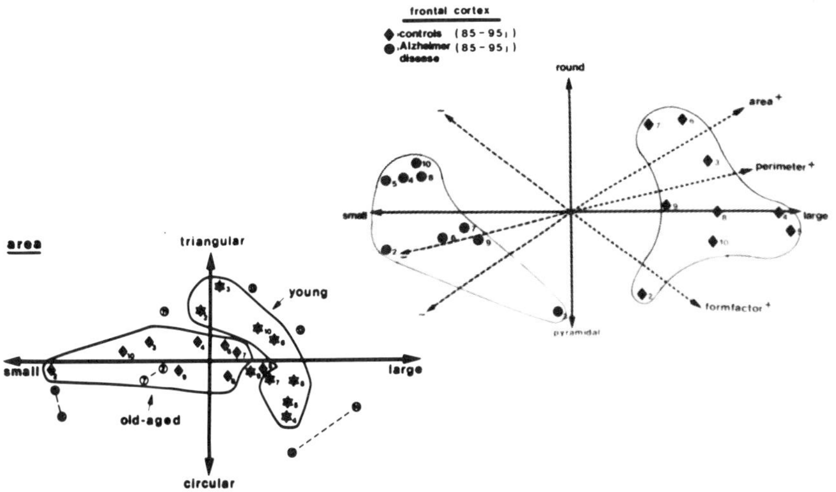

Fig. 5. Multivariate analysis of mean perikaryal values per measured cortex layer (Arabic numerals indicate the consecutive stereologically measured layers: I = 1; II = 2,3; III = 4,5; IV = 6; V = 7,8; VI = 9,10). Left: Normal aging. Old age group (rhombuses) are 85-94 years of age. Young group (stars) are 19-44 years of age. Right: In Alzheimer's disease (black circles) cortex neurons are significantly smaller than in age-matched controls (rhombuses).

In contrast to normal aging we found in Alzheimer's disease a significant decrease in nerve cell size. The comparison between age-matched controls and Alzheimer cases demonstrates a significant decrease of nerve cell size in all brain cortex layers (Fig. 6). Terry et al. (1981) recently also reported that larger neurons in the frontal and temporal cortex are about 40 % smaller in demented cases. Capillary measurements demonstrate a significant shrinkage of the brain cortex which obviously shows that normal aging has no direct link with a dementing brain disease of the Alzheimer type (Fig. 7).

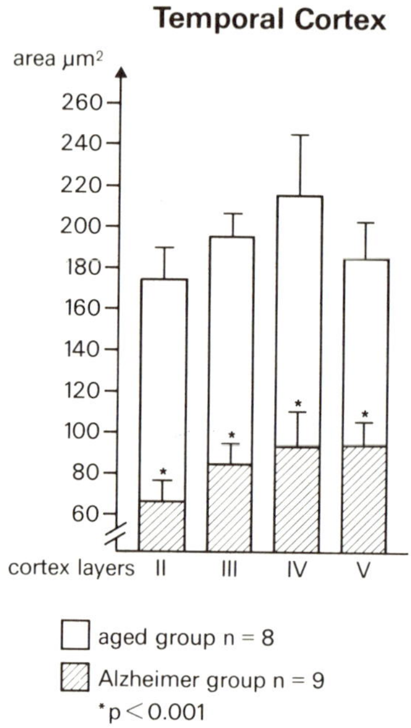

Fig. 6. Changes in neuronal size in cortical layers of the temporal gyrus in Alzheimer's disease and age-matched controls. In the different cortex layers the nerve cells show a significant decrease in size.

In conclusion we may say that normal aging changes the stereological parameters of nerve cells and the capillary net only moderately. It seems that a normal aging brain stays within the functional reserve capacity of the brain. Senile dementia of Alzheimer's type, however, is a progressive brain disease with significant shrinkage phenomena in the nerve cells and the brain cortex.

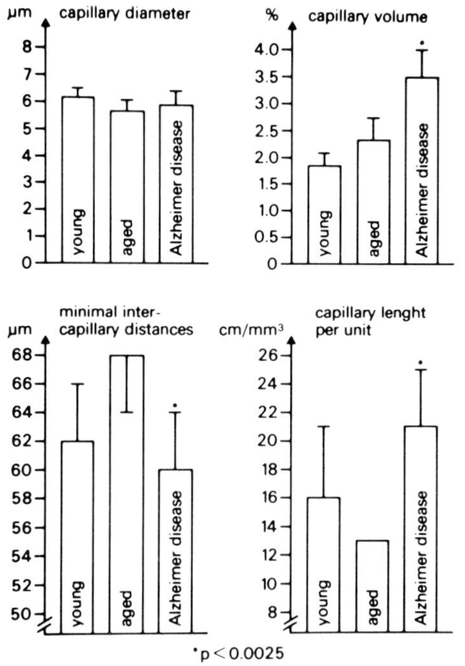

Stereological parameters of capillaries in the frontal cortex of the human brain. Comparison of mean values (± S.D.) between young (19–45 years; n = 6), aged (85–95 years; n = 9) and Alzheimer patients (85–95 years; n = 11).

Fig. 7. Stereologic measurements of the capillaries in the frontal brain cortex in old age and Alzheimer's disease show a significant increase in capillary volume and length in Alzheimer's disease, which indicates a shrinkage of the cortex.

S U M M A R Y

In normal aging brains stereologic investigations show no significant cortical shrinkage phenomena. The decrease in brain volume results from a shrinkage of the white matter. Significant nerve cell shrinkage could be found only in brains over 85 years of age.

Alzheimer's disease is characterised by a significant shrinkage of the brain cortex. The white matter does not show a significant shrinkage. Compared with age-matched controls, stereologic nerve cell measurements demonstrate a significant decrease in nerve cell size, which is more than 40 % in layers II and III.

Brody H (1955). Organization of the cerebral cortex. III. A study of aging in the human cerebral cortex. J of Comp Neurol 102:511

Brody H, Vijayashankar N (1977). Cell loss with aging. In Advances in behavioral biol. 23:15. Plenum Press New York -- London

Buell SJ, Coleman PD (1981). Quantitative evidence for selective dendritic growth in normal human aging but not in senile dementia. Brain Res 214:23

Hall TC, Miller AKH, Corsellis JAN (1975). Variations in the human Purkinje cell population according to age and sex. Neuropath Appl Neurobiol 1:267

Haug H (1967). Probleme und Methoden der Strukturzählung in Schnittpräparaten. In E.Weibel (ed): "Quantitative Methods in Morphology", Berlin-Heidelberg-New York: Springer

Haug H (1972). Stereological methods in the analysis of neuronal parameters in the central nervous system. J Microscopy 95:165

Haug H, Barmwater U, Eggers R, Fischer D, Kühl S, Sass NL (1983). Anatomical changes in aging brain: morphometric analysis of the human prosencephalon. In J.Cervos-Navarro, H.J.Sarkander (eds): "Brain Aging: Neuropathology and Neuropharmacology", series: Aging 21, New York: Raven Press, p 1

Hunziker O, Abdel-Al S, Frey H, Veteau MJ, Meier-Ruge W (1978). Quantitative studies in the cerebral cortex of aging humans. Gerontology 24:27

Hunziker O, Schulz U, Walliser Ch, Serra J (1976). Morphometric analysis of neurons in different depths of the cat's brain cortex after hypoxia. Nat Bureau of Standards (NBS) Spec.Publ. no 431:203

Hunziker O, Schweizer A (1977). Post-mortem changes in stereological parameters of cerebral capillaries. Beitr Path 161:244

Konigsmark BW, Murphy EA (1970). Neuronal populations in the human brain. Nature 228:1335

Konigsmark BW, Murphy EA (1972). Volume of ventral cochlear nucleus in man: its relationship to neuronal population and age. J Neuropathol Exp Neurol 31:304

Meier-Ruge W, Hunziker O, Iwangoff P, Reichlmeier K, Sandoz P (1978). Alterations of morphological and neurochemical parameters of the brain due to normal aging. In Nandy K (ed): "Senile dementia: a biomedical approach", series: Develop Neurosc 3:33. New York - Amsterdam: Elsevier/North Holland Biomedical Press

Meier-Ruge W, Hunziker O, Schulz U, Tobler HJ, Schweizer A (1980). Stereologic changes in the capillary network and nerve cells of the aging human brain. Mechan Ageing Develop 14:233

Miller AKH, Alson RL, Corsellis JAN (1980). Variations with age in the volumes of grey and white matter in the cerebral hemispheres of man: measurements with an image analyser. Neuropathol Appl Neurobiol 6:119

Monagle RD, Brody H (1974). The effect of age upon the main nucleus of the inferior olive in the human brain. J Comp Neurol 155:61

Sandoz P, Meier-Ruge W (1977). Age-related loss of nerve cells from the human inferior olive, and unchanged volume of its grey matter. IRCS Medical Science 5:376

Sokoloff L (1975). Cerebral circulation and metabolism in the aged. In Gershon S and Raskin A (eds): "Genesis and Treatment of Psychologic Disorders in the Elderly", Series Aging Vol 2, New York: Raven Press, p 45

Scheibel ME, Lindsay RD, Tomiyasu U, Scheibel AB. Progressive dendritic changes in aging human cortex. Exp Neurol 47:392

Scheibel ME, Scheibel AB (1977). Differential changes with aging in old and new cortices. Adv in Behavioral Biol 23:39. New York - London: Plenum Press

Schulz U, Hunziker O, Walliser Ch (1976). Quantitative investigations on neurons in the cerebral cortex of hypoxic cats. Z Anal Chem 279:98

Schulz U, Hunziker O, Frey H, Schweizer A (1980). Postmortem changes in stereological parameters of cerebral neurons. Path Res Pract 166:260

Terry RD, Peck A, DeTeresa R, Schechter R, Horoupian DS (1981). Some morphometric aspects of the brain in senile dementia of the Alzheimer type. Ann Neurol 10:184

Treff WM (1974). Das Involutionsmuster des Nucleus dentatus cerebelli. Eine morphometrische Analyse. In Platt D (ed) "Altern", Stuttgart - New York: F.K. Schattauer, p 37

Vijayashankar N, Brody H (1979). A quantitative study of the pigmented neurons in the nuclei locus coeruleus and subcoeruleus in man as related to aging. J Neuropath Exper Neurol, p 490

Senile Dementia: Outlook for the Future, pages 137–149

CHANGES IN BRAIN CAPILLARY STRUCTURE IN AGING AND DEMENTIA

Arnold B. Scheibel, M.D.

Departments of Anatomy and Psychiatry
and Brain Research Institute
UCLA Medical Center, Los Angeles, CA 90024

"A neuron is no better than the vessel that nurtures it."

In the recent renaissance of research interest in the senile and presenile dementias, the structural, functional and chemical changes undergone by neurons have been the focus of primary investigative concern. Relatively little interest seems to have been expressed in supportive systems such as neuroglia and the vasculature even though it is perfectly clear that the enormous neuronal populations are totally dependent on these tissues for their sustenance. During the course of examination of tissue from the brains of a group of very old cats (> 17 years), guinea pigs and a small group of patients with senile dementia and their non-demented controls, it became obvious that there were robust structural changes in the cerebral capillary bed which appeared to correlate positively with advanced age and/or the degree of clinical dementia.

The descriptions that follow are based largely on scanning electron microscopy which has proven particularly effective in visualization of elements of the parenchymal vascular bed and the perivascular environment. Golgi-impregnated material and cresyl violet-stained sections have served as controls.

Cerebral capillaries in the young adult nervous system, in all species studied so far, are characterized by smoothness of external (abluminal) contour, and a sinuous course marked by straight segments and gentle curves. The diameter of the capillary segments (usual range, 3-8 μm) remains relatively constant or tapers gently, the major changes in caliber occurring at bifurcations or branch points. The abluminal surface, made up primarily of basal membrane, bears the bean-shaped swellings of occasional pericyte cell bodies usually oriented along the long axis of the vessel. Cytoplasmic processes may emerge from one or both ends of such cells and extend for varying distances along the vessel surface. Mounds or tufts of somewhat less well circumscribed tissue represent astrocytic expansions (end feet) and when larger, the occasional cell body of astrocyte or oligodendrocyte.

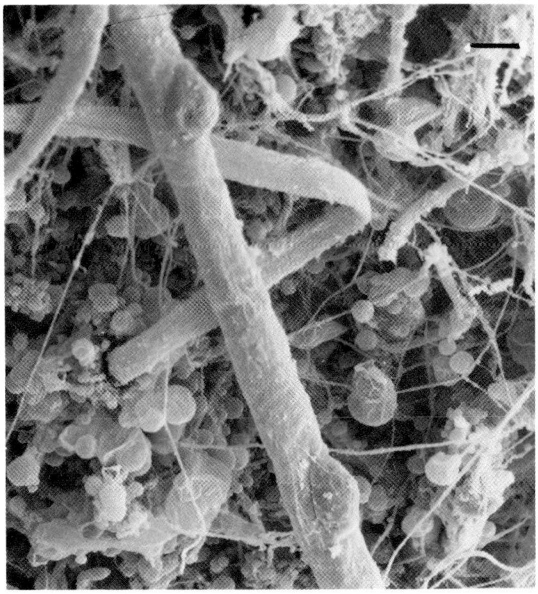

Fig. 1. Scanning electron microphotograph of capillary in upper brain stem of a middle-aged (~45 years) individual showing normal capillary structure. Note two pericytes and fine plexus of neural fibers on the basement membrane covering the vessel and pericytes. Calibration bar: 5 µm. Original magnification: X2500.

Virtually every vessel wall that we have examined is covered by a plexus of very fine (>0.2 µm) fibers, some densely nodulated, others bearing few or no varicosities along those portions of their course that can be followed. Many of these fibers terminate in nodules or expansions which sit directly upon, or are partially buried in, the outer surface of the vessel wall or on the adherent pericytes. The plexus of nodulated fibers strongly resembles the perivascular network of fine catecholamine-positive fibers revealed by fluorescence in the report of Edvinsson and his colleagues (1973). In many cases, the "parent" fiber has apparently been avulsed in the initial tearing procedure which provides the surface for scanning, leaving only a nodule with a short stem or wisp of protruding fiber. These fine fiber systems and their terminal and en passage nodules are indistinguishable from the presynaptic axons and synaptic terminals which we have repeatedly identified on the perikaryal and dendritic surfaces of neurons seen in similar preparations.

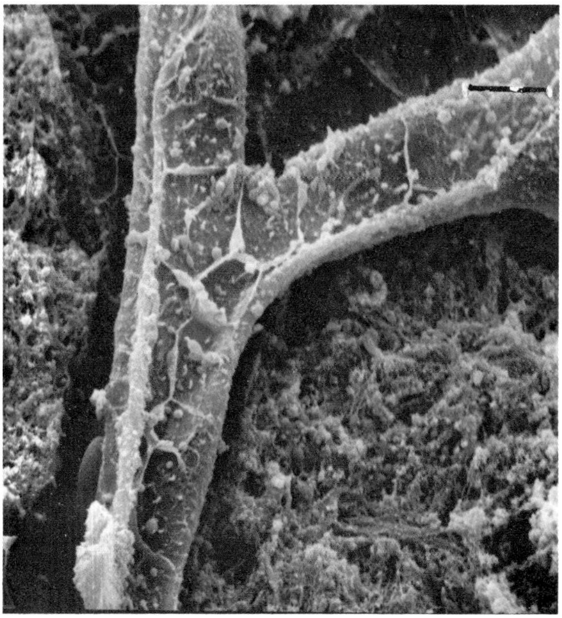

Fig. 2. Scanning electron microphotograph of small blood vessel in cerebral cortex of a guinea pig. Note elaborate plexus of nodulated fibers on the surface of the vessel. Calibration bar: 3 µm. Original magnification: X4500.

We are powerfully persuaded that this perivascular fibrous net represents the innervation of the intraparenchymal capillary system of the brain. The source and chemical signatures of the fibers constituting this axonal plexus cannot, of course, be determined from scanning microscopy alone. However, a weight of evidence is developing which argues for a central origin for many, if not all, of these fibers. Their persistence following bilateral cervical sympathectomy strongly implicates the locus ceruleus as a likely site of origin for the presumed adrenergic components (Edvinsson et al. 1973). In this regard, it is of further interest that transmission electron microscopy reveals that many of the synaptic terminal-like structures on the vessel walls contain medium and large-sized dense core vesicles indistinguishable from those found in adrenergic synapses on neurons (Itakura et al. 1977). The nature and source of a presumed cholinergic system is somewhat less clear, but studies such as those of Rennels and Nelson (1975) and Ando (1981) make a central origin increasingly likely.

We have now examined samples of the capillary bed in a number of portions of the brain including several stations in the neocortex, the hippocampus, the caudate nucleus, substantia nigra, and the pontomesencephalic regions of the brain stem. In all cases, we have found evidence of the neurovascular plexus described above. At least two types of fibers are recognizable on the basis of morphological criteria, one probably adrenergic, and the other, non-adrenergic. The latter group may well represent terminals of a widely disseminated cholinergic system, thereby providing the capillary bed with a dual and presumably functionally opposed innervation. It is, of course, possible that other aminergic transmitters are also represented in the fiber plexus.

Examination of tissue from very old animals and from aged and senile human patients reveals a dramatically different picture. The abluminal surfaces of the capillaries are lumpy and uneven, the basement membrane stretched over rounded protrusions of varying sizes along most of the course of each vessel. In some cases, the protrusions are low, rounded, and quite regularly spaced, resembling a row of loaves of bread placed side by side. In other cases, the protrusions resemble grapes or lozenges protruding at right angles from the vessel (Fig. 3), often becoming

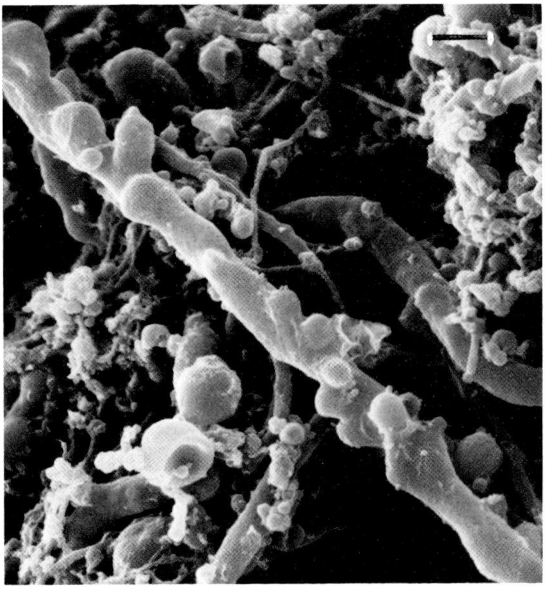

Fig. 3. Scanning electron microphotograph of capillary in upper brain stem of patient dying with senile dementia of Alzheimer type. Note the numerous swellings and extrusions from the vessel wall and the relative absence of a fine plexus of fibers on the surface. Calibration bar: 4 µm. Original magnification: X2500.

swollen, pedunculated, cyst-like structures (Fig. 4). Ultrathin sections through the latter, viewed with transmission electron microscopy, reveal that they are frequently filled with masses of lipid-like material, either in granular form or in small pools. Glial overgrowth may be seen, but this appears variable.

In an earlier report (Scheibel, Fried 1983), we suggested that the multiple abluminal protrusions were the result of massive replication of pericytes. Further study suggests that hyperplasia of the endothelial cells of the intimal lining of the vessel may also be importantly involved in this dramatic structural change in the vessel walls. Although the massive inclusions noted within the swollen cells in our earlier communication (Scheibel,

Fried 1983) might seem more typical of pericytes, endothelial cells are also known to have a phagocytic function (Kristensson, Olsson 1973; Olsson, Hossmann 1970).

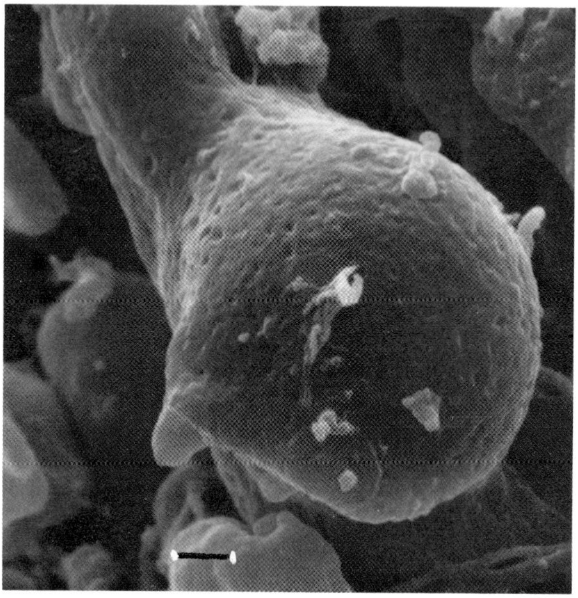

Fig. 4. Scanning electron microphotograph of a globular swelling on the surface of a cortical capillary in a 24-year-old cat. The swelling is either a pericyte or endothelial cell, swollen with lipid-like material. Note the "peau d'orange" appearance of the basement membrane stretched over vessel and cell and the almost complete absence of a fine perivascular fiber plexus. Calibration bar: 1.5 μm. Original magnification: X10,400.

Even more striking is the fact that the tautly stretched basement membrane, often appearing to have a finely pitted "peau d'orange" appearance, seems totally devoid of its neural plexus. This is particularly true in brain material from cats older than 15 years. In human brain tissue, partial loss of perivascular axons and axon terminals becomes obvious in the seventh decade. Although attempts at quantification have only begun, we have the strong impression that the loss is more advanced in patients over 75 years of age, and is especially striking in individuals dying with dementia. These observations are based on examination of brain tissue from six patients with diagnoses of senile dementia Alzheimer type (SDAT) in comparison with a non-demented control group. The total number of observations is accordingly limited so far, but the changes are robust and consistent.

Although these studies are clearly in an introductory phase, several interesting questions are immediately raised.

1) Do the structural alterations in vessel walls previously reported in the literature, and those described above affect cerebral blood flow and transmural exchange mechanisms?

2) Is there a relationship between loss of innervation of the capillary walls and the swelling and overgrowth of the cellular elements of which they are constituted?

1) Age-specific alterations in the vascular bed have been known for some time. More than 40 years ago, Scholz (1938) described "plaque-like degeneration" of blood vessels characterized by narrowing of the lumen of small brain arteries combined with thickening of the walls and radially arranged fibrillary changes in the adventitia. Similar alterations were reported by Morel and Wildi (1952) who called them "dysphoric angiopathy." A variety of structural changes, characterized by looping, twining and braiding of the vessels in individuals beyond 70 were referred to as "glomerular loop formations" and "vascular wicker works" by Hassler (1965), who speculated that they might cause reduction in cerebral blood flow. More recent studies by Fang (1976), and especially by Ravens (1978) emphasize tortuosity of small vessels and perivascular proliferation of connective tissue. Their putative relationship to altered transport mechanisms, disturbance of the blood brain barrier, and encephalomalacia has also been considered by Ravens.

An equally large and often discordant literature addresses the problem of cerebral blood flow in the aged and senile. With the introduction of the intracarotid xenon-133 method of evaluating blood flow and clearance patterns through the brain, it became possible to show that in patients with presenile and senile dementia of the Alzheimer type, there is a decreased proportion of rapid clearance (mainly through grey matter). The diminished cerebral blood flow is more or less proportional to the degree of mental impairment and is, in fact, most marked in frontotemporal areas where pathological changes are also usually maximal (Obrist et al. 1970). More specifically, loss of verbal ability was found to correlate closely with a marked general reduction of blood flow to the dominant hemisphere (Gustafson et al. 1978), while verbal memory decreased when the blood flow in temporal and parietal areas was reduced (Hagberg 1978).

It seems increasingly likely that cerebral blood flow and the selective permeability of the blood-brain barrier may be significantly affected by neuronal control. In addition to structural studies identifying adrenergic and cholinergic innervation of intraparenchymal vessels (Ando 1981; Hartman et al. 1979; Rennels and Nelson 1975; Swanson et al. 1977), a group of reports documents the responsiveness of cerebral blood flow and vascular permeability to manipulations of adrenergic and cholinergic neural mechanisms. Thus, Raichle et al. (1975) showed that electrical stimulation of the locus ceruleus, or administration of carbachol, produced major effects on the intracerebral microvasculature of ganglionectomized monkeys, i.e. a prompt reduction in hemispheric cerebral blood flow and an increase in brain vascular permeability to water. Both effects were reversed by administration of phentolamine, an alpha adrenergic blocker. Hartman, Preskorn and their colleagues (1979) conclude that a significant degree of central adrenergic control is exercised in tonic fashion upon the cerebral blood vessels, "...Neural regulation of cerebral permeability to water provides a rapid mechanism by which the brain can respond to changes in systemic osmolarity and blood pressure." (Preskorn et al. 1979, p. 136). "The permeability of other substances such as electrolytes, amino acids, and glucose may also be under regulatory control." (Hartman et al. 1979, p. 124)

Data from our scanning electron microscopy as well as that of other laboratories using fluorescent (Edvinsson et al. 1973) and transmission electron microscopy (Rennels, Nelson 1975) have succeeded in identifying adrenergic terminals, almost certainly of central origin, not only on pericapillary smooth muscle fibers, but on pericytes and on endothelial cells or the immediately adjacent basement membrane. It is therefore of considerable interest that Owman et al. (1978), using immunohistochemical techniques, have demonstrated the presence of actin and myosin in the structural elements of brain capillary walls, including pericytes and endothelial cells. Actin filament stress fibers have also been demonstrated in bovine vascular endothelial cells in areas subjected to "blood flow of high velocity and turbulence" (Wong et al. 1983). Although these are not usually considered to be among the flow characteristics of the cerebral capillary bed, they undoubtedly occur in areas where sudden decrements in diameter occur as in the case of the deep penetrating vessels where they leave the anterior cerebral and anterior communicating arteries to enter the anterior perforated substance. In any case, the possibility that vascular endothelium and subjacent pericytes may have contractile capabilities at least partly under the control of central adrenergic neurons suggests a reasonable substrate upon which the neural manipulation of cerebral blood flow and transcapillary exchange phenomena can be exerted.

2) At present there is less evidence available which might causally link the loss of innervation of the parenchymal capillary bed which we have described above with the hyperplasia and thickening of the microvascular walls. However, in a series of studies carried out by Gunn et al. (1970), it has been shown that denervation of blood vessels in and around the heart lead to thickening and hyperplasia of the cellular elements of the vessel walls with coincident suppression of lipid mobilization and increase in lipid synthesis. There is significant enhancement (by about 30%, three weeks after denervation) of free fatty acids, sterol esters and phospholipids. The authors conclude that the artery wall "needs the trophic influence of neural stimulation to maintain morphological and functional integrity." (Gunn 1981, p. 58)

Caution must be used in applying the results of experimental denervation of cardiovascular arterial vessels to the cerebral parenchymal capillary bed. However, it is tempting to speculate that similar mechanisms are operative throughout the body wherever neural representation is found along the walls of blood vessels. It is especially interesting in view of the massive lipid loading within swollen pericytes on the abluminal surfaces of the capillaries of very old animals which we reported previously (Scheibel, Fried 1983).

Let us assume for the moment a causal relationship between progressive loss of aminergic and cholinergic innervation of the cerebral capillary bed and the development of structural changes in the vessel walls resulting in increasingly impaired perfusion of the surrounding brain tissue. What alterations peculiar to the aging process might be responsible for this progressive denervation? Loss of axon terminals and preterminal fibers usually follows upon injury or death of the parent neurons. The best documented examples of age-related loss of subcortical cell masses presently available are those of the locus ceruleus (Vijayashankar, Brody 1973) and the nucleus basalis of Meynert (Coyle et al. 1973). In each case, cell loss may vary from 30-70%, and there is some evidence for direct correlation between the degree of subcortical neuronal loss and the extent of clinical deterioration shown by the patient. These are the nuclei of presumed origin for the major adrenergic and cholinergic pathways innervating the cerebral hemispheres. Progressive loss of the neurovascular plexus serving the cerebral parenchymal capillary bed may, accordingly, result from neuronal damage and cell loss in these two subcortical centers. There seems little question that the extensive projections from these two nuclei also supply vast neuronal ensembles, so it is, at present, unclear whether the progressive, age-related denervation of cerebral neurons themselves or of the metabolically supportive non-neural tissue is more critical to the development of the characteristic neuropathological and neuropsychological picture of senile dementia. Equally unclear at the moment is the nature of the process which attacks these critical subcortical centers.

Summary: An extensive series of age-related alterations develop in the walls of the capillary bed of the central nervous system. These changes are characterized by thickening of the vessel walls, swelling and proliferation of endothelial cells and pericytes, and loss of the fine neural plexus which invests the abluminal surface of these vessels. The innervation which includes cholinergic and adrenergic components is almost certainly of central origin and we hypothesize that its progressive disappearance is a function of the now-well-established age-related pattern of neuronal loss in the nucleus basalis of Meynert and the locus ceruleus. It is possible that the loss of vascular innervation is causally related to the alterations in the capillary walls which may, in turn, bear significant responsibility for the extensive neuronal changes of the senile brain.

REFERENCES

Ando K (1981). A histochemical study on the innervation of the cerebral blood vessels in bats. Cell Tissue Res 217: 55.

Coyle J, Price DL, DeLong MR (1983). Alzheimer's disease: a disorder of cortical cholinergic innervation. Science 219:1184.

Edvinsson L, Lindvall M, Nielsen KC, Owman CH (1973). Are brain vessels innervated also by central (non-sympathetic) adrenergic neurones. Brain Res 63:496.

Fang HCH (1976). Observations on aging characteristics of cerebral blood vessels, macroscopic and microscopic features. In Terry RD, Gershon S (eds): "Neurobiology of Aging", New York: Raven Press, p 155.

Gunn CG (1970). Proliferative nature of arteriosclerosis, and Regulators of metabolism and movement. In Wolfe S (ed): "The Artery and the Process of Arteriosclerosis", New York: Plenum Press, see pp 56 et seq., 230 et seq.

Gustafson L, Hagberg B, Ingvar DH (1978). Speech disturbances in presenile dementia related to local cerebral blood flow abnormalities in the dominant hemisphere. Brain Language 5:103.

Hagberg B (1978). Defects of immediate memory related to cerebral blood flow distribution. Brain Language 5:366.

Hartman BK, Swanson LW, Raichle ME, Preskorn SH, Clark HB (1979). Central adrenergic regulation of cerebral microvascular permeability and blood flow: anatomic and physiologic evidence. Adv Exp Med Biol 131:113.

Hartman BC, Udenfriend S (1972). The use of dopamine β hydroxylase as a marker for the central noradrenergic nervous system in rat brain. Proc Nat Acad Sci (Wash) 69:2722.

Hassler O (1965). Vascular changes in senile brains. Acta Neuropathol. (Berlin) 5:40.

Ingvar DH, Gustavson L (1970). Regional cerebral blood flow in organic dementia with early onset. Acta Neurol Scand [Suppl 43] 46:42.

Itakura T, Yamamoto K, Tokyama M, Shimizu N (1977). Central dual innervation of arterioles and capillaries in the brain. Stroke 8:360.

Kristensson K, Olsson Y (1973). Accumulation of protein tracers in pericytes of the central nervous system following systemic injection in immature mice. Acta Neurol Scand 49:189.

Morel F, Wildi E (1952). General and cellular pathochemistry of senile and presenile alterations of the brain. Proc 1st int Congr Neuropathol, Vol 2, Turin: Risenberg and Sellier, p. 432.

Obrist WD, Chivian E, Cronquist S, Ingvar DH (1970). Regional cerebral blood flow in senile and presenile dementia. Neurology (Minneap) 20:315.

Olsson Y, Hossmann RA (1970). Fine structural localization of exuded protein tracers in the brain. Acta Neuropathol (Berlin) 16:103.

Owman CH, Edvinsson L, Hardebo JE, Gröschel-Stewart U, Unsicker K, Walles B (1978). Immunohistochemical demonstration of actin and myosin in brain capillaries. In Cervos-Navarro J et al (eds): "Advances in Neurology", Vol 20, New York: Raven Press, p 35.

Preskorn SH, Hartman BK, Raichle ME, Swanson LW, Clark HB (1979). Central adrenergic regulation of cerebral microvascular permeability and blood flow: pharmacologic evidence. Adv Exp Med Biol 131:127.

Raichle ME, Hartman BC, Eichling JO, Sharpe LC (1975). Noradrenergic regulation of cerebral blood flow and vascular permeability. Proc Nat Acad Sci (Wash) 72:3726.

Ravens JR (1978). Vascular changes in the human senile brain. In Cervos-Navarro J et al (eds): "Advances in Neurology", Vol 20, New York: Raven Press, p 487.

Rennels ML, Nelson E (1975). Capillary innervation in the mammalian central nervous system: an electron microscope demonstration. Am J Anat 144:233.

Scheibel AB, Fried I (1983). Age-related changes in the peri-capillary environment of the brain. In Samuel D et al (eds): "Aging of the Brain", New York: Raven Press, p 81.

Scholz W (1938). Studien zur Pathologie des Hirngefässe II Die drusige Entartung der Hirnarterien und Capillaren. Z Neurol Psychiatr 162:694.

Simard D, Oleson J, Paulson O, Lassen NA, Skinhøf E (1971). Regional cerebral blood flow and its regulation in dementia. Brain 94:273.

Swanson LW, Connelly MA, Hartman BC (1977). Ultrastructural evidence for central monoaminergic innervation of blood vessels in the paraventricular nucleus of the hypothalamus. Brain Res 136:166.

Vijayashankar N, Brody H (1973). The neuronal population of the nuclei of the trochlear nerve and the locus coeruleus in the human. Anat Rec 172:421.

Wong AJ, Pollard TD, Herman IM (1983). Actin filament stress fibers in vascular endothelial cells in vivo. Science 219:867.

Senile Dementia: Outlook for the Future, pages 151–155

INNERVATION OF NEURITIC PLAQUES BY LOCAL NEURONS OF DIFFERENT TYPES: A GOLGI STUDY IN THE HIPPOCAMPUS*

Probst A, Ulrich J.

Department of Pathology, Neuropathology Division
University of Basel, Schönbeinstrasse 40,
CH - 4003 Basel (Switzerland).

Neuritic plaques (NP) are one of the most conspicuous brain lesions found in patients with Alzheimer's disease, though also present in smaller number in normal aged individuals. Electron microscopy has shown abnormal distended neurites to be an essential constituant of NP, amongst amyloid deposits and non neuronal reactive cells (Wisniewski and Terry 1973). Furthermore most of the abnormal neurites correspond to dystrophic axonal terminals although dendritic boutons also may contain pathologic organelles (Gonatas et al 1967). According to Wisniewski et al (1981) a proportion of neurites in NP present a picture reminiscent of Wallerian degeneration, whereas other neuritic profiles present the ultrastructural appearance of regenerating nerves. NP are therefore likely to contain a complex admixture of dystrophic, degenerative and regenerative neuritic changes.

Quite apart from the functional significance of neuritic alterations as seen in NP by electron microscopy, the question of the origin of neurites involved in NP has never been adequately investigated. Although there is some evidence that catecholaminergic (Berger et al 1980) and cholinergic (Struble et al 1982) axonal terminals are involved in neocortical plaques, no information is available concerning an axonal innervation of NP by local cortical neurons. Furthermore a morphologic connection

* This article summarizes work to be published in "Brain Research", where also the Figs 1-3 will be printed (Probst et al 1983). With permission of the editor of "Brain Research".

between neuritic terminals in the NP and their neuronal perikaryon has never been demonstrated until now. In order to demonstrate such a connection, we applied the Golgi impregnation technique(Van der Loos 1956) on human hippocampal and parahippocampal tissues obtained at autopsy from patients having presented severe form of senile dementia of the Alzheimer type.

75 to 100 µm thick sections were cut from unembedded impregnated tissue samples using a vibratome, counterstained as previously described (Probst et al 1983) and mounted. NP were identified as darkly stained patches (Fig 1) disclosing higher cellularity than the surrounding neuropil. NP containing well impregnated neuronal process (es) were photographed and the process(es) traced using a drawing tube attached to a microscope. Impregnated processes (axons and spiny dendrites) could be traced until variable distances from the NP. Some of them were found to be in continuity with the dendritic domain or the axon of pyramidal cells. Other processes could be traced to non pyramidal cells of the hippocampus (Fig 2).

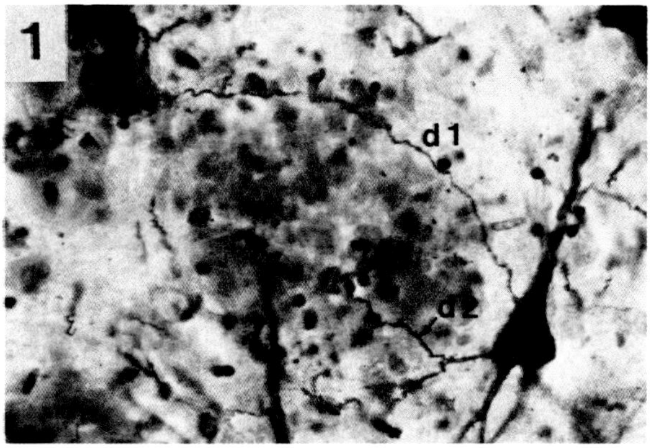

Fig. 1 Neuritic plaque in a 75 µm thick Golgi impregnated section counterstained with cresyl violet. The plaque is an inhomogenous patch staining more deeply than the surrounding neuropil. An impregnated pyramidal cell penetrates the plaque by its horizontal dendrite d_2, whereas the dendrite d_1 seems to be pushed aside by the plaque. x 320

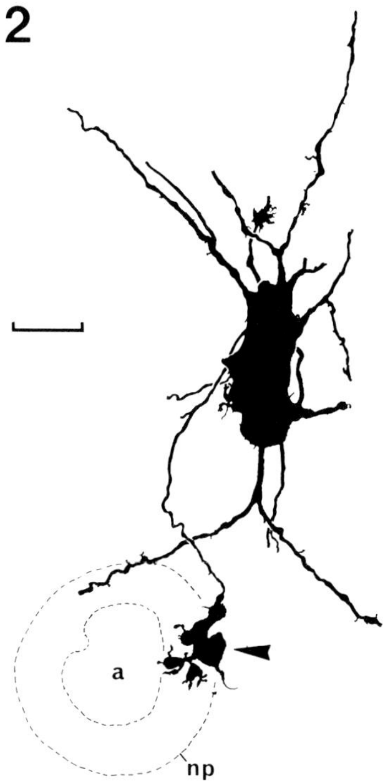

Fig. 2 Non-pyramidal neuron of the entorhinal cortex participating in a small neuritic plaque (np). The process shows an irregularly shaped terminal expansion (arrowhead) in the neuritic corona of the plaque. a indicates amyloid core of the plaque. Note also some filiform processes on the expansion. Bar = 10 um.

The morphology of dendrites and axons within NP was frequently abnormal. Abnormalities included a) pleomorphic outpouchings of terminal and preterminal dendritic and axonal segments wich probably correspond to dystrophic changes. b) filopodia like processes on otherwise unaltered neurites or on terminal outpouchings of dendrites and axons (Fig 2). Furthermore the axon collaterals of some hippocampal neurons branched richly as they entered plaques (Fig 3). A frequent feature consisted of apparently unaltered smooth neuronal processes (probably axons) crossing through the plaques.

Our Golgi observations show that a connection can be established between abnormal neurites in NP and their neuronal perikarya. They confirm furthermore, that NP are innervated by neurons of different types including local circuit neurons and are likely to receive functionally different presynaptic imputs. The finding of an occasional axonal sprouting in NP and of filopodia like neuritic expansions could represent a regenerative process of neuritic elements in response to a primary injury of the nervous tissue in the plaque.

3

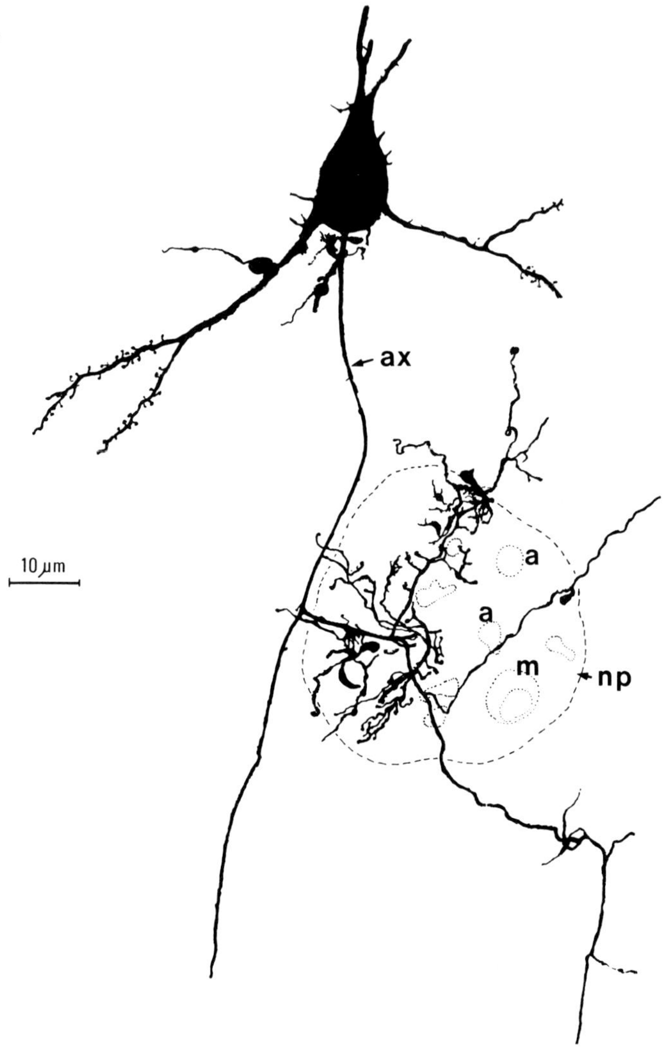

Fig. 3 Camera lucida drawing of a pyramidal neuron of the entorhinal cortex participating in a neuritic plaque (np) by a collateral branch of its axon (ax). The axon shows sprouting soon after its entry into the plaque. a: probable astrocytic nuclei; m: probable macrophagic cell.

Berger B, Tassin JP, Rancurel G, Blanc G (1980). Catecholaminergic innervation of the human cerebral cortex in presenile and senile dementia. Histochemical and biochemical studies. In E. Ysdin, T.L. Sourkes, M B H Youdin (Eds), Enzyme and Neurotransmitters in Mental disease. J. Wiley and Sons, pp. 317-328.

Gonatas NK, Anderson W, Evangelista I (1967). The contribution of altered synapses in the senile plaque: an electron microscopic study in Alzheimer's dementia, J Neuropathol 26:29.

Probst A, Basler V, Bron B, Ulrich J (1983). Neuritic plaques in senile dementia of Alzheimer type: a Golgi analysis in the hippocampal region. Brain Research. In press.

Struble RY, Cork LC, Whitehouse PJ, Price DL (1982). Cholinergic innervation in neuritic plaques. Science 216:413.

Van der Loos H (1956). Une combinaison de deux vieilles méthodes histologiques pour le système nerveux central. Mschr Psychiat Neurol 132:330.

Wisniewski HM, Terry RD (1973). Reexamination of the pathogenesis of the senile plaques. In H M Zimmermann (Ed), Progress in Neuropathology, Grune and Stratton, New York, London, Vol. 2, pp 1-26.

Wisniewski HM, Sinatra RS, Iqbal IY (1981). Neurofibrillary and synaptic pathology in aged brain. In J E Johnson (Ed), Aging and cell structure, Vol. 1, Plenum Publishing Corporation, pp. 105-142.

V. SOCIO-MEDICAL ORGANIZATION AND SENILE DEMENTIA

Presided by T. Arie (Nottingham)

Senile Dementia: Outlook for the Future, pages 159–166

"SOCIAL" SENILITY

Walter M. Beattie, Jr.

Professor, Gerontology and Social Policy
School of Social Work, Syracuse University
Syracuse, New York 13210

Before looking ahead over the next two decades, let us look back to where we have been. In his paper, "Gerontology-Past, Present, and Future," Nathan Shock noted that the first conference on senility, where 34 papers were presented, was held in Kiev, USSR, in 1938. In 1972, when he presented this introductory lecture at the 9th International Congress of Gerontology, he stated, "The papers in 1938 were primarily concerned with disease states in the elderly. Today [some 34 years later] research is directed toward the underlying causes of aging and methods of minimizing the diseases of aging people." "Truly," he stated, "gerontology has come of age." (Shock, 1972, p. 13)

It is important to note the early emphasis on equating aging with disease. In the biomedical areas aging was often seen as pathological and dysfunctional. In the social areas it was classified as social pathology or as a social problem. Indeed, in my earliest teaching days, textbooks on social problems often included aging along with alcoholism, delinquency, and mental illness.

However, in his introductory lecture to the 9th International Congress of Gerontology, Shock, in assessing the then present and future, noted the beginning social science awareness to aging. Aging, until the past decade, had little scientific status and little organized attention among social scientists except for notable pioneers such as Burgess, Havighurst, Shanas, and Neugarten. My thesis is that although it is important and necessary to identify, eradicate where possible, and ameliorate disease states of the aging through biomedical and behavioral research in such areas as Alzheimer's disease, it is equally important to identify, eradicate, and/or ameliorate what may represent equally significant causes of "senility" in the social domain of man's life. In particular, I should like to stress the relationship of sensory deprivation often associated with aging through social-environmental barriers and losses.

James Birren, in discussing research findings related to aging, maladjustment, and psychopathology (Birren, 1964) states that, "...a proper assessment of the many factors contributing to mental disorders of mental life depends upon an accurate description of the physical and social environment of the individual, his present affective and cognitive functioning, and his physiological and psychiatric states." (p. 266, underlining added for emphasis) Although Birren wrote this nearly 20 years ago and this conference is to address the next 20 years, it is evident that little organized social science research related to senile dementia has occurred. An agenda over the next 20 years must identify a social research protocol and support for such research if we are going to reverse present social policies and practices which, in themselves, may contribute to what I have chosen to call "social" senility.

Senility is a slippery term, one of the oldest in use both scientifically and popularly to describe what, until recently, was viewed as an irreversible characteristic of aging, that of mental and physical deterioration. As in most of the early concerns with aging, it was thought that if the disease of old age could be cured, senility would be conquered. This is not to suggest that diseases associated with aging should not be identified but, rather, that perhaps the "cure" for old age lies not alone in the identification, treatment, and eradication of disease, such as Alzheimer's, which is an important and current concern not only of this conference but in countless communities throughout Europe, North America, and the developed world. Rather, it is to suggest, as Lawrence K. Frank, one of the early American pioneers of gerontology and sociology, stated many years ago, "society is the patient." (Frank, 1948)

Indeed, when I began my work in gerontology, more than 30 years ago, one of the recurrent issues I found confronting old people, their families, neighbors, and communities, was what to do with them. Indeed, land use and zoning disputes often related to the location of care facilities where homeowners and others took legal steps to prevent the location of such facilities near their domiciles because the visibility of older persons was perceived to negatively affect their children and themselves.

The issue of the place of older persons in the family, the neighborhood, the community, and the society is yet to be resolved. Ronald Blythe, the British author, in his magnificent book, The View in Winter: Reflections on Old Age, describes this concern in relation to the older person who has come to recognize that he/she must leave the community, perhaps his/her son's or daughter's home, which is not truly his/her home, and move to an institutional setting. He describes this recognition by an older "...man or woman who has come to the point where they have to leave their son's or daughter's family setting, where there are grandchildren, and where there has been a growing recognition that it is not their home and they aren't entirely wanted. Some little house where they can feel the squeeze...the old person feels intrusive and a nuisance. The young people are tolerant, but not loving. They wouldn't hurt him but they don't want him. He isn't FATHER any more, he is their old-age problem." (Blythe, 1979, p. 109)

It was in these days of 30 years ago, at least in my part of the United States, that old people, because they were "different", acted "unusual", or were a "nuisance" were soon shipped off to state and county mental institutions, often without due process of law to protect their civil liberties and rights. It was then that I became aware of the "forgotten old" in the back wards of hospitals comingled with the psychotic young, at times finding old men in cages, stripped of clothes and dignity, to be punished on bread and water for violating rules and regulations. Surrogates of society defined them as "senile" and soon it became evident that this was not solely a clinical or biomedical issue; equally and perhaps more so, it was a civil, legal, and societal issue.

I do not speak from a clinical or biomedical background. My views are drawn from both a sociological/behavioral and a humanistic training. It was through working with the legal, social, and medical structures of the society that I soon learned that aging, if recognized at all, was of little or no priority. This was indeed its status in the academic world as well, with little emphasis on research, training, and professional leadership.

It was against this background that I then began to raise the question of "social" senility which, from my observations, suggested that should one live long enough one could expect what could be called an increasing state of sensory deprivation. Butler and Lewis have defined such deprivation as "...the experience of being cut off from usual external stimuli and the opportunity for perception [which] may occur experimentally or accidentally in various ways, such as in loss of hearing or eyesight, by being marooned, by solitary confinement...and which may lead to disorganized thinking, depression, panic, delusions, and hallucinations. (Butler and Lewis, 1982, p. 437)

It is not unusual in gerontological research to turn to early stages of infant and early childhood development for clues to developmental changes in the later years. It is suggestive to note that some of the first studies of sensory deprivation related to the earliest developmental stages, such as the work of Rene Spitz on "hospitalism" and John Bowlby in the 1950's and 1960's which identified, among other things, long-term physiological and mental damage to infants placed in cribs or in isolated environments with little ongoing interaction with adults or other persons. Indeed, as the aging are removed from social group identities and from familiar environments, there is an accompanying loss of meaningful stimuli. All too often there is physical movement toward a world of decreasing psychological, sociological, and life space. This may be seen in the movement from a home to an apartment or flat, to a room, to a bed. Such changes suggest not only the diminution of physical space but of all the sensory inputs that sustain and give renewal to our daily lives at younger life stages. Even the destruction of or movement from familiar habitats of home and neighborhood, or from one part of a closed-institutional environment to another, has been correlated with increased morbidity and mortality rates among the elderly. (See work of Liberman, Tobin and Slover) The destruction of social continuity and social identity appears to be critical to meaning and purpose among the aging--especially among those who are frail and of advanced years. It is important to note that world-wide the 80 and over population is the most rapidly increasing segment of of all age groups. As Else Melin states,

> To live in an institution often means mental stress to the persons. There is a great danger in the hospitalization process which can cause passivity, isolation and a too good adaptation to the institution. This process also means sensory deprivation. In experiments Heron (1957) has shown the effects of sensory deprivation to the individuals. His subjects, who all were volunteers, were kept from using their hands, seeing and hearing. After a few days the subjects became restless, spoke to themselves, whistled and recited poems. They were alone in their rooms except for meal times, when they were very eager to speak to the person who brought the food. After two days they found difficulties in finding their way to the lavatory and they seemed confused. Many of the subjects got hallucinations and many had great difficulties when they tried to think. After a few days the experiment had to be stopped because of the negative feelings of the subjects. They reported that their ego-identity was disturbed. (Melin, p. 89)

My thesis is not that senile dementia, organic brain syndrome, Alzheimer's disease, and other clinically identified patholgies are not real and do not require continued research as to their etiologies in order to develop appropriate clinical and therapeutic modalities of care, treatment and rehabilitation where possible. Further, it is not to deny the psychological-behavioral dimension of these behavioral changes. Rather, my thesis is that little theoretical and research development has occurred in the sociological domain, which accounts for much of what has been loosely defined as "senility". Perhaps man's most distinguishing characteristic is the fact that beyond his biological nature he is essentially a social animal. Again, as identified by research on the earliest stages of child development, the requirement for social stimuli; touching, feeling, verbal communication, etc., as well as visual and auditory stimuli, are essential to the formation of human nature and human behavior, particularly in view of the tremendous plasticity of the bio-psycho-social organism called man.

While popularly we are all familiar with the losses associated with aging, not all of these are biologically determined. Some may stem from cultural and social values and practices. Such losses, even should they be biological in origin, such as bereavement and loss of spouse or children, are responded to and addressed through socially structured responses and alternatives. Others, such as the loss of work roles through mandatory retirement, which is occurring at earlier ages despite extended life-spans in most of the developed world, represents not only a loss in income. Equally and perhaps more so, the recognition and status which accompany occupational capacity and performance are lost. Such social inventions as retirement result in the movement from independence to the state of increasing dependence and loss of mastery over self and environment for many older individuals. However, loss of work role, as indeed other psycho-social losses, also represents a reduction in social contacts and stimuli such as the loss of work-related friendships and the significance of being engaged each day in a purposeful existence.

One could go on and illustrate similar losses relating to family roles and statuses in the modern world, particularly when increased longevity moves one from the loss of child-rearing roles and traditional concepts of parenting to grandparent, great-grandparent and, in some instances, great-great-grandparent. In these later "great" life stages little in the way of role function and status has been identified or spelled out other than the fact that one has lived long, that one's children are often aged as is oneself, and one is all too redundant in the sense of having significance or identity other than that of longevity. Such losses, including socially recognized roles and their associated purposes and goals, associated with organic and physiological changes and often accompanied by specific disease states, have led to our increasing separation of the old from the generations which follow. Age segregation rather than age integration has become the primary model of care and service provision for older people. Because the majority of our service models are based on treatment modalities which are curative and restorative, and because aging, until recently, has been viewed as only decline and loss with little recognition of growth, it has represented the lowest of priorities and, indeed, in most countries the social dimensions of care have yet to be fully developed and supported. Public policies in many developed countries place the lowest priority, and therefore give the lowest financial support, to meaningful social services, facilities, and programs which would have as their goal the continuing social integration and continuing social support of older persons in the family, the neighborhood, and the community.

Research is indeed needed in a number of areas which will identify ways to prevent sensory deprivation and promote meaningful social integration of the aging. A brief example of such research is that being carried out by one of our doctoral students at Syracuse University, Kathleen Seely, in the area of communication disorders and the aging. She has begun to identify, if only in a preliminary way, the fact that older institutionalized individuals tend increasingly to withdraw from communication with others. It is not they who initiate speech with staff or family. Rather, they respond when spoken to, and usually only in a staccato manner. Others have taken over their decisions. The old have become the recipients or, if you will, the objects rather than the subjects of life. They have lost mastery over their bodily selves and their environments and have become increasingly alienated without the social supports necessary for continued self-actualization.

I recognize, as stated in the beginning, that some of the tragic diseases increasingly associated with the aging, such as Alzheimer's, must be addressed as a high priority concern. At the same time, we must not focus only on one or even a few disease entities as ways of solving the issue of "senility" in aging societies. Rather, we must begin to methodically examine society itself and, if you will, engineer societies so they are structurally responsive to and inclusive of the aging as legitimate social actors who can contribute, participate and identify with the social world in which they exist.

The English-born, American poet, W. H. Auden, in his poem, "The Old People's Home," perhaps best captures the dilemma of the older person in today's modern, industrial society. To be the generation in the march of human history which, as he states, "...is the first to fade...not at home but assigned to a numbered frequent ward, stowed out of conscience as unpopular luggage..." To be set aside from the business of family, community, and society, or perhaps even worse, to be tolerated, is the very stuff of what is meant by "social" senility. We must, therefore, begin to develop a research agenda that recognizes that pathology may not always lie within the individual. Rather, in the specific case of aging, as Frank stated, with society as the patient.

References

Birren JE (1964). "The Psychology of Aging." New Jersey: Prentice-Hall, Inc.

Blythe R (1979). "The View in Winter: Reflections on Old Age." New York: Harcourt Brace, Jovanovich.

Bowlby J (1951). "Maternal Carc and Mental Health." Baltimore: Penguin.

Bowlby J (1953). "Child Care and the Growth of Love." Baltimore: Penguin.

Butler RN, Lewis ML (1982). "Aging and Mental Health." Third Edition, St. Louis: C.V. Mosby Company

Frank LK (1948). "Society As the Patient: Essays on Culture and Personality." New Brunswick: Rutgers University Press.

Melin E (1976). Dependency on Activity Before, During and After Activating Treatment in a Home for Aged People. In Munnichs JMA, van den Heuvel WJA, "Dependency or Interdependency in Old Age." The Hague: Martinus Niijhoff.

Shock NW (1972). Gerontology--Past, Present, and Future. In Chebotarev DF (ed): "9th International Congress of Gerontology." Vol 1, Plenary and Section Sessions, Kiev, USSR.

Spitz R (1972) "Facial Expressions in Children: Three Studies." New York: Arno Press.

Spitz R (1965) "First Year of Life." New York: International Universities Press.

Senile Dementia: Outlook for the Future, pages 167–176

VIEILLISSEMENT DE LA POPULATION ET ALLOCATION DES RESSOURCES DE SANTE PUBLIQUE

Pierre Gilliand

Professeur à la faculté des sciences sociales et politiques de l'Université de Lausanne et à l'institut de hautes études en administration publique, Lausanne, Cité Devant 2 – Suisse

Introduction

Le vieillissement de la population est inéluctable. Il a d'importantes incidences en matière de santé publique : volume et genre de soins; équipements et infrastructure; ampleur et modes de financement des prestations... Ce phénomène démographique concerne tous les aspects de l'organisation de la santé publique et de la sécurité sociale. Or on tarde à en tirer les conséquences. Pourtant, dans ce domaine complexe de la santé, les décisions d'aujourd'hui engagent les générations à venir.

La démence sénile – objet de ce congrès – est l'occasion de mettre en évidence, sur un plan général, la nécessaire réallocation des ressources. Le ralentissement économique a resserré les budgets sociaux. Des effets pervers de mesures prises hier, en période de prospérité, pèsent aujourd'hui sur les coûts de la gestion sanitaire. Demain, pour faire face en quantité et qualité aux besoins de santé, qui croissent avec le vieillissement, il convient de rappeler la signification littérale du mot économie : c'est "ordre dans la maison". C'est dire qu'importe l'orientation du système et du financement de la santé publique, visant efficacité et adéquation; il s'agit de les faire converger avec l'humanisation des soins.

Accroissement du nombre de personnes âgées

Quelle que sera l'évolution du nombre total d'habitants dans un pays industrialisé, il est possible dès maintenant de cerner de façon approximative le nombre des personnes âgées en 2040 : tous ceux et celles qui auront plus de 57 ans à cette date sont déjà nés; et les taux de mortalité par âge se modifieront peu vraisemblablement. En Suisse par exemple, l'accroissement prévu sera de l'ordre de 3/5 à 2/3.

Fort vieillissement démographique

Le vieillissement de la population est un phénomène irréversible : la proportion des personnes âgées va croître fortement dans les décennies à venir. En Suisse, la part des habitants qui dépassent 65 ans est de 14 % en 1980. D'ici 2040, elle atteindra plus de un cinquième (21 %) si se réalise une variante démographique haute (remontée de la fécondité et maintien constant de l'indice conjoncturel au seuil de remplacement des générations); elle atteindra plus du quart (28 %) – proportion énorme – si se confirme une variante basse, la natalité restant stable au très bas niveau actuel (1,5 enfant par femme en âge de procréation, et le nombre total d'habitants diminuant de un cinquième environ).

Années		1980	2040	2040	2040
Variante		—	forte	moyenne	faible
Nombre habitants (millions)		6,3	6,7	5,8	4,9
0 - 19 ans	%	28	26	22	17
20 - 64 ans	%	58	53	54	55
65 ans et plus	%	14	21	24	28

Vieillissement secondaire

Par ailleurs – et cette remarque importe dans le domaine de la gériatrie et en particulier pour la maladie d'Alzheimer –, on assistera à un vieillissement dit secondaire : au sein de la population âgée, la part des grands vieillards a tendance à croître. La durée de vie moyenne étant notablement plus longue pour le sexe féminin, le nombre et la proportion des femmes âgées deviennent prépondérants.

Vieillissement et modification de la pathologie

La morbidité augmente statistiquement avec l'avance en âge. La pathologie liée à la vieillesse est souvent invalidante. La structure des besoins et la demande de soins seront profondément modifiées par le vieillissement de la population.

Des études dans le canton de Vaud et en Suisse illustrent ce phénomène : en 1966-68, Vaud compte 1 habitant sur 8 dépassant 65 ans. Or 2 lits d'établissements hospitaliers sur 5 sont occupés par des personnes âgées. La proportion est supérieure à la moitié des lits, en incluant dans les équipements les maisons de vieillards.

Etude, Vaud 1966-68	
Population de 65 ans et plus (13 %) :	1 habitant sur 8
Part des lits occupés par des malades âgés :	
– hôpitaux généraux et psychiatrie (32 %)	1 lit sur 3
– hôpitaux et lits malades chroniques (40 %)	2 lits sur 5
– hôpitaux, chroniques, homes vieillards (51 %)	1 lit sur 2

Si "toutes autres choses restaient égales", le vieillissement entraînerait une formidable augmentation du nombre de lits d'hospitalisation et d'hébergement. Pour les personnes âgées, ce serait un doublement en une cinquantaine d'années. Ce qui, en forçant l'image, conduirait à une Suisse asilaire, où des malades en nombre grossissant nécessiteraient des infrastructures, des effectifs de personnel et des dépenses sans cesse croissants.

La part des malades très âgés, notamment en psychiatrie, devient énorme dans ces conditions. "Toutes autres choses égales", la démence sénile, dont le taux s'élève fortement avec le très grand âge, occuperait de plus en plus de lits d'hôpitaux et de soignants.

Etat de santé, institutionnalisation et revenus

D'un sondage concernant la situation économique des personnes âgées en Suisse, il ressort que l'état de santé des personnes âgées et le placement en établissement médico-social sont en relation étroite avec l'âge et le revenu.

Parmi les rentiers AVS*, 18 pour cent déclarent que leur santé est "très bonne", 45 pour cent "bonne", mais 28 pour cent l'estiment "passable" et 9 pour cent "mauvaise". 80 pour cent des rentiers sont tout à fait indépendants, sur le plan physique; mais 6 pour cent sont vraiment dépendants, dont la moitié le sont gravement. Et près de 6 pour cent sont placés en institution.

Cependant, avant 70 ans, les proportions des personnes âgées dont la santé est déficiente et qui sont institutionnalisées sont faibles. En revanche, chez les vieillards de plus de 85 ans, environ 1 sur 6 a une santé déficiente; 1 sur 6 également est physiquement dépendant; et plus de 1 sur 4 – c'est beaucoup – est en institution.

Les rentiers pauvres sont plus fréquemment placés dans un établissement : 15 pour cent chez ceux dont le revenu figure dans le dixième inférieur, 1 pour cent seulement pour ceux qui sont à l'aise, situés dans le dixième supérieur. Certes, les rentiers dont les ressources sont les plus modestes sont généralement les plus âgés. Mais à tous les âges, les pauvres sont plus souvent placés en établissement médico-social.

* Personnes âgées de plus de 62 ans chez les femmes, de plus de 65 ans chez les hommes, au bénéfice d'une rente vieillesse fédérale.

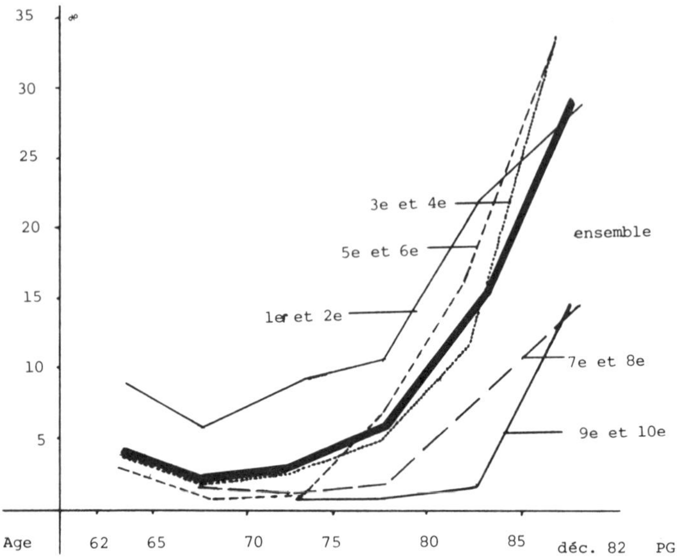

1er et 2ème déciles de revenus : les plus démunis
9ème et 10ème déciles de revenus : les plus aisés

Proportions de personnes en institution, par groupe d'âges et par catégorie de revenu

Analyse des correspondances sur le revenu des personnes âgées

Le revenu économique a des corrélations évidentes avec la qualité de vie pendant la vieillesse : degré de satisfaction, intensité des contacts, maintien à domicile en cas de maladie, etc... Une analyse des "correspondances" sur le revenu est explicite à cet égard. Il y a cumul d'avantages ou d'inconvénients. La vieillesse est une reproduction des conditions antérieures de vie. La retraite amplifie les écarts.

Parmi les retraités, les plus démunis, généralement, n'ont pas de fortune ou disposent d'une mince épargne; ils se caractérisent par le grand âge, l'isolement selon l'état civil (veufs, célibataires, divorcés) et le fait de vivre effectivement seuls, la dépendance physique, l'absence ou la faible intensité des contacts, le fait de ne pas avoir – ou d'avoir juste – le nécessaire pour vivre; ils sont fréquemment en institution hospitalière ou d'hébergement médico-social; c'est surtout le sort de femmes seules, d'ouvriers agricoles, de ménagères ou personnes sans profession, de manœuvres. Le degré de qualification est généralement faible, et c'est parmi ces personnes que la satisfaction de la situation est négative. Etc... Le revenu est déterminant, pour une grande part, des conditions sociales d'existence.

Le vieillissement accroît-il les coûts de la santé ?

La courbe des frais de santé s'élève fortement avec l'avance en âge. Le glissement vers une structure démographique vieillissante entraîne donc des coûts supérieurs (à moins d'accepter une dégradation de la qualité des soins).

Cependant, certains ont contesté que le vieillissement ait un rôle important dans l'évolution des dépenses sanitaires. Certes, pendant le troisième et prospère quart de ce siècle, les progrès de la médecine, l'extension de l'accès aux soins grâce aux assurances sociales, les investissements consentis dans les grands et hauts murs des hôpitaux, ont financièrement pesé davantage que le vieillissement de la structure d'âges. Mais cette vision restrictive du rôle du vieillissement est marquée par l'époque d'observation et par une interprétation statique. En effet, l'hospitalo-centrisme, qui a marqué l'orientation de nombreux pays, et l'insuffisante prise en considération du vieillissement auront des incidences à long terme. Les conséquences de la récession économique et de la stagnation prévisible – voire la régression – du nombre des habitants, n'ont pas vraiment été tirées à cet égard. Or les infrastructures, la formation des médecins et des soignants, les modalités de financement du système de santé – ou plus précisément et sans notion péjorative : de "réparation de la santé dégradée" – sont orientées vers des structures de population relativement jeunes. Et les comportements ne sont pas encore adaptés au fort vieillissement à venir.

Poids direct et indirect du vieillissement

Actuellement en Suisse se côtoient – entres autres – un grand secteur hospitalier, surdoté et coûteux; un secteur ambulatoire de médecine privée, qui s'étend à un rythme accéléré et qui multiplie les équipements et les actes (doublement de la densité médicale en 15 ans, triplement vraisemblable d'ici 2010); un secteur ambulatoire peu développé de services de maintien à domicile de malades chroniques et handicapés; ces services sont nettement moins onéreux que le placement institutionnel; mais les lacunes et les modes actuels de financement en vigueur découragent le recours à de tels services et pénalisent ceux qui se dévouent pour garder un proche à la maison.

Ainsi, de manière directe et indirecte, le vieillissement et sa faible prise en considération dans la politique de santé sont des causes primordiales d'accroissement des coûts.

"Toutes choses ne restent jamais égales"

Mon but n'est pas ici de développer ces distorsions et paradoxes, qui ne sont pas propres à la Suisse. Il tend à signifier aux responsables de l'organisation sociale de la santé l'urgence d'une autre allocation des ressources. Des économies sont certes possibles à court et moyen termes en matière de gestion; mais à long terme, ce sont des structures inadéquates qui provoqueront gaspillages et coûts difficilement supportables. "Efficacité productive" certes; plus encore "efficacité allocative".

Il ne s'agit pas de passer de l'"hospitalo-centrisme" à l'"extra-hospitalo-centrisme", selon l'expression du professeur J. Wertheimer. Mais de mettre de l'ordre dans l'immeuble santé, où de nombreux appartements doivent être réaménagés !

Des exemples brièvement décrits soulignent le propos.

Sectorisation psychiatrique, canton de Vaud

"Toutes autres choses égales", le secteur hospitalier de psychiatrie aurait dû, en ce canton, augmenter la quantité de lits à disposition d'une population fortement vieillissante. Or l'adoption de la sectorisation il y a 17 ans, la décentralisation hospitalière et le développement des services psychiatriques ambulatoires, conjointement aux progrès de la médecine et de l'accompagnement médico-social, ont permis une notable diminution de la dotation en lits : moins un quart environ. Exemple parmi d'autres, exemple d'un intérêt évident.

Soins de longue durée à domicile : humanisation et économie

Une étude de l'activité du "Centre lausannois des soins à domicile" dégage ceci : le maintien à domicile répond à la volonté d'un grand nombre de malades âgés. Grâce à l'entourage – le conjoint notamment –, des malades peuvent rester chez eux lorsque des services adéquats de soins et de soutien à domicile sont à disposition. Cela correspond généralement au souhait de l'entourage. Bien sûr, il y a des limites au maintien à domicile : l'institutionnalisation est préférable quand les déplacements sont trop nombreux ou quand survient la fatigue de l'entourage, souvent âgé lui aussi.

La comparaison entre le coût des soins et soutien à domicile et le coût de l'institutionnalisation est difficile à établir de façon stricte. Le dévouement et l'aide bénévole ne sont pas quantifiables. Et la séparation de conjoints qui ont vécu de nombreuses années ensemble, de même que l'aggravation de la dépendance physique et psychique qui peut résulter d'un placement en institution, ne sont guère chiffrables.

Les ordres de grandeur sont toutefois patents, dans les conditions de Lausanne (chef-lieu du canton de Vaud, 140 000 habitants) : les soins à domicile, avec l'appui des services d'aide, évitent, raccourcissent ou diffèrent des hospitalisations et surtout des placements de longue durée en établissements médico-sociaux. Les malades sont généralement des "cas lourds". L'économie en lits correspond à 14 lits pour 10 000 habitants, soit plus du dixième d'une norme globale retenue il y a une quinzaine d'années. Le coût comparatif du maintien à domicile est trois fois inférieur à l'institutionnalisation. Le seul service de la dette (intérêts, amortissement) pour les lits médico-sociaux d'établissements qu'il faudrait construire sans ce service de soins, équivaut... au coût du fonctionnement du Centre !

La comparaison économique est nettement à l'avantage du maintien à domicile. A elle seule, l'humanisation des soins pour ceux qui veulent et peuvent rester dans leur cadre de vie habituel, avec le compagnon ou la compagne de vie, justifie le développement de ces services.

Il n'est pas de mon ressort de centrer cette contribution sur les maladies liées à la sénilité. Les exemples ci-dessus sont illustratifs et permettent d'élargir le propos à l'organisation sociale et prospective des services de santé, en particulier en relation avec le vieillissement de la population.

Nouvelle donne gérontologique : tout se joue "en amont"

Une nouvelle donne gérontologique est à mettre en œuvre. Elle est partie intégrante de la politique de santé; elle commande même une organisation médico-sociale adéquate. En bref, quelques points, qui font l'objet de discussions dans ce pays, en vue d'une autre allocation des ressources.

- D'abord s'impose un principe de *complémentarité.* Les institutions de santé ont trop souvent des buts sectoriels et sont justaposées. Une meilleure coordination et une flexibilité d'utilisation sont grosses d'améliorations et d'économies.
- La *comparaison et l'évaluation* des services de santé, selon une vue d'ensemble, sont des préalables à la prise de décisions cohérentes.
  Les recherches concernant les services de santé peuvent ainsi devenir des investissements rentables.
- Il y a des listes d'attente dans plusieurs établissements médico-sociaux; mais il y a, en Suisse, surdotation manifeste en lits d'hôpitaux.
  Une *conversion des missions* (hôpitaux de jour, établissements pour malades chroniques...) représente une économie d'investissements en constructions; une économie de gestion aussi, car des "lits vides" sont administratrivement onéreux.
- Des personnes âgées passent une grande partie de leur temps, et parfois tout leur temps, dans leur appartement. Aussi importe-t-il de *construire des logements adéquats et d'abaisser les "barrières architecturales"* des appartements existants.
- Pour un malade chronique âgé ou handicapé dépendant, être soigné à domicile – si c'est son souhait et si les conditions le permettent – est un besoin aussi fondamental que se nourrir, se vêtir et se loger. *L'extension des services de soins et de soutiens à domicile* – qui disposent actuellement d'une portion congrue du financement de santé publique – est prioritaire.
- Des "investissements" supplémentaires en *personnels pour ces services décentralisés* seront largement compensés par la diminution des investissements dans les murs des hôpitaux. Dans une société fortement vieillissante, l'économie grâce aux soins et soutiens à domicile est si grande qu'elle en est impérieuse.

- Un soutien accru à ceux qui gardent un proche à la maison offre sécurité, allège inquiétude et fatigue, favorise le maintien à domicile. *L'aide à l'entourage qui aide* est un principe essentiel.

Entourage, services de soins et soutiens à domicile, bénévoles, médecins, établissements médico-sociaux, hôpitaux, sont des éléments complémentaires du système de santé, si importants pour la population âgée.

Un recentrage est nécessaire, car avec la spécialisation des équipements et des fonctions, on court le risque de sélectionner les destinataires et de renforcer les cloisonnements.

Ces mesures – dont l'énumération n'est pas exhaustive – évitent ou retardent des placements institutionnels et le déracinement. Elles visent à rompre la solitude dans laquelle s'enferment en silence maints vieillards. Souffrances tues et cachées.

Cependant, le "succès de toutes les politiques sociales se joue sur tous les âges et sur tous les fronts". (Vieillir demain, Documentation française, 1980, p. 176). Le but est l'autonomie de la personne. L'action utile déborde le cadre de la santé publique. La retraite correspond encore à une mise à l'écart, une perte des rôles et un sentiment d'inutilité chez beaucoup.

- *La précarité des conditions d'existence induit des placements* en institutions, qui sont ainsi des refuges de la pauvreté. Les vieux les plus démunis sont en effet plus fréquemment institutionnalisés.
- *L'élévation des revenus des citoyens les plus modestes résorbe la pauvreté.* Elle limite l'incertitude matérielle, voire la crainte du lendemain, ainsi que la décompensation psychique, le repli et la dégradation de l'image de soi, qui souvent l'accompagnent.
- L'amélioration sélective des revenus les plus bas conduit à de *moindres dépenses d'aide sociale et d'hébergement* en institution, à charge des assurances et des pouvoirs publics. Cela s'est manifesté de façon patente en Suisse lorsque, en 1966, les rentes de l'assurance vieillesse fédérale ont été sensiblement améliorées et des prestations complémentaires introduites pour garantir un "minimum vital".
- *Des mesures indirectes* agissent dans le même sens : prise en charge sélective, totale ou partielle selon les revenus, des cotisations d'assurance; abaissement du coût du loyer; appareils auxiliaires, etc.
- Le *passage graduel de la vie professionnelle à la retraite* facilite la transition vers un temps libéré dûment aménagé : activités et loisirs choisis.
- Les disparités des conditions de travail et des revenus professionnels retentissent sur le développement personnel et, par reproduction, conditionnent l'existence pendant la vieillesse. Plus que des correctifs "en aval", une *réduction "en amont" de l'éventail des revenus primaires* apparaît préférable.

- La ville est inhospitalière aux personnes âgées. Le tissu urbain souvent éclaté, la priorité implicite à la circulation automobile dense et rapide, le manque de lieux de rencontres, l'absence d'espaces calmes, conduisent à l'exclusion de maints vieillards. Aussi l'intégration des personnes âgées et la prévention passent-elles également par des *aménagements des infrastructures et de l'environnement.* Pour toute la population, il s'agit de *réapproprier les espaces* publics, afin de bien vivre dans la cité.
- Les personnes âgées peuvent contribuer au *mouvement de vie associative*, où jeunes, actifs et vieux trouvent les termes de nouveaux échanges, d'entraide, de solidarité et de relations conviviales.
- Les personnes âgées peuvent devenir "*promoteurs de leur propre avenir*", en organisant mieux leur temps libre. A cet effet, la satisfaction du besoin de sécurité est nécessaire à l'expression du besoin de liberté.

Finalité : un bon état de santé de la population

Le vieillissement de la population implique une "médication" sur le plan des structures et de l'organisation de la santé publique. A la concentration implicite des investissements dans les "murs" pendant le troisième quart de ce siècle, il faut dorénavant accorder une priorité explicite aux investissements en personnels qualifiés. A l'"explosion" désordonnée des dépenses doit succéder une "implosion" planifiée des ressources du système de santé, pour modifier l'allocation des montants et les orienter vers des structures et une gestion économes, efficaces et de qualité.

La finalité n'est pas la "réparation de la santé dégradée", nécessaire mais non suffisante. C'est le maintien et la promotion d'un bon état de santé de la population. Des actions et une politique sociale centrées sur la santé, le revenu, le travail et l'habitat sont des moyens de prévention intervenant "en amont". Elles ouvrent une voie à l'intégration sociale des personnes âgées et des grands vieillards, en si grand nombre demain. Dans cette option de qualité de vie en société, les services de santé à la population prennent valeur de sens. On ne règle pas par une arithmétique économique ce qui relève des valeurs.

Quelques références bibliographiques

Vieillissement démographique et planification hospitalière. P. G. Dpt Intérieur, Lausanne 1969.

Démographie médicale en Suisse. P. G. et al. Office de statistique, Lausanne 1976.

Vieillir aujourd'hui et demain. (P. G., recueil de contributions). Réalités sociales, Lausanne 1982.

Soins à domicile. L. Ramel, C. Willa, P. G. Réalités sociales, Lausanne 1982.

Rentiers AVS : une autre image de la Suisse. P. G. Réalités sociales, Lausanne 1983.

Senile Dementia: Outlook for the Future, pages 177–188

SENILE DEMENTIA - SOCIO-ECONOMIC ASPECTS, PREVENTION AND MASS DETECTION

Doctor Deboise

Physician Responsible on the National Level of the U.C.C.M.A.
Paris, France

My Dear Colleagues,
The theme chosen for our Conference is both difficult and fascinating. It is difficult because we have to deal with an illness that keeps the secret of its pathology and for which we are relatively unprepared. It is fascinating because the scientific mind always wants to pierce the mysteries of the unknown.

My presentation will be neither that of a clinician nor of a fundamentalist. Rather, it will be that of a social physician entrusted by the M.S.A.[x] with the collective health protection of the 2.8 million retired agricultural workers.

In France the M.S.A. is the organisation for the compulsory social protection of all agricultural workers and their families, whether they be farmers, hired workers or retired. Except for its appointed duties the M.S.A. has always developed a medico-social policy based on preventive medicine.

In the domaine of geriatry we have given priority to the maintenance of physical and mental autonomy, which has led us to set up a system of prevention and detection of the principal causes of illness among the aged.

[x]M.S.A. (Mutualité Sociale Agricole)

Among these causes senile dementia has occupied our attention. My task will be to present why and how we have perfected a way of fighting against mental illness and in particular against senile dementia. I point out the fact that we are talking about a collective action that takes place before and after the illness; the diagnosis and treatment belonging to curative medicine.

Thus, we believe that we can master the increase of this illness in spite of the predictable ageing of the population from now to the year 2000.

I - AGEING OF THE POPULATION AND THE SOCIO-ECONOMIC WEIGHT OF SENILE DEMENTIA

Senile dementia being one of the major consequences of ageing, it is evident that the larger the elderly population in the future the greater the number of cases of senile dementia that will exist.

Only a fundamental discovery in the area of treatment or prevention of this illness could change this probability. Today, based on actual conditions, everything presupposes a progressive and marked accentuation of ageing of the French population in the twenty years to come, and consequently of the socio-economic weight of senile dementia.

1 - Ageing of the French Population (statistics 1982 from the INSEE and the INED)

. of the 54 million French we count 10 million people aged 60 years and older, of which 7.5 million are over 65 (14% of the French population).

. among those over 65 we count 3 million aged 75 years and older of which 700,000 are over 85.

All of the prospective demographic studies forsee a progressive accentuation of the phenomenon of ageing and in particular of the number of people who are quite old. For the year 2000 it is expected that there will be nearly 4 million people of 75 years and older, of which 1 million will be over 85.

2 - The Greatest Ageing among the Agricultural Population

The agricultural milieu is particularly touched by ageing since of nearly 7 million under the jurisdiction of the M.S.A. we count 2.8 million retired. This particular ageing is the direct result of the industrialisation and mechanisation of modern agriculture which uses less and less manual labor. The young people leave to work in the city and the older people stay in the villages.

These few figures justify the importance that we attach to our gerontological policy.

3 - The Place of Senile Dementia in Mental Illness

All the statistics concerning senile dementia are taken from general data about mental illness. If our information about specialized establishments is precise it is even more exact about non-specialized establishments, but very fragmentary about the ill who live at home. However, we can determine the truth with the following facts:

a) Senile dementia in specialized services. (1981 statistics from the Ministry of National Solidarity and the Ministry of Health concerning psychiatric establishments both public, and private functioning as public, for the year 1979)

. 284,807 ill admitted during the year for 36,544,000 days of hospitalisation, representing 13% of the total hospitalisation budget in France.

. On December 31, 1979, 101,964 ill were hospitalised for a total capacity of 122,050 beds.

. Among those hospitalized 35% were 60 years and older as compared to 24% in 1953 - document of CREDOC).

. According to the statistics of the INSERM, senile dementia represents 10% of those hospitalized or approximately 11,000 people of which 10% were 75 years and older. Their cost in 1981 was approximately 1.3 billion francs.

b) Senile dementia in non-specialized services. These services have as their goal to take the aged who can no longer stay in their homes for medical or social reasons. Three types of establishments are to be considered: long term, hospices and medical retirement homes. Their total capacity is approximately 300,000 beds.

. Long term establishments: receive elderly people who are dependent for different reasons. 220,000 beds.

According to the statistics of Professor Forette - Director of the National Foundation of Gerontology, the population of these services is distributed in this manner:

. 36% mentally ill, half of which are senile dementia,

. 33% physically handicapped,

. 14% chronically ill,

. 17% those who are there for social reasons - essentially isolated people.

Thus we can estimate at more than 30,000 the number of mentally ill housed in these services. It is certainly a good solution, medically and humanly speaking to keep them in non-psychiatric surroundings, as long as they do not disturb the proper functioning of the establishment.

. Hospices: I mention them only for memory's sake since the new hospitalisation laws will do away with them, and replace them with long term establishments for those persons who are dependent and by medical retirement homes for those persons who are able-bodied. In these hospices which still exist we find 10% of those with senile dementia, or approximately 3,000 persons.

. Medical Retirement Homes: are created to receive the aged who are autonomous. However, in practice, because of the pressing demands of families, they take a certain number of mentally ill on condition that their mental deterioration does not bother the others.

It is difficult to know the exact number of these people, but it can be estimated at 5% from the surveys taken in certain establishments, or approximately 3,000 mentally ill.

c) Senile dementia at home. Although it is very difficult to identify all of the mentally ill who live at home, we are certain that they are not very numerous. In fact this situation requires the conjunction of conditions which are difficult to bring together: an aged person whose mental deterioration is not too advanced, a solid, well motivated family and permanent medico-social help.

II - A PRIORITY IN GERIATRY : THE KEEPING OF AUTONOMY

Responsable for the health protection of the agricultural population, the medico-social policy of the M.S.A. is committed to fight against the principal causes of illness and death of this population. Three actions which have priority direct this policy: prevention of the illness, its early detection and finally its follow-up. Each of these actions is of course adapted to the age group concerned.

For the elderly we have given the priority to the fight against debilitating illnesses, considering that the main goal of a gerontologic policy is the maintenance of physical and mental autonomy. Before going into the details of the fight against senile dementia, I would like to resume briefly the spirit of these three actions:

. Prevention of the illness. It is health education. It is a question of informing the public about the principal risks of the elderly so that each one will be aware that he is partly responsible for the quality of his old age in order to adopt the proper behavior to ensure good health.

. Early detection of the illness. It has as its objective a systematic search, every five years - each person 65 years and older, for the existence of debilitating illnesses in order to treat them as early as possible.

. Follow-up of the illness. This is addressed to elderly people who have a debilitating illness, in order to fight against the results and relapses, with a social reinsertion in sight each time possible.

In the case of senile dementia the possibility of re-education and rehabilitation is unfortunately illusory. Our role comes down to ensuring that the mentally ill person is treated under the best of conditions necessitated by his mental state.

I am now going to give you the details of the three programs used to fight against the mental deterioration of the aged.

1 - Prevention of Mental Deterioration

I will stay within the domain of collective prevention, being persuaded that the change from an active life to the life of a retired person is a fundamental rupture which contains certain psychological elements which create a climate for mental deterioration. We will consider two:

. The feeling of uselessness. It is particularly felt in a society where man's worth is found in his work. The retired person has nothing left to offer; no one expects anything more of him; he has become a negative social element who is there only to collect his retirement pay. As a result there is a social situation which is depressing for the retired person who will have a tendancy to withdraw and loose interest in the outside world.

. Relational isolation. This is the consequence of the brusque mutation of the traditional family structure which from patriarchal has become parental in two or three generations. In 1981, according to the results of a survey taken by the M.S.A. in the agricultural world, 70% of those aged 65 years and older live alone (older couples, widows, widowers, singles). For people who have known an active family and professional life, this isolation is sometimes difficult to bear, and more so as they are frequently deprived of their ancestral role as grandfathers and grandmothers.

Outside of organic causes, which are at the origin of 30% of these mental illnesses, the feeling of uselessness and isolation are the two factors which weigh heavily on the mental deterioration. To remedy this we have counted on the development of an associative life.

Ten years ago we instigated the creation of associations for the aged, to permit them first to meet each other, and then to become aware of their existence and the role that they could have in our society.

Today, the development of these associations has gone beyond anything that we could have expected. In fact, of the 16,000 associations for the elderly in France, 11,000 are rural associations grouping more than 1.5 million people. Their enthusiasm has led them to form federations in each department in France and then a national association. Going farther in their desire to know and be acquainted with, they created, three years ago, the International Federation of Associations for the Elderly (FIAPH) to which twelve countries already belong and which has been recognized as O.N.G. at the O.N.U.

Thus old age, which seemed to have the greatest difficulty integrating into our modern society, comes out of its position of retirement to re-occupy the place that it had abandoned and which belonged to it just two or three generations ago. The associative life has given the elderly the possibility of taking care of themselves and rediscovering the joys of life, the desire to know, the taste for undertaking and the spirit of solidarity.

We have witnessed in less than fifteen years a phenomenon of social adaptation that most certainly constitutes the best prevention of senile dementia.

What is more, for the M.S.A., each one of the 11,000 rural clubs of elderly people is an ideal place to inform the public on the health education of the elderly. Preoccupied by the consequences of ageing, the retired demand information on health. We meet their demands, and our physicians and social workers go to different areas to lead meetings on health education which are always well attended, not only by older people but also by the young. The preservation of mental autonomy is one of the most asked for themes.

2 - The Early Detection of Mental Deterioration

I will certainly surprise you by saying that this detection is done only by the interpretation of a questionnaire that is distributed, sector by sector, to all the elderly, that they must fill out themselves, or if they cannot, someone else in their entourage must do so.

We have adopted this new technique of detection after having made certain conclusions from 100,000 traditional check ups (including complete laboratory tests adapted to the elderly and a systematic clinical examination) and observing that they did not reach their goal. In fact:

. they almost always do the same work as curative medicine since 95% of those questioned were already being followed by a physician, that 65% of them were under medical treatment and that 55% had had paraclinical examinations in the same year.

. They do not allow knowledge of the social situation of those concerned, although in geriatry social difficulties can have a determining effect on the health and particularly mental health.

. They have a low effectiveness as compared to their cost because they reveal only 3% of unknown pathologies for an individual cost of over 300 F. Actually they are useless in 97% of the cases.

a) These facts have lead us to conceive a more Global Approach to the Problems of the Elderly. When it is a question of a population of almost three million persons, the essential is not to make a precise individual diagnosis, but to identify only those persons who have need of diagnosis and treatment in order to direct them as rapidly as possible to medical help which will take care of them.

This questionnaire has three parts:

. medical, to find the principal pathologies of the aged,

. autonomy, in order to know the degree of physical, sensorial and mental independence of each person,

. social, destined to identify the persons who seem to have difficulties of a social order.

b) The Interpretation and Follow up which are given to each questionnaire rest on the concordance or lack of concordance between the responses to the closed questions and responses to the open questions. As of this moment the statistical exploitation of the first 40,000 questionnaires received has permitted us:

. to identify 3% of the unrecognized pathologies, that is to say as many as with the check ups, but for a cost of four times less,

. to know the persons who have an alteration of physical, sensorial or mental autonomy,

. to know the social difficulties of each one. This knowledge permits us to act on an individual level, but above all it reveals the collective needs to us.

c) The Detection of the Alteration of Mental Functions is arrived at by interpreting the answers to the specific questions about mental autonomy as well as to the questions relative to their relationships in daily life. The time given to me does not permit me to give the details of this questionnaire, but we can talk about them during the discussion.

Since it has to do with mass detection, which is essential, it is not for making a precise psychiatric diagnosis, but for identifying each person who seems to have mental problems in order to send him to a physician who can treat him or who can refer him to a psychiatrist.

To be sure that the person is followed by a program of curative medicine, we verify what happens, and when we are in possession of the precise diagnosis we continue to follow up the person.

3 - The Follow up of those with Senile Dementia

Once a diagnosis of senile dementia is established, our role is to see that the person receives a treatment corresponding to his state. Depending on the degree of his mental deterioration we have three possibilities:

. At the beginning of the illness we prefer to keep the person at home if the family is in agreement and if it is possible to have medical help in the home. As we have already seen these conditions are hard to obtain even though keeping the person at home is the best solution to stopping the evolution of the illness.

. At a more advanced stage, placing the mentally ill person in an institution may be necessary. This is the time to make a decision which will impose a traumatising situation on the ill person whose possibilities of adaption are greatly lessened.

To lessen the consequences of the rupture, it seems to us preferable to place them in long term non specialized services, on the condition that they not be a hindrance to the proper functioning of the establishment.

Placed in an open environment, meeting invalids and different handicapped people, they find themselves in a non-psychiatric milieu where geriatric physicians give them the best chances to regain their existing potential and to fulfill the possibility of recovering their equilibrium.

. It is only when the preceding possibilities are excluded that a hospitalisation in a psychiatric environment is decided upon. The ideal would be a geronto-psychiatric service but we do not have enough of them, and it is the general psychiatric hospitals that remain the last resort. It is above all for the protection of society, as we all know that a long psychiatric hospitalisation finishes by dependence, passivity and the ill person giving up.

III - CONCLUSION

To conclude, I will go back to the theme of our Conference which asks us a question about the future: "Will the socio-economic weight of senile dementia increase in the years to come?"

Today, given the facts in our possession, the answer is yes. In fact, how could it be otherwise when on one hand we are sure that the ageing of the population will continue to grow in our western world, and on the other that we are not yet prepared to control an illness whose evolution is inevitable.

Given these conditions, collective prevention and early detection are certainly the best ways to hold off mental deterioration as long as possible and to slow down the evolution of this formidable illness in the years to come.

However, these are only temporary measures and often they have not stood up to the success of medical discoveries. I hope and I am convinced the the work shown us during this Conference by our colleagues will invalidate these temporary measures.

Senile Dementia: Outlook for the Future, pages 189-200

L'organisation médico-sociale de la démence sénile

GOMMERS A.

Responsable du Centre d'Etudes Gérontologiques
Faculté de Médecine
Université de Louvain - 1200 Bruxelles-Belgique

Un des plus graves problèmes médico-sociaux et économiques auxquels notre société se trouve confrontée est le problème de la démence sénile. Cette opinion de M. Aronson (1981) se justifie tant par le nombre de vieillards atteints que par le retentissement de la maladie au niveau de la personne, de sa famille et de la communauté.

La nécessité d'apporter une réponse aux besoins nés de cette situation a suscité des réalisations sanitaires et sociales variables en fonction des politiques de santé et du comportement des populations. Mon propos n'est pas d'en présenter un impossible inventaire exhaustif mais plutôt d'alimenter notre réflexion.

Examinons, dans un premier temps, les solutions institutionnelles et, ensuite, les conditions d'un éventuel maintien à domicile.

Quelle que soit la région étudiée, on constate que les déments séniles peuvent être pris en charge dans des établissements de statuts fort variables : hôpitaux généraux ou psychiatriques, centres de gériatrie ou de gérontopsychiatrie, maisons de retraite avec ou sans reconnaissance d'un forfait pour les soins. Il apparaît que, trop souvent, ce sont les circonstances, plus que la pathologie, qui décident du lieu d'hébergement ou de traitement : d'une part, l'entrée dans le circuit d'hospitalisation se fait très souvent dans des situations d'urgence ou de pseudo-urgence et, d'autre part, ce sont davantage les situations locales (la présence ou l'absence des structures adaptées ou de places disponibles) qui déterminent le suivi thérapeutique.

Ainsi, le vieillard en état d'agitation ou d'agressivité angoissante pour l'entourage et le médecin de famille sera dirigé soit vers l'hôpital général, soit vers un établissement psychiatrique, institutions où n'existent pas toujours des unités propres à accueillir ce genre de patients. Ceci constitue une rupture de la vie relationnelle et de l'environnement du malade et ne doit donc se faire qu'à bon escient. Deux questions se posent : 1) cette hospitalisation lourde de conséquences, décidée comme intervention de crise, est-elle toujours nécessaire ? 2) une institution non différenciée (c'est-à-dire s'adressant à l'ensemble de la population) est-elle adéquate pour résoudre une situation psychogériatrique complexe ?

Dans leur Manuel de Psychogériatrie, les professeurs Müller et Wertheimer (1981) soulignent que si la perturbation du comportement du malade est le centre vers lequel converge toute l'attention, cependant la crise ne se limite pas à l'individu : "elle emporte aussi dans son tourbillon ceux qui gravitent autour de lui, famille, amis, voisins, médecins, personnel soignant ou travailleurs sociaux. Cette constellation est étroitement impliquée dans l'équilibre du vieillard et par conséquent, aussi, dans le déséquilibre dont il est victime, ainsi que dans la recherche de remèdes à la crise. En situation aiguë, il est donc important de repérer la cause de la demande d'intervention." Si les facteurs précipitants de la crise sont généralement mal connus, il reste que l'appel à l'aide extérieure provient d'un entourage qui ne se sent pas -ou plus- capable de supporter le comportement pathologique. L'angoisse, la crainte, le sentiment d'impuissance l'emportent. Une bonne information sur la maladie et les mesures susceptibles de répondre au mieux à la situation de crise et un soutien psychologique permettraient peut-être d'éviter un recours trop rapide à l'institution. Cette action de prévention relève du médecin de famille. Encore faut-il que sa formation, tant médicale que psychologique et morale, l'ait préparé à assumer cette tâche et à ne décider une hospitalisation que si celle-ci s'avère indispensable.

Dans ce cas, où convient-il d'adresser le malade ? L'hôpital général permet une approche pluridisciplinaire; il dispose d'un ensemble de moyens techniques aptes à différencier les syndromes démentiels. Cependant, le diagnostic de démence sénile établi, si l'institution ne dispose pas d'unités spécifiquement vouées à la gériatrie, il faut craindre un rejet du patient et une demande de placement rapide dans la première structure d'accueil disposant d'une place.

L'admission du vieillard présentant des troubles de type démentiel dans un établissement psychiatrique peut donc paraître plus indiquée. En France, le Rapport du groupe de travail "Prospective des Personnes Agées"(1982) révèle que, d'après les statistiques médicales de l'INSERM pour 1978, 14 % des patients présents dans les hôpitaux psychiatriques figuraient sous le diagnostic : "état d'affaiblissement de la sénilité et démence pré-sénile". La même année, 19.858 admissions étaient motivées par ce diagnostic. Des situations comparables existent dans la plupart des pays occidentaux. Il est évident que l'hospitalisation en milieu psychiatrique permet une bonne évaluation de l'état démentiel -ceci toutefois à condition qu'elle se fasse avec la collaboration d'internistes- et un traitement adéquat des manifestations aiguës de la maladie.

Que penser d'une prise en charge thérapeutique prolongée dans un type d'établissement qui, ces dernières années, tente une reconversion en services ouverts et actifs ? Trois sortes de risques existent : 1) le désintérêt des psychiatres pour une dégradation psycho-organique considérée comme irréversible, 2) la méconnaissance des affections somatiques associées ou le poids de leur traitement pour le personnel (lutte contre les escarres et le grabatarisme, par exemple), 3) l'inadaptation du milieu en tant que lieu de vie pour la personne âgée. Ces écueils sont évidemment évités si l'hôpital psychiatrique comporte un département réservé à la gérontopsychiatrie, disposant d'un personnel médical et paramédical spécialisé et motivé.

Ainsi, quel que soit le cadre administratif -variable de pays à pays et même de région à région- dont relève le malade, c'est à un milieu hospitalier à vocation gériatrique et plus précisément psychogériatrique qu'il convient de l'adresser si l'hospitalisation paraît indispensable. La dénomination de ce service, sa place dans le système institutionnel, son mode de fonctionnement (durée plus ou moins longue du séjour, financement par la Sécurité Sociale, etc...) diffèrent selon les législations, elles-mêmes d'ailleurs en perpétuelle évolution. Mais il doit exister un dénominateur commun à ces sections psychogériatriques : la certitude que la démence sénile est accessible au traitement avec, comme corollaire, une attitude positive et dynamique. La mission de ces hôpitaux, départements ou unités sera :

- établissement par une équipe pluridisciplinaire du diagnostic qui, non seulement doit porter sur le degré de détérioration mais fera également l'inventaire des capacités restantes et des potentialités à développer
- mobilisation de toutes les ressources thérapeutiques : médicaments, psychothérapie, sociothérapie, activités occupationnelles et ludiques, etc...
- évaluation régulière des résultats en présence de tous les intervenants
- climat d'accueil et adaptation des lieux à la désorientation du malade
- intégration de la famille aux objectifs thérapeutiques
- coordination avec les établissements résidentiels ou les organisations de soins à domicile pour assurer une continuité thérapeutique lors du transfert du patient.

La complexité des tâches, le nécessaire recours à des spécialistes de différentes disciplines, la charge en personnel infirmier et paramédical, exigent que ces départements relèvent des structures hospitalières et non des services médico-sociaux comme les maisons de soins, par exemple. Faut-il préconiser le développement de sections spécialisées dans l'hospitalisation de vieillards présentant des symptômes de détérioration psycho-organique ? Il nous a été donné d'en connaître plus particulièrement deux, vouées par choix ou par accident aux déments séniles. La motivation, le dynamisme de l'équipe et les résultats présentés sont assez convaincants. Signalons l'initiative remarquable de l'un d'entre eux : l'initiation et la participation du conjoint bien portant à la dynamisation de l'époux malade, en vue d'un retour à domicile.

Dans le désastre économique actuel, le coût de telles sections psychogériatriques risque de faire obstacle à la poursuite d'une politique institutionnelle efficace. Des pays, comme la Belgique, envisagent de retirer ces malades du secteur hospitalier. C'est méconnaître le changement d'optique intervenu ces dernières années dans l'approche médicale des patients séniles et leur dénier le droit à un traitement actif suffisamment prolongé pour être efficace. Par ailleurs, une gestion saine des dépenses de santé peut-elle se limiter à l'immédiat et négliger le bénéfice à moyen et à long terme d'une action qui se veut préventive et revalidante ?

On peut se poser la question du bien fondé d'un maintien définitif en psychogériatrie active de déments légers ou même graves qui n'exigent plus qu'un traitement d'entretien pour ne pas rétrograder. En Grande Bretagne, la tendance semble être de multiplier des unités d'admission urgente et d'évaluation à durée d'hospitalisation limitée. De là, les patients sont dirigés, selon les cas, soit vers leur domicile avec l'assistance de services communautaires soit vers des sections psychogériatriques de long séjour ou des homes pour vieillards atteints de maladies mentales (Dublin, Coventry).

L'hôpital, en effet, -sous peine de dévier de ses objectifs- ne peut devenir un substitut du foyer personnel. Le cadre de vie qu'il propose n'est d'ailleurs guère approprié à un séjour prolongé, non plus que la rigidité de ses règlements et de son organisation. Les maisons de retraite, et ce que les Anglo-saxons dénomment "Nursing Homes" peuvent-ils assurer la prise en charge prolongée ou définitive des vieillards déments qui, pour l'une ou l'autre raison, ne peuvent séjourner dans leur foyer ? En fait, on trouve dans ces établissements résidentiels une proportion non négligeable de ces malades. L'atteinte pathologique est généralement légère ou moyenne. Beaucoup de ces séniles trouvent place dans des homes privés, à but lucratif. Dans ces maisons, comme dans les établissements sociaux, les soins d'hygiène de base peuvent être bons et l'atmosphère, familiale. Mais il est évident que faute de personnel assez nombreux et compétent, il ne peut y être question de dynamisation des facultés restantes. Un autre problème crucial est celui du faible seuil de tolérance aux comportements anormaux, ceci tant de la part du personnel que des autres personnes âgées. L'appel fréquent à l'hospitalisation au moindre incident et le recours massif aux sédatifs sont sources d'aggravation de la pathologie.

La transformation d'anciens hospices en maisons de santé et de cure médicale, la création de homes de soins par le transfert de certains lits hospitaliers vont-ils permettre de répondre plus adéquatement aux besoins

complexes des vieillards déments ? Oui, sans doute, mais à différentes conditions, parmi lesquelles on peut citer :
- nombre suffisant de places disponibles
- objectif de resocialisation plutôt qu'excès de médicalisation
- adéquation du personnel (quantité, qualification)

Ceci suppose que les ressources financières mises à la disposition de ces institutions soient en rapport avec les exigences de la population hébergée. Le risque évoqué par F. Jandrot-Louka et J.M. Louka (1979) de créer des "parcages" dans des structures à bas prix est réel si l'administration de soins de base ne s'accompagne pas de mesures de stimulation à l'autonomie et de sociothérapie. Or, dans l'état actuel des choses, il est bien évident que les soignants n'ont pas reçu une formation leur permettant l'investissement relationnel nécessaire à ces malades. Le vieillard atteint de troubles mentaux fait peur : l'angoisse devant un comportement aberrant s'ajoute à la difficulté de vivre avec ces patients. Un meilleur enseignement de base et, peut-être, le recours à la psychothérapie de groupe seraient sans doute susceptibles de remédier à cette situation.

La spécialisation de certaines maisons de soins en résidences pour déments séniles pourrait également, malgré des avis contradictoires sur le sujet, constituer une heureuse solution. Elle assurerait mieux que les homes polyvalents l'adaptation du milieu à la pathologie démentielle, ce qui permet d'influer positivement sur le cours et l'expression des manifestations morbides. Il existe quelques réussites remarquables à cet égard, comme par exemple, la maison de Essen, à la frontière belgo-hollandaise, basée sur la liberté des "habitants" et la totale intégration des professionnels à l'ensemble des activités , quelle que soit leur qualification initiale. Mais ici aussi, la compétence du personnel et sa motivation sont primordiales. La présence d'un infirmier psychiatrique paraît capitale. En formons-nous assez ?

D'autre part, les objectifs d'économie qui ont souvent présidé à la création de maisons de soins sont-ils compatibles avec la nécessité de tout un personnel paramédical (kinési- et ergo-thérapeutes), d'assistants sociaux et si possible, de psychologues ?

Le placement en institution n'est heureusement pas le sort réservé à tous les déments séniles. Une étude de l'O.M.S. rapporte qu'à Newcastle (Angleterre), 80 % des

des personnes atteintes de troubles psycho-organiques vivent chez elles, tandis qu'à Copenhague, on trouverait 65 % de déments graves dans leur foyer (WHO, 1982). Ceci signifie sans doute, comme le constate le groupe de travail cité, que "les raisons qui déterminent le maintien d'un patient à son foyer ou son admission en institution n'ont souvent aucun rapport avec son état et tiennent au degré de motivation de son entourage, au degré d'efficacité de l'organisation des soins à domicile, au degré d'adéquation du logement et à des facteurs économiques." Ajoutons à ces éléments l'existence de solutions temporaires d'hébergement et le soutien apporté aux familles par la communauté.

Garder à son domicile un vieillard dément n'est pas chose facile. Disons d'ailleurs que le maintien à tout prix n'est pas souhaitable. Pour certains gérontologues, la contrainte essentielle serait d'ordre financier. Nous ne le croyons pas. Car s'il ne semble pas y avoir a priori de contre-indication médicale (voir les réponses des médecins au questionnaire relatif à l'Action sanitaire et sociale en France : Rapport du groupe"Prospective Personnes Agées" Préparation du 8ème plan, 1980), par contre, les capacités de résistance de l'entourage ont des limites. Dans la plupart des cas, c'est la défaillance de la famille ou des amis qui est à l'origine des placements en institution, justifiés ou non. La vie du dément sénile dans la communauté dépend donc en partie de l'organisation médico-sociale de soutien qui est mise à sa disposition.

La famille constitue le pivot des solutions alternatives à l'institutionnalisation. Partout, dans le monde -et cela malgré les stéréotypes souvent négatifs sur le sujet- elle reste la principale source de services aux personnes âgées : selon les études de Shanas (in Brody, 1981), les proches assureraient 80 % des soins de santé aux vieillards non placés et certains enfants adultes y consacreraient l'équivalent d'un travail full-time au moins. Dans le cas du dément sénile vivant à domicile, le fardeau est non seulement physique mais, plus encore, psychologique.

Même du seul point de vue économie de la santé, les politiques de la vieillesse devraient être axées sur des programmes d'aide aux familles. Comme le signale Butler (1977) pour les U.S.A., si seulement une partie des sommes investies dans les Nursing Homes étaient utilisées pour soutenir les familles, nous verrions diminuer le nombre de ces institutions coûteuses et, dans ce pays surtout, très éloignées d'offrir des conditions optimales de soins aux personnes âgées.

L'aide aux familles peut prendre de nombreuses formes : financière, matérielle, psychologique.

Un apport financier (réduction des impôts pour prise en charge d'un vieillard handicapé, allocation supplémentaire pour soins fournis, etc...) peut faciliter la tâche de la famille en permettant de faire appel à des aides extérieures pour le ménage ou la garde momentanée des vieillards. Le Conseil municipal de Stockholm, par exemple, fournit un salaire imposable aux membres de la famille qui assurent des soins constants ou partiels à un parent âgé malade. L'équivalent du prix horaire d'une aide-ménagère, ainsi que les avantages sociaux liés à cette fonction sont également accordés. Il ne s'agit pas de payer le dévouement : même si le montant est parfois relativement élevé, il ne représente cependant qu'une compensation très partielle à la perte d'emploi qu'entraîne la décision de rester à la maison pour s'occuper du vieillard.

Les charges qui pèsent sur les proches assurant la vie quotidienne du dément à leur foyer doivent également pouvoir être allégées par l'appel à des services communautaires ou par le recours à différentes formes d'hébergement ou de garde temporaire.

Les services de soins à domicile et d'aides-ménagères existent dans tous les pays industrialisés. Mais ils ne peuvent malheureusement faire face à tous les besoins. Dans de nombreux cas, les prestations ont dû être limitées aux économiquement faibles et aux vieillards isolés. Or, les déments séniles se trouvent généralement en famille. Ces malades devraient donc également être inscrits comme prioritaires pour l'attribution de ces services. Quant à l'hospitalisation à domicile, formule qui a fait ses preuves en France, elle aussi se heurte à un réel problème lorsqu'il s'agit du traitement de séniles : c'est celui de l'irréversibilité de la pathologie avec, comme corollaire, la durée illimitée de la demande d'intervention.

Intermédiaires entre l'institution et le domicile, les Hôpitaux ou Centres de jour présentent le double avantage d'assurer au malade un traitement polyvalent dans des conditions optimales et de soulager sa famille par une décharge temporaire. Né en U.R.S.S. en 1932, l'hôpital de jour, eut à l'origine, un objectif psychiatrique. La formule s'est ensuite considérablement développée en faveur des personnes âgées en Grande Bretagne et dans les pays scandinaves. Pour J. Keet (1979), "l'hôpital de jour est considéré comme un élément fondamental de la gériatrie anglaise" et son orientation serait principalement psycho-gériatrique. Les "clients" de ces établissements sont des malades au sens strict du terme, qui réclament un personnel et un équipement hospitalier capables d'assurer un large éventail de soins.

Le Centre de jour serait davantage axé sur les aspects psycho-sociaux. Comme le dit le Dr Balier (1978), qui en fut l'initiateur dans le 13ème arrondissement à Paris, il constitue une "unité thérapeutique de quartier, complémentaire des soins dispensés par les médecins traitants. Il prend en charge dans la journée des personnes âgées souffrant de maladies diverses qui, de plus, cumulent des difficultés d'ordre psychologique et social. Outre une surveillance de la santé, le centre de jour offre des thérapeutiques à base de techniques de rééducation et de réadaptation. Organisées dans le cadre d'une vie collective, elles permettent de réintégrer les personnes âgées dans la vie du quartier et de retrouver un rôle et une existence sociale". En fait, il semble qu'une certaine confusion ait toujours régné et que la distinction entre les deux types d'établissements, hôpital et centre de jour, soit plus théorique que réelle. Elle peut cependant avoir son importance, dans la mesure où, comme en France, des administrations différentes (Ministère de la Santé pour l'un, des Affaires Sociales pour l'autre, par exemple) en assureraient la gestion, avec les problèmes de coordination qui peuvent en résulter.

D'autres formes d'hébergement temporaire existent : les Hôpitaux de nuit dans divers pays, les "Nursing Day Homes" au Danemark, sortes d'annexes aux maisons de soins, qui assurent les traitements aux malades regagnant leur domicile le soir. Dans les pays où le volontariat est florissant, on peut voir des bénévoles mais aussi des familles participer régulièrement aux activités thérapeutiques (cf expériences de Aarhus, Danemark).

Pourquoi ces formules, si dynamiques dans certains pays, semblent-elles échouer dans d'autres ? La revue française Gérontologie et Société consacrait en 1978 un cahier entier au thème : les Centres de jour en question. Un certain nombre d'hypothèses ont été avancées : absence de cohésion entre services sociaux et services de santé, lourdeur des procédures administratives de fonctionnement, manque d'information de la population, insuffisance de collaboration des médecins généralistes qui craignent la concurrence, décalage entre les objectifs idéalistes de l'équipe et la réalité sociale. Il existe cependant des expériences réussies, comme à Grenoble et à Montargis, par exemple. Il serait instructif de pouvoir analyser les raisons de leur succès.

D'autres solutions originales sont proposées dans les pays scandinaves et anglo-saxons, une fois de plus pionniers en la matière : prises en charge pour le week-end, pour les vacances, lors de situations de crise, non seulement dans des institutions mais aussi chez des personnes privées qualifiées (voir à ce sujet le Liverpool Personal Service Society). Le fait de pouvoir à tout moment disposer d'un lieu de séjour provisoire est une puissante incitation à garder des parents séniles dans leur foyer.

Le support psychologique aux familles, dont le fardeau moral est bien plus lourd que la charge physique, connaît un développement rapide un peu partout en Europe et en Amérique du Nord. Des programmes de soutien sont offerts soit par les municipalités, soit par des volontaires : psychothérapie individuelle et de groupe pour libérer la tension et déculpabiliser les proches épuisés, information et éducation afin de mieux faire face aux manifestations de la maladie, groupes d'entraide et d'auto-assistance, bénévoles servant de "Granny sitters" momentanées. Signalons l'existence, aux U.S.A., d'une organisation nationale, l'Alzheimer's Disease and Related Disorders Association (ADRDA) qui a pour objectifs de réunir les familles affectées par la maladie, de promouvoir des programmes de support et de conseil mutuels et d'encourager la recherche.

Notre tour d'horizon est loin d'être complet. En cheminant ainsi à travers le dédale des réalisations, nous avons rencontré des formules heureuses et des lacunes évidentes. Pouvons-nous conclure que certains types de politique (par exemple, sectorisation de la gériatrie, regroupement sous une même direction des structures sanitaires et sociales) seraient de nature à favoriser les unes et à éliminer les autres ? Il ne semble pas qu'on puisse proposer un modèle idéal pour tous les pays mais il apparaît que certains impératifs doivent être respectés si l'on veut réaliser une organisation valable au niveau de la démence sénile :

- considérer le vieillard non comme individu isolé mais comme membre d'un groupe familial et social
- refuser toute législation qui défavoriserait financièrement les familles assurant le maintien à domicile
- promouvoir une collaboration pluridisciplinaire
- améliorer l'information et la formation des médecins et du personnel paramédical
- favoriser le développement des solutions originales en leur donnant le temps et les moyens de faire la preuve de leur efficacité.

Cependant, quelle que soit la politique choisie, elle ne répondra au problème de la démence sénile que si elle est réalisée dans la souplesse et animée par des personnes créatives et motivées.

Aronson MK, Liokowitz R (1981). Senile dementia, Alzheimer's type : the family and the health care delivery system. J Am Geriatr Soc 29:568-571.
Attias-Donfut Cl (1981). Vie et mort des Centres de jour. INSERM 101:265-274.
Balier C (1978). Définition des Centres de jour. Gérontologie et Société 7:8-16.
Brody EM (1981). Health and its social implications. In Aging : a challenge to science and society (Gilmore AJJ, Svonborg A, Marois M, Beatties WM, Piotrowski J eds) Oxford University Press 2:189-201.
Butler RN (1977-78). Public interest report # 24 : Nursing home care : an impossible situation unless.. Int J Aging and Human Develop 8:291-294.
Jandrot-Louka F, Louka JM (1979). Hospice et Psychiatrie : un mariage d'oraison. Gérontologie et Société 11:28-57.
Keet J (1979). L'hôpital de jour gériatrique en Grande Bretagne. Gérontologie et Société 9:89-98.
Müller Ch, Wertheimer J (1981). Psychogériatrie. Masson SA, Fribourg et Paris.
Rapport du groupe "Prospective Personnes Agées" (1980). Vieillir demain. La Documentation Française, Paris.
Secrétariat d'Etat chargé des Personnes Agées (1982). Tarification et fonctionnement des établissements pour personnes âgées. Ministère des Affaires Sociales et de

la Solidarité Nationale, Paris.
World Health Organization (1982). Epidemiological studies on social and medical conditions of the elderly. Regional office for Europe, WHO, Copenhagen.

Senile Dementia: Outlook for the Future, pages 201–209

DEMENTIA: IMPLICATIONS FOR SERVICES

Tom Arie, M.A., F.R.C.Psych., F.F.C.M., F.R.C.P.

Professor of Health Care of the Elderly
University of Nottingham; Sherwood Hospital,
Hucknall Road, Nottingham NG5 1PD, U.K.

Dementia in old age seems likely to be among the central issues for health services in developed countries during the working lifetimes of all present members of the health professions - and one might add, of all present members of governments. I propose briefly to consider its implications under five headings:

1. Need for long term care and for acute intervention
2. Pressure for institutional solutions
3. "The Staff Factor"
4. Organisation and Style of Services
5. Education

Dementia alone of all diagnoses - and I use it in the sense of a single condition for convenience here - is without question the greatest consumer of health resources. The reason for this is not difficult to understand, but it may be worth spelling out. Its characteristics are such that it generates both need for constant surveillance, and, at the same time, it generates crises. Therein lies my first point: dementia is often acknowledged as the supreme consumer of long term care and so indeed it is; but it impinges on health and social services at almost every point also by creating need for acute interventions. Let me elaborate a little.

Dementia reduces the individual to a condition approaching that of a small infant. The demented, along with the young and immature, lack the capacity for self care which derives from judgement and insight. They are, in greater or lesser measure, unable to minister to everyday changing needs, to avoid common dangers, to learn dependably from mistakes, to avoid causing distress to other people, and above all to monitor their own needs; that they may lack control of elimination and other bodily functions is a further similarity.

This means that between planned contacts with other people they cannot be relied upon to summon intercalated care when need arises - a crucial difference between the demented and those who are severely physically disabled. The demented, further, like small infants, are not only without the capacity to avoid common dangers, but they actually bring disasters on themselves - by wandering in front of passing cars, or by the trite hazard of gas taps left on - in the case of the infant through playing with them, in the case of the dement through forgetting to turn them off.

Not only are demented people prone to cause crises due to deficient surveillance, but they are specially susceptible to crises due to acute exacerbations of unwanted behaviour, most often due to acute or subacute confusional states precipitated by relatively minor physical disturbances.

Finally, crises arise from sudden breakdown of the balance between disability and tolerance, due to changes in either or both, or to external factors.

In many of our countries the law punishes those who leave small children unattended; whereas current practice applauds attempts to maintain even the otherwise unattended dement alone at home. There is scope therefore for scrutiny of some of the assumptions underlying our current philosophies of "community care" (Hawks 1975). It is important when doing so to disentangle the various interests which we pursue when making decisions - the interests of the old people; the interests of their carers and neighbours; and the interests of services themselves - the three often pointing in contrary directions, and it is as well for us to be clear which direction we are pursuing in each component of the policies which we propound.

Let me briefly demonstrate by analogy the extent of the dependence of the demented by contrast with what might be regarded as a vastly more disabled group. Consider a person totally paralysed by virtue of poliomyelitis - his motor activity confined, say, to the ability to blink the eyelids. He subsists in a respirator - many I believe are still in this condition in Britain.

One could scarcely be more disabled; and yet such a person is more capable of being left unattended for extended periods than is an even moderately demented old person. A neighbour or nurse can attend to his needs at intervals, and this *episodic* care is possible because with simple technology, and with the crucial fact that intelligence is intact, he can summon intercalated help if difficulty arises between intermittent episodes of care. For instance, by blinking his eyelids he can cause a bell to ring in some place where contingency help is located. This is the very thing that the demented cannot do - namely, *to act as their own monitor*. It is not surprising therefore that demented people are such huge consumers of the most expensive commodity which the state has to offer in any setting - around-the-clock care.

A study in Newcastle gave some empirical support to this view (Bergmann et al 1978). Here demented people were followed up after intensive domiciliary and day hospital support had been sustained throughout a year. At the year's end only one fifth of demented people living alone were still in their homes - the rest had either been institutionalised, or had died; for those living with families the figure was just under one half still at home; whilst those living with only an aged spouse had an intermediate outcome. Although these were not rigorously matched groups followed prospectively, yet the implication is clear: the outlook for even the well supported solo dement at home is poor; whilst support for families may go much further. It may be that conventional priorities in the disbursal of scarce resources for home support should be reconsidered, and that solo dements, so far from being given intensive support at home, should be fairly readily moved to settings where they receive the care they need, when their disabilities are great; for attempts to support them with scarce resources may be no more than the fruitless sending of good money after bad.

"THE QUIET EPIDEMIC"

A leading article in the British Medical Journal (BMJ 1978) coined this excellent phrase, which is apposite in more senses that one. The sense in which the British Medical Journal used it was both as an undramatic condition quietly pressing upon society and upon individual families, but also as an epidemic so vast that it is often even unnoticed. By the same token, it is the diagnosis most commonly omitted from our record systems. Thus the demented old lady is admitted to hospital with a fractured femur but appears in hospital records as "fracture of the proximal femur" - with no mention of the dementia which was the underlying cause of her fall; similarly the terminal dement admitted with bronchopneumonia features as "bronchopneumonia", again without reference to dementia on the discharge sheet or the official diagnositic record. It is a case of the Emperor's Clothes - no-one mentions the obvious.

Therefore it is difficult to measure precisely the cost of dementia to services. By way of example, an important article by the then Chief Scientist to our Department (or Ministry) of Health a few years ago attempted to estimate the burden on the health service of individual conditions; dementia was not even one of those on the list (Black, Pole 1975).

Yet it is possible to put together some approximate estimate of the cost of dementia in cash, though I will spare this audience the arithmetic. Emily Grundy and I (Grundy, Arie 1983) recently attempted such a review of "Resources for Dementia" and we noted that in 1979 the cost of dementia in the United States had been estimated at 12 billion dollars, whilst in England expenditure on health and social services alone had in the same year been estimated at £300 million. Such figures omit both the extra income support involved, the direct cost borne by families, and the "opportunity costs" which are borne chiefly by the traditional army of female carers at home (an army unlikely to continue always to be willing to be mobilised on the scale that has so long been taken for granted). Such costing omits the uncostable accounting of emotional, marital, and physical burden on families.

GROWING EXPECTATIONS

These costs are compounded by growing pressure in modern societies for institutional solutions to the care of the elderly. With successive censuses in my country the institutionalisation rates of the very aged (over-80s) have been increasing dramatically (Grimley Evans 1977). The growth in the number of over-80s would in itself be expected to increase the *number* of very aged people in institutions, but the increasing age-related institutionalisation rates must be due to factors other than mere increase in numbers.

The main explanation is likely to be the general increase of expectations in our society. These derive from higher standards everywhere, and along with them higher expectations of well-being and of relief from the burdens of caring for the elderly; and specifically relief from *direct* responsibility for the unremittent care of very dependant old people. The fact that women, the prime care givers throughout the centuries, are no longer so available for direct personal care, both because their life horizons have broadened, and because they are more likely to be out at work, is another factor. In short, a *second* major consequence of dementia for health services is in the dramatic increase in the rate and number of demented old people for whom institutional solutions to their care are being sought; and the same high expectations demand much higher quality of material and personal care in these institutional settings than has previously been the rule; indeed shabby care followed from deliberate policies based on the principle of "less eligibility" which was long a feature of social policy, as well as from neglect. Preoccupation with quality and appropriateness of care in institutions is likely to exercise planners - and the public - for the rest of this century, as it is indeed already doing (Jolley 1981).

THE STAFF FACTOR

A *third* major implication is the growing need, in a

society with generally higher expectations of job and life satisfaction, for growing numbers of people to be involved in the "care industry" - in the business of giving direct personal care to the demented in non-domiciliary settings. The issues of job satisfaction, of status, and of the esteem in which this work is held are ones that are going to preoccupy societies such as ours for the next few decades. Research on the sources of job satisfaction, and the factors that enhance it and make for high staff morale in these settings is still in its infancy, though clearly it is of the profoundest consequence. So far in the planning of services the "staff factor" (Arie 1977) has been much neglected.

THE ORGANISATION OF SERVICES

This has become a major area of study and it is not possible to review it in a few minutes; it is my fourth theme, and it subsumes the others. It is probably the most prolific field of writing on the subject of dementia in Britain at the moment - exceeding even the happily great volume of publications on the biological aspects. The development of a new specialty of geriatric psychiatry in recent years, documented in a recent survey from my department (Wattis, Wattis, Arie 1981), is only one factor in this process. The codification of the basic elements of services is now well established - acute admitting units in hospitals, longer stay and rehabilitation units, day hospitals, and the whole apparatus of outreach and support services for people at home, and for those who care for them.

Similarly recognised (though much less often implemented) is the crucial function of early detection and intervention - of case-finding, and of surveillance of those in trouble or at risk (Williamson 1981).

But what has been much less discussed is the "style" of services - those characteristics of services, over and above minimally adequate levels of provision, which determine whether services actually work (Arie, Jolley 1982). This concerns the ways in which professional skill and resources may be most productive in enhancing the will and capacity to cope on the part of non-professional agencies and of the main carers themselves -

the family. The exercise is one of building confidence and elsewhere I have discussed in some detail the _modus operandi_ which seems most likely to give such confidence.

In this exercise of confidence building, it is important to remember that there are at least three main "constituencies" to be satisfied - the public on the one hand; colleagues in associated professions on the other (and not least fellow physicians); and finally to the staff of one's own service. The fact that the expectations of one's service differ between the three groups - indeed often point in contrary directions - makes this a particularly delicate and tricky business. Promptness of intervention, willingness to respond on the terms of urgency declared by those who call for help rather than on the objective merits of the case, readiness to take the service to people's homes, readiness to use one's staff, and indeed oneself, in an undefensive and unhierarchical way - these are a few of the tactics that I have in mind.

The post-war period in particular has seen the growth of geriatric medicine and of developments in psychiatry, both institutional and extramural. These movements have defined the types of resources and the types of staff we need - and they have established the principle of teamwork both within a service, and between services. But now we need to move further and look in detail at the style in which the service is deployed, to the end that it gives maximum confidence to those involved with it. For this is our best bet for diminishing the inexhaustible demand for help, and for containing the bulk of the problem within the framework of the family and the neighbourhood rather than encouraging vain fantasies of transposing it wholly to institutional settings. And we must never forget that about 30 per cent of the very aged have no family.

The _last_ consequence of dementia for services to which I wish to draw attention, is in the field of education. Education certainly of the public itself; but I am concerned here particularly with education of professional staff. The care of the very aged has featured too little, and still does, in the education of the professions most concerned with dementia. Major redeployment of emphasis within curricula is essential if these are to match the novel commonplaceness of extreme old age among the concerns of the health professions.

May I end my talk with a brief account of our teaching department in Nottingham, where we have two unusual things; first, a joint department of physicians and psychiatrists working together; and second, an intensive contribution to medical student education in the form of a month's full-time attachment to our department for all students. This is a standard part of the curriculum in Nottingham, and (as I can happily quote from a recent statement by the Medical School to our University Grants Committee) the course "has proved extremely successful and is highly valued by students".

Our course is aimed specifically at the problems of the very aged: dementia receives great emphasis, both in its biological and its social aspects, and most particularly in its impact on services and the way in which services can respond. Most importantly, the students are involved in an apprenticeship to all aspects of our work, which is non-selective and based on care for all old people with the whole range of medical and psychiatric disorders in a defined community. A formal programme of teaching, and the execution on the part of each student of a project in this field under the supervision of a staff member, complements the more traditional apprenticeship to our clinical services.

The most important part of society's response, and that of services, to the Everest of a problem that is dementia, lies in education: therein lies the seedcorn for the future and therein are our best hopes of reordering political priorities and personal attitudes, and thus of providing better formal and informal services. With more investment of money and talent we should be able to capitalise on the present glimmerings of hope that we shall in our time make progress with effective treatments, and even prevention, of the Alzheimer and other common dementias; but at present it is wisest in my view not to bank on that. Better services remain our best bet.

REFERENCES

Much of the material in this talk was originally explored in my Fotheringham Lectures at the University of Toronto, which are still to be published.

Arie T (1977). In Exton-Smith N, Grimley Evans J (eds): "Care of the Elderly: Meeting the Challenge of Dependency". London: Academic Press, New York: Grune & Stratton.
Arie T, Jolley D (1983). In Levy R, Post F (eds): "Psychiatry of Late Life". Oxford: Blackwells.
Bergmann K, Foster EM, Justice AW et al (1978). Management of the Demented Elderly Patient in the Community. British Journal of Psychiatry 132:441.
Black DAK, Pole JD (1975). Priorities in Biomedical Research: Indices of Burden. British Journal of Preventive and Social Medicine 29:222.
British Medical Journal (1978). "The Quiet Epidemic". Leading Article 1:1.
Grimley Evans J (1977). In Exton-Smith N, Grimley Evans J (eds): "Care of the Elderly: Meeting the Challenge of Dependency". London: Academic Press, New York: Grune & Stratton.
Grundy E, Arie T (1983). Resources for Dementia. In Exton-Smith AN, Weksler M (eds): "Practical Geriatric Medicine". London: Churchill Livingstone. In the Press.
Hawks D (1975). Community Care: An Analysis of Assumptions. British Journal of Psychiatry 127:276.
Jolley DJ (1981). In Arie T (ed): "Health Care of the Elderly". London: Croom Helm; Baltimore: Johns Hopkins Press.
Wattis J, Wattis L, Arie T (1981). Psychogeriatrics: a national survey of a new branch of psychiatry. British Medical Journal 282:1529.
Williamson J (1981). In Arie T (ed): "Health Care of the Elderly". London: Croom Helm; Baltimore: Johns Hopkins Press.

Senile Dementia: Outlook for the Future, pages 211–217

RESPONSIBILITY FOR CARE OF VICTIMS OF SENILE DEMENTIA IN A SECTORIAL STRUCTURE OF PSYCHOGERIATRICS

Pierre Schwed

Médecin Directeur-adjoint
Hôpital psycho-gériatrique
Prilly, 1008 - Suisse

Switzerland is a confederation of 27 cantons and half-cantons. While the Federal Government is in charge of such matters as foreign affairs and national defense, the cantons have a primary responsibility for educational, religious, social and of special interest to us here, health organizations.

This system is advantageous in that it provides local solutions for public health problems, especially in the field of gerontology. In this paper accordingly, we shall deal with solutions in the canton of Vaud, which are different from those in other cantons not only political terms but also for geographical and economic reasons.

In 1980, the resident population of Vaud totaled 528'747 persons, of whom 15% were over the age of 65 years and 3,1% over the age of 80.

Psychogeriatric developed in a framework of psychiatric sectors based on the location of the hospitals in the canton. There are four such sectors : the Centre (250'000 inhabitants) which is responsible for the Lausanne area and also for a mountainous region near the French border, and the three other sectors, designated as West, North and East, each with a population of about 80'000. Psychogeriatric cases are assigned to adult and child psychiatric teams in the hospitals and consultation centres in the East and North sectors. In the

Centre sector, which includes university services, adult psychiatry, child psychiatry and psychogeriatrics are totally indepedent from one another, both administratively and medically. In the West sector, between Lausanne and Geneva, both hospitalization and outpatient care of aged patients are under the charge of one or the other of two organisms: an adult psychiatry team and a psychogeriatric hospital connected with the university psychogeriatric service, which itself is located in the Centre sector.

The history of the Lausanne University Psychogeriatric Service is as follows :

The Prilly Psychogeriatric Hospital was inaugurated in 1963 as an element in the University Psychiatric Clinic of Cery. Its responsibility at that time was to meet the needs of the whole canton. Very soon, it became impossible to accomplish this. An outpatient centre had to be created, to work in close cooperation with the hospital and avoid unnecessary admissions by providing home care or consultations. The centre also had to plan for the discharging of patients, by providing for sustained extramural care. The Lausanne Psychogeriatric Centre (CPG) was established in 1968, It then became necessary to provide for intermediate structures, day hospitals, working in the same spirit of giving more effective service to the community, upstream and downstream from the Psychogeriatric Hospital. The first of these day hospitals has been operating since 1973 at the Prilly Hospital, the second since 1974 as an annex to the CPG in the city. Finally, in order to increase the availability of beds for the Service, the vaudois authorities in 1977 assigned to it responsability for a psychogeriatric hospital 30 kilometers from Lausanne at Gimel, in the West sector, resulting in the first supra-sectorial psychiatric organization in the canton. In the course of this long process of structuration, psychogeriatrics became autonomous.

First, there was a separation of the medical direction, which had been provided up to 1972 by the University Psychiatric Clinic. In 1979, there was an administrative separation vis-à-vis the same clinic. Finally, in 1980, the Psychogeriatric Service became a part of the University.

Since that time, the structure of the University Psychogeriatric Service has been as follows :
Under the authority of the Director, there are:

1. The Prilly Psychogeriatric Hospital, together with a day hospital.
2. The Gimel Psychogeriatric Hospital, with a team of extra-hospital consultants
3. The Lausanne outpatient psychogeriatric centre, together with a day hospital.

These institutions work in such close cooperation that transfers of responsibility for cases can be made without red tape.

The Prilly and Gimel hospitals have, respectively, 154 and 150 beds. Their responsibility is to take in all patients over the age of 65 who are in a situation of psychiatric crisis and also younger patients suffering from presenile dementia.

These patients may either come from home, from a medico-social institution or by transfer from a general hospital. Admission may be at the request of the patient's own doctor, of a doctor representing the administrative authorities in the case of a contested admission or on the advice of the outpatient team of the Psychogeriatric Centre. Departure may be either a return to the patient's home, placement in a specialized institution, in rare cases transfer to a general hospital, or the death of the patient.

What is the sequence of events in this structure for taking charge of a patient with senile dementia ?

The Psychogeriatric Centre is often the first to be notified in the event of a deterioration in the situation in the patient's home, in a medico-social institution and more rarely in a general hospital. It may be called either by the family, by a private doctor or by a social service. A multidisciplinary team, the composition of which varies according to the needs, which are briefly described by telephone, evaluates the situation it finds and makes an initial decision: to leave the patient at home, to hospitalize him in a specialized service or to place him directly in a medico-social institution.

In 1981, a total of 297 cases were examined by the CPG team. An analysis was made of the new patients taken in charge during the first 6 months of that year, 155 in all, of whom 41 (26,5%) suffered from more or less serious degenerative psycho-organic syndromes.

The analysis showed that 68% of the calls came from the patients homes, but with the doctors (51%) making the calls more often than the families (12%). The CPG was also called upon very often simply for advice by general hospitals (7%) and medico-social institutions (19,5%).

What becomes of the patients after the Centre intervenes ?

With respect to patients seen at home, it was found that half of them could remain there for various periods, up to a maximum of 12 months, depending on the method of evaluation. Hospitalization (25%) or placement in a medico-social establishment (18%) took place after a stay at home of one or two months, often because of lack of space, and the delay might be as long as three months for the medico-social establishments. Keeping patients in serious condition at home necessarily calls for a substantial organization to take charge of support and care.

Among the 41 serious cases for which the CPG assumed responsibility, 8 came from medico-social establishments. Thanks to supervision by the CPG,

4 of them could remain in these places, an indication of the stabilizing effect of the Centre.

What assessment can we make of the results of the work of the psychogeriatric hospital and its effects on the condition of patients suffering from a more or less severe psycho-organic syndrome?

The objectives of the hospital are to make a precise diagnosis, to evaluate the general functional conditions of the patient and attempt rehabilitation on the basis of residual capacities. The measures taken are medical, physiotherapeutic, ergotherapeutic and occupational. The specific responsibilities assigned to the nursing personnel play a very important role in certain agitational states and in resocializing the patients.

In 1981, there were 364 admissions to the psychogeriatric hospital, including every type of cases. In the same year, there were 304 discharges, 122 of which were of patients with more or less advanced senile dementia. If we compare cases of senile dementia with the population of patients hospitalized for other psychiatric conditions, we find, considering both the diagnosis and prognosis, that the mortality rate is four times higher among the dements and the probability of going back home four times lower. The frequency of placements (about 40%), however, is equal for both groups. Among the dements, nevertheless, there was a small group of patients who could return to their homes (11%).

It seemed interesting to consider what particular factors might explain why such a patient could be sent home or placed in an institution. For this reason, we analyzed 62 of the 71 files of patients who left our services (14 men and 48 women suffering from degenerative or mixed psycho-organic syndromes).

Ten patients (16%) returned to their homes. What were the reasons ?

Two of them were discharged from the hospital on the request of their families, against medical advice. In one of these cases, there was no catamnesis. In the other case, it was possible to maintain the patient at home for 6 months, after which rehospitalization was necessary due to cerebral vascular accidents. The evolution in the service was favorable enough so that 8 patients, including a couple, could be followed at home, due to help employed by the family and assistance by various social services and the CPG. Of these 8, 2 were rehospitalized after 3 months.

It is quite clear that the cases which are least deteriorated and in the best physical condition are the ones which can best be maintained at home.

The reasons for transfer of 4 cases (6%) to another hospital were fractures of the neck of the femur in 3 instances. The largest group of patients were those placed in medico-social institutions (77%).

Of the 40 patients hospitalized from their homes, 29 were later placed in such institutions (72%). In many of these cases, hospitalization had been due to agitation, hostile behavior or anxiety. The multi-disciplinary care provided in the hospital often improved or stabilized the condition of the patients, but the remaining deficits were such that placements were necessary. Such placement is a delicate matter, requiring great attention by the social service to make sure that the patient is placed in an environment suited to him.

It is interesting to note that 20 patients were admitted to the psychogeriatric hospital from medico-social institutions in a state of psychic and sometimes physical decompensation. Of these 20, none could return to their homes. Two had to be transferred to a general hospital because of falls. The other 18 could be sent back to medico-social estalishments; 6 of them to the one they had come from and 12 to different ones. In general, these latter cases were too deteriorated to be handled in the initial institutions. It should be emphasized that the average age of the patients in the latter group was 81,5 years and of the 10 who could go back home 81,2 years.

In conclusion, we find that hospitalization in a psychogeriatric institution is not a final step. It is often possible to send senile dements to a less hospitalized environment, if there is continuity in care and supervision, provided by a hospital and extra-hospital system which is flexible and adaptable.

The sectorial organization makes possible such solutions, which have the advantage of being well suited to the handling of local psychogeriatric problems.

REFERENCES

Les consultants du centre ambulatoire de psychogériatrie de Lausanne 1968-1971. Etude de l'Office de statistique et de l'hôpital psycho-gériatrique. Office de statistique de l'Etat de Vaud. Septembre 1974.

Wertheimer J, Le-Dinh T. Organisation sectorielle psychogériatrique: Le Service universitaire de psycho-gériatrie de Lausanne. Colloque international de Limoges (France). Octobre 1982 (à paraître).

VI. CLINICAL ASPECTS OF ALZHEIMER'S DISEASE: PART ONE

Presided by R.N. Butler (New York)

Senile Dementia: Outlook for the Future, pages 221–237

RISK FACTORS IN LATE LIFE DEMENTIA[1]

Donna Cohen, Ph.D.
Carl Eisdorfer, Ph.D., M.D.

Montefiore Medical Center
111 East 210 Street
Bronx, NY 10467

INTRODUCTION

Alzheimer's disease and related disorders have been referred to as the "silent epidemic of the next century" and, indeed, their prevalence makes them one of the most serious public health problems we face throughout the world. Our present knowledge about the etiology, pathogenesis, treatment, and prevention of Alzheimer's disease and related disorders remains limited and only now that we are sensitized to the increasing prevalence of the disorder(s) have we begun to agressively pursue research into etiology and prevention. In our attempt to understand the cause(s) of Alzheimers type of dementia, risk factor analysis becomes a powerful strategy.

How should we proceed in the light of so little data? First, we should be wary of the fallacy of the concept of a purely age-related risk for any disease. The United States Surgeon General's Report on Healthy People (1979) reported that many young children have elevated cholesterol and high blood pressure, two of the risk factors for stroke in later life. Thus, age per se is hardly the only cause of stroke and vascular disease in persons who are vulnerable.

[1]The authors gratefully acknowledge the help of the Potamkin Prize Fund and the Morrell Foundation in support of the work cited in this report.

Second, we should take advantage of the large body of work on measuring risks that has gone on before. Therefore, the first part of this paper will briefly introduce the reader to several statistical concepts of risk. The second section will review our current knowledge about specific risk factors in stroke and multi-infarct dementias in the aged. The third part will examine the available evidence for risk factors for dementias of the Alzheimer type. The latest data from our laboratory will be presented. The final section will briefly describe several promising research designs which may be used to determine whether an antecedent condition increases the risk for Alzheimer's disease or a related disorder.

THE STATISTICAL CONCEPTS OF RISK: DEFINITIONS OF THE DATA WE WANT

Estimation of the risk for disease in persons with different characteristics and past experiences is a statistical area where models are undergoing significant change. Gruenberg (1980) proposed at least five statistical models which may be useful to consider for the measurement of risk: Individual risk, contingency risks, relative risks, attributable risks and lifetime risks. Each of these concepts provide different approaches to understand the data we need to accurately define risks for developing the dementias of later life.

Individual Risk: The concept of individual risk refers to the probability that a single individual is likely to experience a specific event or succumb to a specific illness or disease. One example is the well established fact that the risk of women having a child with Down's syndrome rises exponentially with advancing maternal age (Collman, Stoller 1962). Another example is the probability of surviving without dementia, estimated by Sluss (1980) as follows:

Years	Probability
60	1.00
70	0.97
75	0.93
80	0.83
85	0.71

This way of presenting the probabilities clearly identifies the importance of advancing age as a predictor for dementing disorders. Therefore, the age variable must be taken into account in the search for other risk factors. One strategy to control for chronological age when trying to examine the relative contribution of another risk factor is to divide a cohort of individuals into two groups and follow them over time to determine whether the risk for one group with a suspected risk factor, e.g., a gene marker, is higher than the other group. This example is important because it highlights another confounding variable in risk factor research, i.e., death. Death introduces an ascertainment bias resulting from the early mortality of gene carriers who might otherwise display a dementia in later life.

Contingency Risks: The model of contingency risk allows us to estimate the probability of an event or disease which is contingent upon the presence of one or more conditions. One example to illustrate contingency risk is the increased likelihood of a person with a previous psychiatric hospitalization being rehospitalized in the future compared to an individual without such a history (Table 1).

How might this model be applied in the study of Alzheimer's disease and related disorders? Contingency risks would be useful for insurance companies to calculate premiums which could be applied to insurance policies for health problems such as Alzheimer's disease or long-term care in general. Hypothetically, if exogenously-incorporated Alzheimer's disease were a factor, an individual living in an aluminum-rich area of the country who also has a parent diagnosed with Alzheimer's disease may have a higher risk for Alzheimer's compared to a person with the same genetic history but not living in an aluminum-rich area. Furthermore, an unmarried, childless individual with a familial history of Alzheimer's disease may have a higher risk for institutionalization compared to another individual with a comparable genetic history but married with a living spouse and five adult children.

Relative Risk: Relative risk is defined as the incidence of disease in an exposed population divided by the incidence of disease in an unexposed group. Cornfield (1951) first defined relative risk as an odds ratio (the cross-products of ac/bd in Table 1). A simple application of the relative risk model is the attempt to understand the

	WITH CONDITION E.G., STRESS	WITHOUT CONDITION E.G., NO STRESS
RISK FACTOR PRESENT E.G., PREVIOUS HOSPITALIZATION	A	B
RISK FACTOR ABSENT E.G., NO PREVIOUS HOSPITALIZATION	C	D

Table 1. A four-way contingency risk table. The probability that a person under stress and a prior psychiatric hospitalization will be rehospitalized (A) is higher than that of another person matched for all other characteristics except previous psychiatric hospitalization (C).

health consequences of cigarette smoking. It is important to emphasize that the relative risk model can only be useful when the data collection methods provide representative samples of diseased and nondiseased persons. The relative risk model could be used to measure the degree to which risk factors such as hypertension or arrhythmias increase the probability of a disease outcome such as multi-infarct dementia.

Attributable Risk: The concept of attributable risk evolved because the relative risk model leaves an important question unresolved. Using the example of smoking-related risks, the question is, "If everyone stopped smoking, what change would there be in the occurrence of lung cancer deaths?" This model will be particularly useful in the study of preventative trials such as antihypertensives for multi-infarct dementias.

Lifetime Risk: The lifetime risk model has been particularly valuable in psychiatric research. Calculating the lifetime expectancy of a disease condition developed from a need to estimate risk in families where a genetic component to a disease was suspected. A great deal of information was needed about those persons who were alive and dead to calculate the risk that a first-degree family member would develop a disease. The mathematical result was the Hardy-Weinberg formula.

Our knowledge about lifetime risks for the major disorders is improving. Myrna Weissman and her colleagues (1978) have estimated that the lifetime risk for major depressive disorders is 26 percent. Sluss' (1980) data suggest that the lifetime risk for the nonreversible dementias is 29 percent. Prospective studies are needed to clarify whether there are differential lifetime risks for the various dementing disorders of later life.

In summary, there are many theoretical paradigms to identify what data are needed to accurately and reliably establish the validity of a risk factor. Unfortunately, the data we want are not the data we have, as is summarized in the next section.

RISK FACTORS FOR MULTI-INFARCT DEMENTIAS

Multiple strokes appear to have a primary etiological role in 15 - 25 percent of persons with nonreversible dementias and a synergistic role in conjunction with Alzheimer's dementia in another 10 percent. Multi-infarct dementias refer to disorders in which the cognitive impairment and personality changes are the result of brain tissue destruction due to multiple small infarcts, and not the result of a chronic ischemic state due to changes in the large blood vessels of the brain.

Although there is considerable information about risk factors in patients with strokes, the risk factors for multi-infarct or lacuner state dementias are not known. It is possible that the risk factors for multiple infarcts may be the same as those for a single major stroke, but they do not necessarily have to be identical. At the moment, our best information on risk factors in stroke is derived from the Framingham study where the subject population has been studied for more than thirty years. The risk factors for cerebrovascular disorders are hypertension, impaired cardiac functioning (e.g., coronary heart disease, arrhythmias, congestive heart failure), diabetes, high normal hemoglobin values, elevated serum cholesterol, and cigarette smoking (Kannel 1971; Kannel et al. 1972; Dawber et al. 1977; Wolf et al. 1977, 1978). The risk for stroke appears to increase with the number of abnormalities present in an individual.

Individuals with hypertension develop approximately seven times as much cerebrovascular disease as normotensives. The presence of cardiac impairments also increase risk independent of hypertension. Three out of four patients with cerebrovascular diseases have one or more cardiac impairments. A study by Librach, et al. (1977) demonstrated that in persons without heart disease, hypertension increased the annual rate of stroke from 3.8 to 11.5/1000 persons, whereas in normotensive individuals with heart disease, the annual rate of stroke was 26/1000 persons. Friedman, et al. (1968) matched his subjects for blood pressure, and still found that cardiac disease was a potent predictor of stroke. The presence of atrial fibrillation resulted in a six-fold increased risk.

Cardiac arrhythmia may be an important risk factor for multi-infarct dementia (Abdon 1977), although it is possible that arrhythmias are secondary to cerebrovascular disease (Schwartz et al. 1978). Arrhythmias are common in the aged, but unless there is serious symptomatology, they are usually not treated. If there is a relationship between arrhythmias and the occurrence of multi-infarct dementias, the use of pacemakers and other interventions may be appropriate.

In the Framingham study, persons with high normal hemoglobin values developed twice as much cerebrovascular disease (Kannel et al. 1972). Diabetic individuals had a two to three fold increased risk (Wolf et al. 1978). Obesity appeared to increase the risk for stroke only slightly (Kannel 1971). The risk for male smokers was significant in those persons who also had hypertension and diabetes. No relationship was observed between smoking and stroke in women.

Clearly, a great deal could be learned about risk factors for multi-infarct dementia by a prospective study of older persons. The potential risk factors could be measured by a thorough physical examination which included the following tests: resting electrocardiogram, 24 hour Holter monitoring, serum lipids, serum renin, urinary sodium, hemoglobin, fasting blood sugar, chest roetgenogram, and blood pressure determinations.

RISK FACTORS FOR DEMENTIAS OF THE ALZHEIMER TYPE

The risk factors for dementias of the Alzheimer's type are substantially less well understood than even those for multi-infarct dementias. At the moment, family history appears to be the best documented risk factor. The probability of manifesting the familial form of the disease may be analyzed in two ways: (1) the probability of carrying the gene; and (2) the probability of the gene showing penetrance (Sinex, Myers 1982). If we assume an autosomal dominant mode of transmission in a first-degree relative of the Alzheimer patient, the probability of carrying the gene is 0.50. The probability of the gene showing penetrance is a function of age, other risk factors, as well as accurate diagnosis.

Heston, Mastri, Anderson, and White (1981) have confirmed the work of Larsson, Sjogren, and Jacobsen (1963) who estimated that approximately 12 percent of the population carry the "Alzheimer gene." In the early onset form of the disease (pre age 65), half of the children of an affected parent and half of all siblings should have the disease. With later onset this probability should decrease unless nongenetic factors are important.

The limited epidemiologic data suggest that sporatic Alzheimer's dementias are more common than the familial Alzheimer's dementia, and here we have no conclusive evidence for any risk factors. Only advancing age appears to have some predictive value. The risk for the dementing disorders of later life appears to increase at least through age 80 or 85. There may be some heuristic value to study the contribution of genetic and nongenetic factors in Alzheimer dementia by evaluating the characteristics of patients in three groups classified by age of onset: onset prior to age 65, onset between 65 - 80, and onset after 80 (Table 2).

Recent evidence suggests that Alzheimer's disease, or perhaps one form, may be an HLA-associated disease (Renvoize et al. 1979; Sulkava et al. 1980; Walford, Hodge 1980; Whalley et al. 1980; Wilcox et al. 1980). In four out of the five studies HLA B7 was increased, and Walford (1982) has argued that individuals with HLA B7 have a 50 percent greater chance of developing Alzheimer's disease. Our laboratory recently reported that Alzheimer patients with HLA B7 had significant deficits in selective attention compared to patients negative in HLA B7 (Cohen, Eisdorfer, Walford 1982). We interpret this observation as evidence that there may be several forms of Alzheimer's disease.

A NEW HYPOTHESIS: PARENTAL AGE AS A RISK FACTOR FOR ALZHEIMER'S DEMENTIA

The genetic association and similarities between Alzheimer's disease and Down's syndrome have generated a number of questions about their relationship (cf review, Sinex, Merril 1982). These two diseases may share aspects of the same pathogenesis such that older maternal age might be observed in Alzheimer's disease as seen in Down's syndrome. Our laboratory first suggested that there may be

RISK FOR MANIFESTING ALZHEIMER'S DEMENTIA	AGE OF ONSET 65	65-80	80
GENETIC			
Probability of Carrying the Gene			
Probability that Gene Shows Penetrance			
NONGENETIC			
Probability of Exposure to Environmental Factors			

Table 2. Contributing Risk Factors for Dementia of the Alzheimer Type May Vary as a Function of Age of Onset.

a subset of children who develop dementia of the Alzheimer type in later life who are at increased risk as a result of being born to older mothers (Cohen, Eisdorfer, Leverenz 1982). An examination of the records of 80 clinically diagnosed cases of Alzheimer's disease revealed an increased maternal age at birth for these patients (median maternal age, 35.5 years) relative to the general population (median maternal age, 27.0 years). However, the diagnosis was presumptive, based upon whether subjects met clinical research diagnostic criteria for dementia of the Alzheimer type (Eisdorfer, Cohen 1980). Since clinical diagnoses are always subject to questions, we undertook a more rigorous test for the existence of a maternal age effect (Leverenz, Cohen, Eisdorfer submitted).

We selected twenty cases with Alzheimer's disease from the files of the neuropathology division of the University of Washington School of Medicine between 1971 and 1981. All cases had to meet the following pathological criteria for selection: Histopathological changes consistent with Alzheimer's disease; no evidence of infarcts; and no evidence of Parkinson's disease or other co-existing neurological disorders. In addition, clinical records had to exist to document cognitive impairment and decline.

Another twenty age-and-sex-matched controls who died between 1971 - 1981 were also chosen from the same neuropathology files. Cases were selected as controls if the individual died in an accident or from any form of cancer except a brain tumor. Cases with any evidence of progressive nervous system degenerative disorder, e.g., Parkinson's disease, multi-infarct dementia, multiple sclerosis, Pick's disease, alcoholism, and Creutzfeldt-Jacob disease were excluded. The median year of birth was 1909 for both the Alzheimer cases and the controls.

In order to be included as an Alzheimer case or a control, written documentation was required to verify the date of birth and the mother's age at birth from vital statistics certificates, records of funeral parlors, cemeteries, or family documents, e.g., family bibles, dated family pictures. This requirement limited the number of cases for this study.

The Alzheimer patients had significantly older mothers at birth compared to the neuropathology control cases as well as the 1907 Washington State population. The median age of our Alzheimer cases was 30.0 years compared to 25.5 years and 26.0 years for the respective control samples ($p = 0.05$). Paternal age of the Alzheimer cases was not significantly different for either of the control groups ($p = .10$). The relative risk for mothers over age 26 was 5.57 using the neuropathology control group (95 percent confidence interval of 1.5 to 20.9) and 3.17 using the vital records control group (95 percent confidence interval of 1.3 to 8.0).

Figure 1 shows the age distribution of mothers at childbirth by five year age groupings for the following populations: the 20 control and 20 autopsy verified Alzheimer cases, the 80 clinically diagnosed Alzheimer patients reported previously (Cohen, Eisdorfer, Leverenz 1982), the 590 1907 Washington State vital records group (Cohen, Eisdorfer, Leverenz 1982), and the 1920 United States caucasian population. The Collman and Stoller (1962) date for Down's syndrome are included for comparison of maternal age. The age distribution of mothers (at childbirth) from the 1907 Washington records closely parallels the 1920 United States Census data. The peak of the age distribution of the mothers of Alzheimer cases falls between the mothers' of the controls and the Down's cases.

At least one other laboratory has reported a slight but significant increase in both maternal ($p = 0.005$) and paternal ($p = 0.01$) age in 69 autopsy-validated cases of Alzheimer's disease compared to 207 controls (Whalley et al. 1982). Maternal age at birth for probands averaged 30.6 years compared to 28.6 years for controls, while paternal age at birth for probands averaged 33.2 years compared to 30.8 years for controls. There was no correlation with order of birth.

Maternal age is the most recent in a series of possible associations found between dementia of the Alzheimer type and Down's syndrome. The basis of a maternal age factor clearly requires further investigation. Certainly the possibility exists that mothers giving birth in a later reproductive period have an altered reproductive physiology which impacts on the child's subsequent

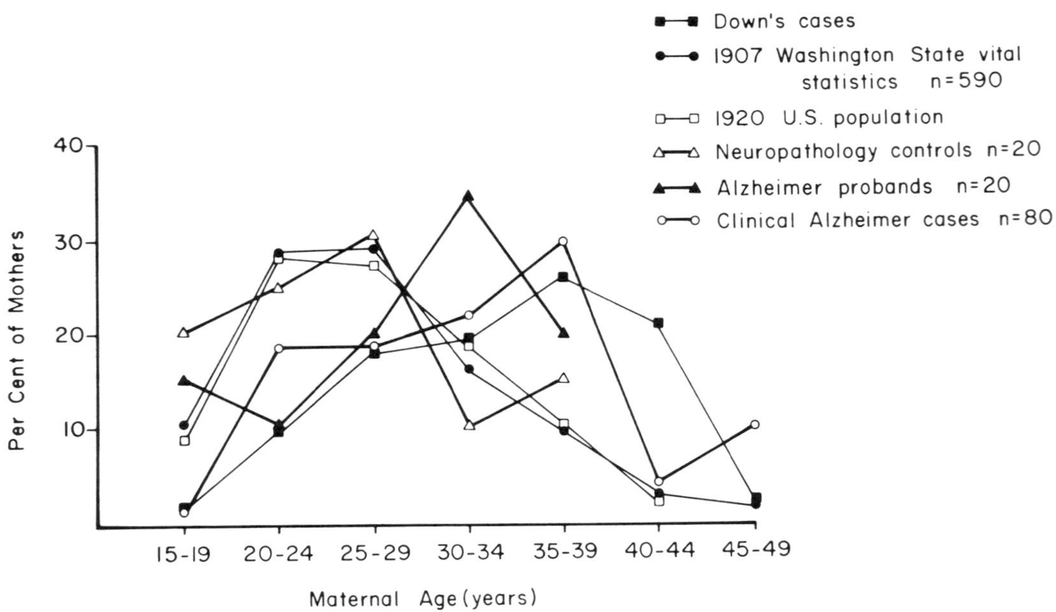

Fig. 1. Percentage of Mothers by Five Year Age Groups for Alzheimer's disease, Control Populations, and Down's Syndrome.

development. The higher mutation rate in the chromosomes of older men (Jones et al. 1975) may be a mechanism to increase the child's vulnerability to disease in later life.

STUDY DESIGNS THAT PROVIDE DATA ON RISK

It should be clear that a significant body of data are needed to identify the risk factors for Alzheimer's disease and related disorders. Several study designs may be used to generate the data we need: Natural experiments, preventative trials, prospective studies, and case control studies.

Adolf Meyer referred to every psychiatric patient as an experiment of nature which could teach the clinician something new about variability in human behavior. In the study of Alzheimer's disease and related disorders, there are many natural experiments which have much to teach us. One example is a large family pedigree containing multiple probands with histopathologically confirmed Alzheimer's disease. Our laboratory has just begun immunologic studies of a Canadian family with 51 members affected with Alzheimer's disease out of 531 identified family members in six generations. These studies are in collaboration with a research team at the Clinical Center, National Institute of Health, who worked up the pedigree (Nee et al. 1983).

Preventative trials are methods used to protect the population when the risk factors are known and the preventative measure is known to be safe and effective, e.g., innoculation with the Salk vaccine to prevent polio. Preventative strategies are valuable research methods because they provide the investigator with the opportunity to manipulate the hypothesized independent variable. They also provide direct measures of attributable risk. For example, anti-hypertensive medications have been used to effectively reduce the frequency of strokes and coronary heart disease (Surgeon General 1979). Preventive trials are more likely to improve our understanding of multi-infarct dementia rather than Alzheimer's disease because we know more about vascular antecedent of strokes.

A prospective study is a potentially valuable research design to identify the antecedent condition for multi-infarct dementia. A prospective study requires that a population with defined characteristics, including hypothesized risk factors, e.g., hypertension, arrhythmia, stress, be followed over time to measure the frequency with which multi-infarct dementias occur. Again, our paucity of knowledge about Alzheimer's disease at this time makes a prospective study an expensive low yield experiment.

A case-control study is the design of choice to investigate risk factors for Alzheimer's dementia. A population of Alzheimer cases must be identified and matched carefully to a group of controls. The selection of comparable controls is important in order to make an accurate comparison of the frequency of occurrence of suspected risk factors for Alzheimer's dementia, e.g., exposure to cattle and sheep, diet, use of alcohol, life stress, HLA markers, family history, etc. Controls should probably be carefully selected for age, sex, education, social class, occupational history, health and family history.

NEED FOR A PUBLIC HEALTH APPROACH TO LATE LIFE DEMENTIAS

The dementias of later life are probably one of our most significant public health problems. Indeed, throughout the world we are witnessing an increase in the prevalence of the major mental disorders and other chronic conditions, including schizophrenia, major affective disorders, epilepsy, as well as the dementias (Kramer 1980). A significant research investment is needed for population studies to develop a sorely-needed data base and implement appropriate and safe prevention strategies.

Alzheimer's disease and related disorders pose another significant problem for our society. They create a population "at risk" for significant health problems. The chronic stress of caring exacts a profound emotional and economic toll on the family (Cohen 1983; Eisdorfer, Cohen 1981). Primary caregivers are at risk for significant depression and physical illness, whereas the entire family experiences emotional distress over what one family member called the "death of the mind, the most horrible death imaginable."

The challenge for the future is clear. Research efforts need to be intensified to learn more about the etiology of late life dementias. In the meantime, those individuals already afflicted with Alzheimer's disease and related disorders need our support to enhance their health, functional effectiveness, dignity and quality of life. The families caring for their relatives need our clinical care and support since it is only with their help that we can most effectively maintain the patient in the supportive environment of their own homes.

REFERENCES

Abdon NJ (1977). Unrecognized intermittent bradycardias in patients treated for senile dementia. In Watanabe Y (ed): "Cardiac Pacing, Proceedings of the Fifth International Symposium, Excerpta Medica International Congress Series No. 395," Amsterdam: Elsevier.

Cornfield J (1951). A method of estimating comparative rates from clinical data: Application to cancer of the lung, breast, and cervix. J Nat Cancer Inst 11:1269-1275.

Cohen D (1982). Psychological issues in the diagnosis and treatment of patients with dementing disorders. In Eisdorfer C, Fann E (eds): "Treatment of Psychopathology in the Aging," New York: Springer.

Cohen D, Eisdorfer C, Leverenz C (1982). A hypothesis: Maternal age and Alzheimer's disease. J Am Ger Soc 30:656-659.

Cohen D, Eisdorfer C, Walford RL (1982). Histocompatibility antigens (HCA) and patterns of cognitive loss in dementia of the Alzheimer type. Neurobiol Aging 2:277-280.

Collman RD, Stoller A (1962). A survey of mongolism and congenital anomalies of the central nervous system in Victoria. N Z Med J 61:24-32.

Dawber TR, Wolf A, Colton TH, Nickerson RJ (1977). Risk factors: comparison of the biological data in myocardial and brain infarctions. In Zulch KJ, Kaufman W, Hossmann A, Hossman V (eds): "Brain and heart infarct," Berlin: Springer-Verlay.

Eisdorfer C, Cohen D (1981). Management of the patient and family with dementing illness. J Fam Prac 12:831-837.

Eisdorfer C, Cohen D (1980). Research diagnostic criteria for primary neuronal degeneration of the Alzheimer type. J Fam Prac 11:553-557.

Friedman GD, Loveland DB, Ehrlich SP Jr (1968). Relationship of stroke to other cardiovascular disease.

Circulation 38:533-541.
Gruenberg EM (1980). Implications of viewing stress as a risk factor. Manuscript.
Heston LL, Mastri AR, Anderson VE, White J (1981). Dementia of the Alzheimer type: Clinical genetics, natural history and associated conditions. Arch Gen Psychiat 38:1085-1090.
Jones KL, Smith DW, Harvey MAS, Hall BD, Quan L (1975). Older paternal age and fresh gene mutation: Data on additional disorders. J Pediat 86:84-88.
Kannel WB (1971). Current status of the epidemiology of brain infarction associated with occlusive arterial disease. Stroke 2:295.
Kannel WB, Gordon T, Wolf PA, McNamara P (1972). Hemoglobin and the risk of cerebral infarction: The Framingham study. Stroke 3:409-420.
Kramer M (1980). The rising pandemic of mental disorders and associated chronic diseases and disabilities. Acta Psychiat Second Suppl 285 62:382-397.
Larsson T, Sjogren T, Jacobson G (1963). A clinical, sociomedical and genetic study. Acta Psychiat Second Suppl 167:1-259.
Librach G, Schadel M, Seltzer M, Hert A, Yellin N (1977). Stroke: incidence and risk factors. Geriatrics 32:85-91, 94-6.
Nee LE, Polinski RJ, Eldridge R, Weingartner H, Smallberg S, Ebert M (1983). A family with histologically confirmed Alzheimer's disease. Arch Neurol 40:203-208.
Renvoize EB, Hambling MH, Pepper MD, Rajah SN (1979). Possible associatin of Alzheimer's disease with HLA - Bw15 and cytomegalovirus infection. Lancet i:1239.
Schwartz PJ, Brown AM, Milliani A, Zanchetti A (eds) (1978). "Perspectives in cardiovascular research, Vol. 2, neural mechanisms in cardiac arrythmias," New York: Raven.
Sinex EM, Merrill CR (1982). "Alzheimer's disease, Down's syndrome, and aging," New York: New York Academy of Science.
Sluss TK (1980). "A method for investigating a risk factor for senile dementia-Alzheimer type in the Baltimore longitudinal study," unpublished doctoral thesis, Baltimore: The Johns Hopkins University.
Sulkava R, Koskimies S, Wikstrom J, Palo L (1980). HLA antigens in Alzheimer's disease. Tiss Ant 16:191-194.
The Surgeon General's Report on Health Promotion and Disease Prevention (1979). "Healthy people," Washington,

D.C.: U.S. Department of Health, Education, and Welfare, DHEW (PHS) Publication No. 79-55071.

Walford RF (1982). Immunological studies of Down's syndrome and Alzheimer's disease. In Sinex EM, Merril CR (eds): "Alzheimer's disease, Down's syndrome, and aging," New York: New York Academy of Sciences.

Walford RL, Hodge SE (1980). HLA distribution in Alzheimer's disease. In Terasaki PI (ed): "Histocompatibility Testing, 1980" Los Angeles: UCLA Tissue Typing Laboratory.

Weissman MM, Myers JK (1978). Affective disorders in a U.S. urban community: The use of research diagnostic criteria in an epidemiological survey. Arch Gen Psychiat 35:1304-1311.

Whalley LJ, Carothers S, Collyer S, DeMey R, Frackiewicz A (1982). A study of familial factors in Alzheimer's disease. Br J Psychiat 140:249-256.

Whalley LJ, Urboniak SJ, Darg C, Peutherer JF, Christie JE (1980). Histocompatibility antigens and antibodies to viral and other antigens in Alzheimer pre-senile dementia. Act Psychiat Scand 61:1-7.

Wilcox CB, Caspary EA, Behan PO (1980). Histocompatibility antigens in Alzheimer's disease: A prelimary study. Eur Neurol 19:262-265.

Wolf PA, Dawber TR, Thomes HE, Colton T, Kannel WB (1977). Epidemiology of stroke. In Thompson RA, Green JR (eds): "Advances in Neurology, Vol. 16," New York: Raven.

Wolf PA, Kannel WB, Dawber TR (1978). Neurological epidemiology: Principles and clinical applications. In Schoenberg BS (ed): "Advances in Neurology, Vol. 19," New York: Raven.

Senile Dementia: Outlook for the Future, pages 239–251

DIAGNOSIS AND TREATMENT OF THE AGED WITH MENTAL DISTURBANCES

Masaki Yoshikawa, M.D.

Professor emeritus, University of Tokyo
Director, Tokyo Metropolitan Police Hospital
2-10-41 Fujimi, Chiyoda-ku, Tokyo, Japan 102

Correct diagnosis and treatment is not only essential of medical practice but also the basis for gerontological, holistic approach to the aged. This consideration is to be emphasized specifically, when the aged has some mental disturbances. This report consists of, first the demographic and medical statistics in Japan, secondly the diagnosis of the aged patient and thirdly the treatment of the aged with mental disturbances.

I. Demographic and medical statistics in Japan

Table 1 shows the life expectancy of the Japanese population from 1920 to 1980. Average length of life in 1980 for male is 73.32, and for female is 78.72. Average length of life of Japanese population has been about 40 until 1920, and in 1950 that for male was 56.57 and that for female 62.97, namely about 60 for both groups. The rapid increase of average length of life from the middle of this century to recent years has been considered primarily due to rapid decrease of the mortality of new-born and children, and also due to the marked decrease of mortality of young adults due to pulmonary tuberculosis during these period. However, relatively large differences of life expectancies over 60 between 1970 and 1980, and also the similar differences in life expectancies over 65 between 1970 and 1980 seem to indicate that in recent years the average length of life has been increasing not only due to the decrease of the mortality rate of young generations, but also due to the real increase of life expectancy of aged people.

	Average Length of Life (0 -)		Life Expectancy over 60		Life Expectancy over 65	
	Male	Female	Male	Female	Male	Female
1921 - 1925	42.06	43.20	11.87	14.12	9.31	11.10
1935 - 1936	46.92	49.63	12.55	15.07	9.89	11.88
1950 - 1952	59.57	62.97	14.36	16.81	11.35	13.36
1960	65.32	70.19	14.84	17.83	11.62	14.10
1970	69.31	74.66	15.93	19.27	12.50	15.34
1980	73.32	78.72	18.28	21.84	14.52	17.63

Table 1. Life Expectancy of the Japanese Population

The Report of the Consultative Meeting on the Problems of the Aged (April 1980 - July 1982), The Policy Headquarters for the Aged, Prime Minister's Office

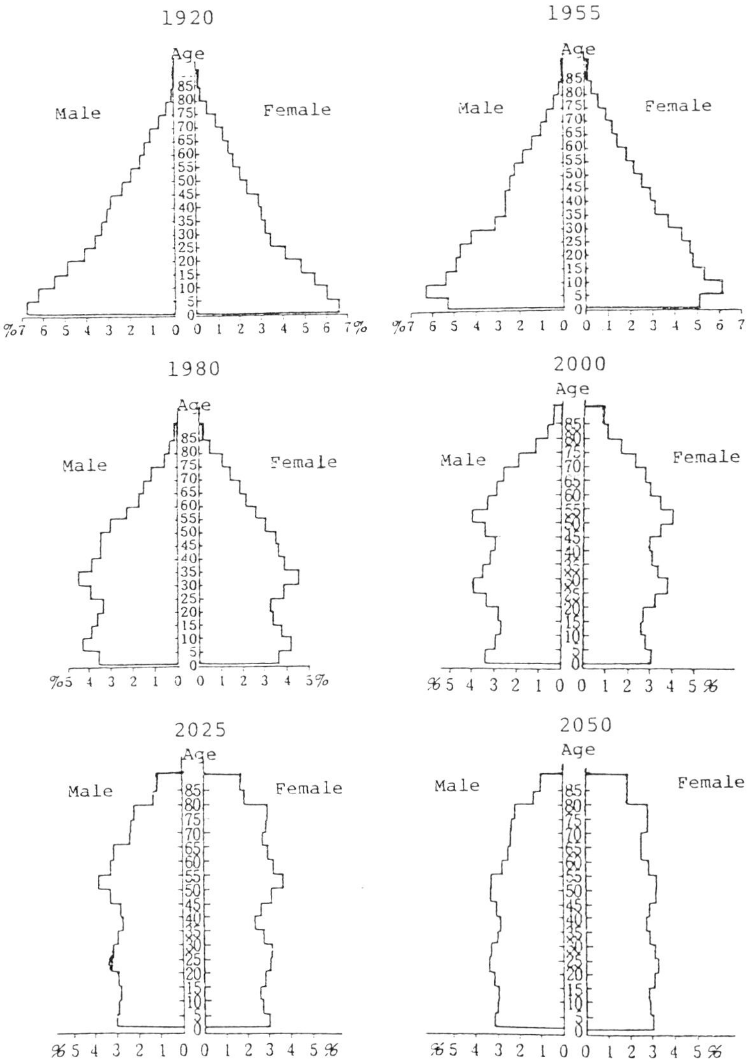

Prime Minister's Office,
The Policy Headquarters for the Aged

Figure 1. The Population Pyramid in Japan

Figure 1 shows the socalled population pyramid in Japan from 1920 to 2050. In 1920 and also in 1955, the shapes of pyramids have been somewhat similar to the shape of Mt. Fuji in Japan due to the relatively large mortality rate of young generations. Recently, in 1980, the pyramid is having the shape of a bottle just as shown here and it is anticipated that in 2000, 2025 and 2050, the shapes of pyramid would become taller. The ratio of population of 65 and over at present in Japan is considered about 10 percent of the whole population and it is anticipated that in the 21 century the ratio of 65 and over in Japan will reach to about 20 percent of whole population, and that the older group of the aged will increase more markedly compared with the younger group of the aged,just similar to the circumstances in the United States and in Europe.

Table 2 shows the divisions of the middle and old age. People in middle age from 40 to 59 is important in geriatrics and gerontology, because they have already some symptoms of normal aging and are often liable to the diseases related to the aging. Senior or old age is divided into two groups, namely, young-old in 60 to 79, and old-old in 80 and over. These divisions seem to be useful in a geriatric and gerontological approach to the old people, although this expression of young-old an old-old is somewhat more chronological compared with the concept of Professor B.L. Neugarten who has maintained the expression of young-old and old-old from more sociological point of view.

Age	Division	
40 - 59	Middle age	
60 - 79	Young-old	Senior or old age
80 -	Old-old	

Table 2. The Divisions of the Middle and Old Age

Table 4 shows the main causes of death in 1980 in Japan, namely 3 years before now, 10 years after previous table 3. Main 3 causes of death in 1980 is just the same as in 1970 in order, namely cerebrovascular diseases first, malignant neoplasms second, and heart diseases is third. However, the number of deaths and death rate has shown some change during these 10 years, namely, in the transition that cerebrovascular diseases are decreasing, and malignant neoplasms and heart diseases are increasing as shown in both tables. In the order of from 4 to 10 in 1980, the liver-cirrhosis 8, renal diseases such as nephritis and nephrotic syndrome are appearing as 10. Although tuberculosis has disappeared in the ten items of table 4 in 1980, the tuberculous diseases is remaining yet as important disease of the aged in Japan. Malignancy, arteriosclerotic diseases, infection such as pneumonia and bronchitis, livercirrhosis and hepatitis, and renal diseases are being thought to be the rather stable important causes of death perhaps until the 21 century in Japan, perhaps similar in the United States and most countries in Europe.

	Cause of death	Number of deaths	Death rate*
	Total number	712,962	694.4
1	Cerebrovascular Diseases	181,315	176.5
2	Malignant Neoplasms	119,997	116.8
3	Heart Diseases	89,411	87.0
4	Accidents & Adverse effe-cts(Injury & Poisoning)	43,802	42.6
5	Senility without mention of psychosis	39,277	38.2
6	Pneumonia & Bronchitis	35,142	34.2
7	Hypertensive Diseases	18,303	17.8
8	Tuberculosis	15,899	15.5
9	Suicide	15,728	15.3
10	Livercirrhosis	12,898	12.6

* per 100,000 - population

Ministry of Health and Welfare

Table 3. Main Causes of Death in 1970 in Japan

	Cause of death	Number of deaths	Death rate*
	Total number	722,801	622.0
1	Cerebrovascular Diseases	162,317	139.7
2	Malignant Neoplasms	161,764	139.2
3	Heart Diseases	123,505	106.3
4	Pneumonia & Bronchitis	39,241	33.8
5	Senility without mention of psychosis	32,154	27.7
6	Accidents & Adverse effects(Injury & Poisoning)	29,217	25.1
7	Suicide	20,542	17.7
8	Chronic Liver Diseases & Livercirrhosis	16,490	14.2
9	Hypertensive Diseases	15,911	13.7
10	Nephritis, Nephrotic Syndrome & Nephrosis	10,180	8.8

* per 100,000 - population
Ministry of Health and Welfare

Table 4. Main Causes of Death in 1980 in Japan

II. Diagnosis of the aged with mental disturbances

Although the diseases of main causes of death is very important in geriatrics, there are many other diseases and syndrome which are not fatal in themselves but are to be considered seriously in their nature of continuous restriction in the life of the aged.

Table 5 shows the classification of diseases of 1,520 cases in the Department of Geriatrics, University of Tokyo, in 1978. We have adopted the index of international classification of diseases, 1975 division, published by WHO. This index is well prepared and has the value due to its international character, although in some parts, the classifications had better be revised according to the establishment of new clinical concepts. In table 5, we can see not only the diseases shown in table 3 and 4, but also many clinical cases such as diabetes mellitus, diseases of digestive system, biliary tract and pancreas, respiratory system, genitourinary system, musculoskeletal system and others. These circumstaces are perhaps similar also in United States and in Europe. Omitting the description of more detailed data, I should like to emphasize here only the importance of diagnosis of the aged which should be performed not only on the diagnosis of clinical entity but also on the diagnosis of pathologic-physiology and the diagnosis of treatment.

Table 5. Classification of Diseases

	(Total 1,520)	%
1. Infectious Diseases (Tbc, Syphilis included)	109	7.2
2. Neoplasms	279	18.4
3. Endocrine and Metabolic Disorders	153	10.1
4. Diabetes mellitus	241	15.9
5. Diseases of the Blood and Blood-forming Organs	88	5.8
6. Mental Disorders	56	3.7
7. Diseases of the Nervous System and Sense Organs	148	9.7
8. Heart Diseases	240	15.8
9. Hypertension	258	17.0
10. Cerebrovascular Disorders	223	14.7
11. Arteriosclerosis and Arteritis	124	8.2
12. Diseases of the Respiratory system	220	14.5
13. Diseases of the Digestive System	160	10.5
14. Diseases of Liver, Biliary Tract and Pancreas	227	14.9
15. Diseases of the Genitourinary System	194	12.8
16. Diseases of the Musculoskeletal System	142	9.3
17. Diseases of the Skin and Subcutaneous Tissues	24	1.6
18. Congenital Anomalies	43	2.8
19. Symptoms Signs, and Ill-defined Conditions	84	5.5
20. Others	28	1.8

(Department of Geriatrics, University of Tokyo 1978)

Non-demented
(46 cases)

		INV	
	Grade	0-Slight	Severe
CVD	0 ~ Slight	43 (94%)	2 (4%)
	Severe	1 (2%)	0 (0%)

Demented
(54 cases)

		INV	
	Grade	0-Slight	Severe
CVD	0 ~ Slight	3 (5%)	22 (41%)
	Severe	16 (30%)	13 (24%)

Table 6. Incidence Related to the Degree of Involutional Changes (INV) and Cerebrovascular Diseases (CVD)

Table 6 shows the neuropathological diagnosis of vascular and involutional changes of the brain. We have studied in autopsies the brains of 54 cases who had indicated clinically the symptoms of dementia. As shown in table 6, 22 cases, 41 percent, had the severe involutional changes of Alzheimer type with no or slight vascular involvement. Sixteen cases, 30 percent, had the severe vascular changes, but with no or slight involutional involvements, and in addition, there were 13 cases, 24 percent, who showed both severe vascular and involutional changes simultaneously. It is well known that the vascular dementia and involutional dementia of SDAT are the main causes of dementia syndrome, and recognition of the fairly frequent presence of mixed type is important also for the correct diagnosis as the basis for the reasonable management of the aged people.

There are many cases of the aged with other types of mental disturbances in addition to or without dementia. Depression and paranoid states are important groups which are classified as the functional psychiatric diseases of the aged. In addition to these well established clinical entities of organic brain damage and functional psychiatric patients, there are many cases who have various complaints of subjective and psychiatric symptoms. Their complaints are caused by many medical diseases in addition to normal aging. Although the severity of their mental disturbances is usually relatively slight or moderate, they are also important in our medical practice and health care of the aged, because they consist of the large number of patients on the spectrum between normal aging and the advanced typical cases of dementia and functional psychiatric diseases, and because they are individuals having the capacity of the response to adequate medical treatment or nursing care.

III. The treatment of the aged with the mental disturbances

The essentials of the treatment of the aged with the mental disturbances are the same as the principles of the medical treatment as general. The basic importance should be given to the adequate advice or psychotherapy to the reasonable life style, especially on the habit of diet with the consideration of physical exercise of the individual.

Table 7 is an example of the diet of average Japanese people which consists of 6 sorts of tables, units of diet, three main nutrients of protein, fat and carbohydrate, their quantities in grams and calories, and their ratio. Table 1 and 2 in this dietary table 7 are meals mainly of carbohydrate, table 3 and 4 of protein, table 5 oil and fat, and table 6 of vegetables and seaweeds. One unit contains 80 calories, and the number in parenthesis under each meal is grams corresponding one unit in individuals item. The ratios of calories to total are 27 percent in fat and 17 percent in proteins. This relatively low intake of fat in Japanese population is thought to be one of the causes of relatively low incidence of the arteriosclerotic heart disease in Japan which is now gradually increasing as shown in demographic table 3 and 4. The high incidence of cerebrovascular diseases is considered to be caused mainly due to hypertension, of which high intake of sodium salt is thought responsible as the most important factor.

On the basis of these guidances on life and diet, various methods of pharmacotherapy, surgical therapy, and rehabilitation should be administered in consideration of the diagnosis of the aged with the overview of the physical and mental status of the patient as a whole.

Figure 2 shows the result of our recently performed double blind test which have compared the effects of 6 and 3mgs of dehydroergotoxine methylate. The dosis of 6mg was superior to 3mg in the effects on subjective and psychiatric symptoms. In this sort of drug which may be classified as vasodilating, cell metabolism enhancing group among the drugs for the nervous system, the effect is mild and side effects are rare and not serious. These characteristics are making their clinical administration more easy, but being liable to the criteria that the effect might be caused or confirmed with more subjective influence of patient and doctor, although there are some experimental and biochemical data suggesting on the mechanism of clinical effects in the human. The blind test performed by many specialists on many clinical cases of adequate indication have given us the objectively confirmed results on the superiority of 6mg compared to 3mg of this drug.

As conclusion, the correct diagnosis and treatment made by coordinated consideration of the whole status of individual patient may be said essentials of the care of the aged with mental disturbances.

Group	Table	Food*	Breakfast	Lunch	Supper	Total units	Protein (gram)	Fat (gram)	carbo-hydrate (gram)
I	Table 1	Cooked Rice, (55) Bread, Buck Wheat (30) Noodle, (Soba) (70) Potato (70–100)	3	3	4	10 } 12	20	—	180
	Table 2	Fruits	1		1	2	—	—	40
II	Table 3	Meat of Animals, Poultry & Fish, Cheese (60) (70) (25)		1	1	2 } 7.3	36	36.5	—
		Egg (50)	1			1			—
		Bean Curds (140)			1	1			—
	Table 4	Milk, Yogurt, Powdered Milk (140) (100) (20)	1.3	1	1	3.3	13.2		13.2
III	Table 5	Oil and Fat (9)	0.5	0.5	1	2	—	18	—
IV	Table 6	Vegetables and Seaweed	0.4	0.2	0.4	1	5	1	13
Appendix		Bean paste (50) Sugar (20)	0.2	0.2	0.3	0.7	3.5	0.7	9.1
Total			7.2 (units)	5.7 (units)	10.1 (units)	23 (units)	78 (grams)	56.2 (grams)	255 (grams)
Calories			576 (cal)	456 (cal)	808 (cal)	1840 (cal)	312 (cal)	506 (cal)	1022 (cal)
Calories (%)			31%	25%	44%	100%	17%	27%	56%

* Figures in ( ) for food indicate grams per 1 unit.

Table 7. An Example of Food Constituents of a Diet containing 1800 Calories or 23 Units

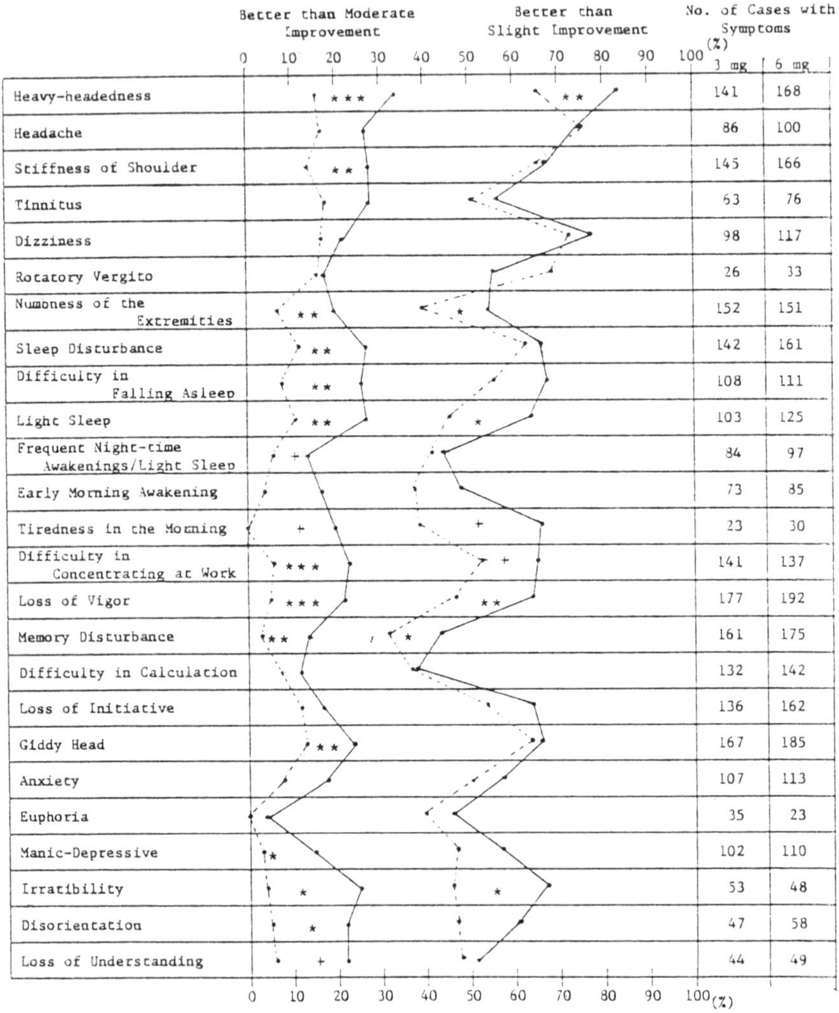

Figure 2. Improvement rating of subjective and psychiatric symptoms. (2 × 2 χ^2 test. P = 0.10; * = P 0.05; ** = P 0.01; *** = P 0 – – – – = 3 mg group; ——— = 6 mg group).

National Report of Japan for the United Nations World Assembly on Aging, May, 1982, The Government of Japan (Prime Minister's Office, The Policy Headquarters for the Aged)

Aging in Japan, 1978 Tokyo, Japan, (Under the auspices: Japan Institute for Gerontological Research and Development)

B.L. Neugarten: Social implications of life extension in Recent Advances in Gerontology, Excepta Medica, 1979, Amsterdam, (Proceedings of the XI International Congress of Gerontology Tokyo, August 20-25, 1978), Page 669-674

Yoshikawa, M., Hirai, S., Aizawa, T., Kuroiwa, Y., Goto, F., Sofue, I., Toyokura, Y., Yamamura, H. and Iwasaki, Y.: A Dose-response Study with Dihydroergotoxine Mesylate in Cerebrovascular Disturbances, Journal of the American Geriatrics Society 31(1): 1-7, 1983. 1

Yoshikawa, M. and Hirai, S.: Chronic Cerebrovascular Insufficiency, Practical Geriatrics: 193-209, Karger, Basel, 1975

Morimatsu, M., Hirai, S., Muramatsu, A. and Yoshikawa, M.: Senile Degenerative Brain Lesions and Dementia, Journal of the American Geriatrics Society XXIII (9): 390-406, 1975

Yoshikawa, M.: Problems in the Clinical Aspects of Geriatric Medicine, Japanese Journal of Medicine 12(4): 225-230, 1973.10

Yoshikawa, M., Okano, K., Nakai, R., Tomori, T. and Takenaka, M.: Aging and Nutrition, Asian Medical Journal 21(5): 359-378, 1978

Senile Dementia: Outlook for the Future, pages 253–265

CURRENT APPROACHES TO TREATMENT OF THE PSYCHOLOGICALLY HANDICAPPED ELDERLY: Clinical Imperatives Identifying Geriatric Psychiatry as a Sub-Specialty in its Own Right

J. RICHARD, P. DROZ, L. BIZZINI Service Universitaire de Psychiatrie Geriatrique, University of Geneva

The classical sequence in clinical medicine is : first diagnosis, then treatment. In geriatric psychiatry, however, it is becoming increasingly apparent that just the reverse may give better results, particularly in the management of declining mental performance. What follows is the description of a novel frame of reference for understanding the psychological concomitants of advanced age, and an appeal for its broader use as a model of medical care for the mentally impaired elderly.

I. PSYCHIATRIC SIGNS AND SYMPTOMS

a. Clinicians sometimes make a distinction between signs and symptoms. In the strict sense, signs are objective findings, in other words indications of a disease or condition which the clinician can perceive without the active assistance of the patient; symptoms,on the other hand, are non-objectifiable phenomena which the patient reports to the physician.

The purpose of medical examination is to detect clinical signs, the objective manifestations of a disease or condition. Any combination of two or more clinical signs, occurring simultaneously, is known as a syndrome. For diagnostic purposes, the absence of certain signs may be just as important as the presence or specific combination of others.Under ideal circumstances, signs enable a physician to confirm health or to diagnose illness and, where feasible, to prescribe appropriate treatment.

Although the respective rôles of patient and physician may vary widely from society to society, they share a universal expectation common to all cultures: the patient is he who seeks - the physician is expected to provide - relief. Geriatric psychiatry does not fit this universal mold. In nearly all cases, the identified patient does not seek relief and the request for treatment originates with a third party. Indeed, the patient may have no active interest whatsoever in the consultation or its outcome, no expectation, no request. Expectations are usually defined by the clinician, who weaves the cloth of knowledge in a pattern he simultaneously learns and creates. Because of these special circumstance, geriatric psychiatrists may find more professional satisfaction and benefit their patients to a greater extent, by pursuing humanitarian goals more assiduously than strictly scientific aims.

Medical intervention therefore begins with an evaluation of signs and their comparison to a standard set of known syndromes. In the process, it is wise to bear in mind that the simultaneous occurrence of two or more signs does not always necessarily have the same clinical significance. It is, after all, quite possible for two or more unrelated signs to develop independently of each other. There are also recognized clinical signs which, taken separately, can indicate any of several underlying conditions - or even no identifiable condition at all!

Not infrequently, psychiatrists are uncertain as to whether they can safely rely on a uniform interpretation of clinical findings or, indeed, whether the ease and efficiency gained through standardization will facilitate or hamper the management of impairment. They are frequently at a loss to predict which clinical signs will ultimately prove significant and which irrelevant. They are painfully aware that they may themselves inadvertantly induce the signs the observe. Moreover, many behavioural traits are meaningless in themselves and only take on clinical significance when they appear in recognizable configurations. In each instance, these configurations must be organized into a coherent vhole even though there may be no valid criteria for their interpretation. In some cases, we still lack the basic scientific knowledge necessary to understand our clinical findings. This state of affairs bears witness to the overwhelming complexity of interpersonal relationships and their clinical interpretation.

Of necessity, geriatric psychiatry has rapidly ajusted to the uncertainties of clinical diagnosis. In the process it has developed a resourcefulness which challenges current concepts of diagnosis and classification, has far-reaching implications for epidemiology and clinical management, and might well serve as a model for other branches of medicine.

b. Defined as "the act of deciding the nature of a diseased condition by examination of the (signs and) symptoms" (Webster's New World Dictionary, 1978 edition), diagnosis would appear to depend solely on the presence and recognition of certain clinical signs or sets of signs. There are, however, several possible approaches to diagnosis. Positive diagnosis relies exclusively on unmistakable, pathognomonic signs. Differential diagnosis, on the other hand, proceeds by deductive reasoning aimed at confirming the most probable - or, ideally, the only possible - diagnosis from among all remotely possible diagnoses. The operational concept of disease makes use of these diagnostic models as well as of its etioligical and pathophysiological underpinnings. Although explanatory models have their drawbacks, awareness of their limitations has neither done away with diagnosis based on clinical signs, nor prevented geriatric psychiatry from recognizing and reaching beyond the flaws inherent in traditional clinical methods to propose a daring new definition of medical objectives.

Geriatric psychiatry has never hesitated to avail itself of the more reliable methods of clinical psychiatry and other medical specialties. Despite the useful contributions from other fields, the routine practice of geriatric psychiatry compels recognition of the fact that care - more often than cure - must still remain the ultimate aim of medicine. This plain reality dictates the sequence we must follow in planning care for the mentally impaired elderly :

1. the preservation and enhancement of residual capacity, including but not limited to the rational exercise of all unimpaired physical and psychological abilities;

2. the modification or reduction of the premorbid need associated with these faculties;

3. finally, whenever (but only when) feasible, the elimination or reduction of impairment.

Care requires first and foremost that the practitioner understand the subjective experience of the ailing individual living with his illness in a given environment. It demands subordination of scientific curiosity to genuine and humane concern for the quality of life. It compels respect for adaptive medicine, for optimal adjustment of the patient to his illness, for prevervation of his integrity and dignity.

It means helping patients to make better use of their abilities and to compensate for their impairments. It should be pointed out that this attitude in no way implies fatalistic resignation; it is entirely compatible with and, indeed, should always be coupled with the simultaneous implementation of all realistic ways and means to effect a cure. For the principal aim of medical care is to train patients to contribute to their own well-being by showing them how best to use the assistance available through family, friends and health professionals. To achieve this aim, health professionals should be equipped to teach patients how to maintain and improve their health, how to keep their impairments from damaging good relations with others. This means that the assistance which is an integral part of care should not be allowed to degenerate into a mutual dependency between patient and health professional. It means that whenever possible patients should assume responsbility for themselves to the full extent of which they are capable. It also means that while patients must be free to choose those from whom they receive care, care-givers have no right to pick and choose among patients.

To give care precedence over all other considerations is to view diagnosis in a new light. Some clinical experience challenges the view that diagnosis should always precede and determine treatment. Therapeutic techniques may be used to determine diagnostic approach, as in family therapy when an entire group is treated according to principles derived from general systems theory without regard to diagnosis.

To take another example, it is sometimes possible to treat, successfully, a condition which is unknown or imperfectly known. Treatment can show how to modify or control behaviour which is considered undesirable. Often, the only benefit desired from explanation is the comforting reassurance it provides clinicians by lending their practices an aura of scientific authority. As the history of hysteria shows, explanation is not necessarily of benefit to the patient. CHARCOT's analysis of the signs of hysteria contributed greatly to their recognition, but did little to help us understand their nature or to relieve distress.

Nor does recognizing and defining a clinical entity in such a way as to attibute a specific etiology to it necessarily furnish guidelines for rational care which, more often than not. must be based on other criteria in geriatric psychiatry.

The avowed goal of medicine is to eradicate disease. This goal is not always compatible with the objectives of care. Because we can anticipate that new clinical entities will be increasingly identified among the elderly, we can also expect a corresponding increase in the gap between scientific knowledge and the ethical requirements of care.

The practice of geriatric psychiatry convinces clinicians that diagnosis is knowledge which sanctions treatment, including but not limited to understanding of the disease process itself. Medicine is an open field. Many clinical entities remain to be described. Clinicians should therefore not only cull through all available information each time they treat a patient, but also seize every opportunity to advance science by adding new knowledge to the acquired store. Medicine is a science which not only "scans the known and identifies" but also "grows by constantly challenging its own limits" (Y. PELICIER, 1972).

There is also a diagnostic approach which seeks to determine the conditions uder which certains types of undesirable behaviour may be eliminated. Obviously, the less undesirable behaviour a patient exhibits, the greater his chances of acceptance by others and of adjustment to community living. Behaviour modification might therefore well be the first step in personal as well as interpersonal adjustment. The same treatment objective underlies identification of signs or symptoms, learning how to make them appear and disappear at will, studying ways and means to mask them, to control the conditions under which they appear and to evaluate the consequences of their modification.

In any event, the right to diagnose carries with it an obligation to treat. It is axiomatic that any health policy which creates a functional or architectural distinction between those who diagnose and those who treat, particularly in institutional settings, ultimately results in the "warehousing" of patients. Custodial facilities, less costly than hospitals worthy of the name, often fail to provide the bare minimum of medical care. The diagnostic approach we recommend implies that it is just as unacceptable to limit diagnosis and choice of treatment to physicians as it is to identify nurses solely as care-givers. Diagnosis and treatment are the legitimate concern of both. Nurses, ergotherapists, sociotherapists, psychologists,physiotherapists, psychomotricians, orthophonists and social workers need diagnoses as much as physicians, but for different purposes.

Although the signs and symptoms of psychiatric conditions are empirically derived from careful and repeated observations and are therefore devoid of broader implications, there is a distinct tendency among clinicians to engage in theoretical speculation about them. But while theories may be useful for the interpretation of clinical data,they may also obscure the significance of clinical observations for treatment. Indeed, the importance of behaviour, the primary concern of the clinician, may be obscured just as readily by lofty theories as it is by fuzzy thinking - sometimes even moreso.

II. CLINICAL SIGNS OF MENTAL DETERIORATION

Although it is still debatable as to how widely it is justifiable to apply the concept of "lesion" to states of dementification, these conditions are regularly associated with more or less well-defined pathology of the central nervous system.

a. For nearly two centuries care for the mentally impaired elderly has been fettered by the myth of incurability and of the uselessness of treatment, perpetuated by a fatalistic view toward the psychological events of aging. This widespread, tenacious pessimism constitutes the main obstacle to the implementation of rational care for the elderly patient with mental impairments.

E. ESQUIROL (1816) was the first physician to draw a sharp line of distinction between congenital and acquired mental impairments. As he put it : "...in dementia,men appear as if deprived of something they once possessed...," "... they are comparable to formerly wealthy men who have fallen on hard times," whereas "idiots have always dwelt in mental misfortune and misery.". He also recognized that there are acute as well as chronic forms of dementia with entirely different prognoses. E. ESQUIROL and E. GEORGET (1820) termed the acute form of dementia "stupidity". As pointed out by P. CHASLIN (1895), patients suffering from this type of dementia "may recover just as completely as those affected by maniacal delirium, contrary to the dementia from which there is no recovery." It is interesting to note, in passing, that in the Nineteenth Century, clinicians tended to focus their attention on the illness and to neglect the patient as a human being. But emphasizing impairments while over-looking residual capacity fosters defeatism and promotes a do-nothing attitude. In the past, such pessimism has resulted in the virtual rejection and abandonment of countless patients. But even more distressing, it is an attitude which has rebounded in gerontological circles over the past few years due to the circulation of misleading information. PHILIBERT (1981) has exposed some of these false notions for the threadbare rationalizations they are, particularly those equating dementia with aging and advanced age with decline and death.

There can be no doubt that assessment of residual capacity must take precedence over pedantic preoccupation with the identification of impairments. If impairments are to be investigated in minute detail, then sound clinical practice demands that equal attention be devoted to residual capacity. Assessments affording patients every opportunity to demonstrate maximum performance and ability to acquire new skills imply an entirely different clinical and therapeutic intent than evaluations limited to the assessment of impairments. Moreover, inferring residual capacity from observed impairments is not the same as isolating impairments from residual capacity. In other words, it is preferable to determine impairments from residual capacity and not residual capacity from impairments.

b. Rational evaluation of the psychological events of aging is further hampered by a medical attitude which too often approaches etiology with a narrow notion of causality and abusively quantifies behaviour without due regard for its qualitative significance to overall performance.

The ambiguity which still permeates psychiatric diagnosis is due not only to our inability to demonstrate organicity clinically, but also to the practice of establishing diagnoses exclusively on the basis of mental impairment. An example of this is the confusion of dementia with mental deterioration. Mental deterioration is by no means a synonym of dementia. Melancholics may temporarily lose use of their cognitive abilities without for all that being demented. This important point was beclouded in the last century by the inclusion of the so-called vesanias in the prevalent classificatory system (it will be recalled that in this concept, the more advanced phases of certain chronic mental disorders such as mood disorders and delusional states were considered true dementias) as well as the concept of dementia praecox prior to its dynamic reinterpretation by E. BLEULER (1908). The attention paid more recently in geriatric psychiatry to the regressive states of the elderly, wrongly considered as states of dementification, has promoted distrust of loose terminology and prompted many to shun certain expressions such as "sinking into (a state of) dementia," which are likely to distort clinical thinking and thus to prevent establishment of a valid correlation between psychopathological reactions and organic lesions.

The etiology of dementia challenges the very foundations of clinical diagnosis and of the relevancy of causality to medical practice. From an etiological or physiopathological standpoint, the purpose of medicine is to decrease or eradicate the incidence of disease. From the viewpoint of adaptive medicine, it is to promote more immediate, individualized aims.

Attempts to quantify mental events hark back to F. GALTON (1876). The influence of his work on behavioural science is evident in the rapid development of differential psychology initiated by STERN (1900). Differential psychology greatly increased clinical focus on impairments. By placing the accent on this aspect of clinical examination it sanctioned the segregation of certain psychiatric patients. It contributed to the denial of rehabilitation for the mentally impaired because it only took overall performance into account, completely disregarding the appropriate strategies developed by patients in their unsuccessful efforts to achieve adequate performance. By overrating the value of the intellectual quotient, it created arbitrary categories and served as a pretext for inadequate care. It brought about the almost total equation of mental disorders with organicity, even though there is still no known organic basis for many mental disorders.

c. Conservatism constitutes yet a third obstacle to the scientific clinical study and effective treatment of the psychological events of aging. Standard medical procedures will have to be discarded, when the time comes, to make way for new knowledge and clinical approaches in a particular field capable of serving as models for new practices. There is also a need to defer certain questions, which should be postponed or reformulated because their impact is still too remote to contribute tangibly to current needs.

The use of models in geriatric psychiatry has been a necessary step in the accumulation of sound knowledge of the mental phenomena of advanced age. The SOMATOMORPHIC model helped establish psychiatry as a medical discipline. Thus, in dealing with states of dementification, clinicians may use the same reasoning as that applied in internal medicine. It is, however, quite obvious that mental disorders cannot be explained by linear causality alone.

The INFANTOMORPHIC model allows comparison of the behaviour of the elderly with behaviour appropiate to various develepmental phases.

For the brief time before it was discarded, the NORMOMORPHIC model identified everything that was non pathological as "normal". This model is also responsible for the distinction drawn between senescence and senility, a view which offers little hope for the immediate or future solution of the problems posed by states of dementification. Even though there are as yet no well-defined indicators of biological age in adult life, reference to age (which can still only be chronological) and to aging can only take on meaning in a developmental perspective, which extends to later life the observations recorded for infants, adolescents and young adults.

Throughout the history of psychiatry there has been a pronounced tendency for clinicians to feel that solutions to specific problems must await the final settlement of such broad general issues as "heredity versus environment", "psychogenesis versus organogenesis", or "normal versus abnormal". Such lofty considerations have little practical value for routine clinical practice. Indeed, it would be tantamount to dereliction of duty for clinicians to await the final word on such issues before making the practical decisions the well-being of their patients requires.

Still another way of looking at the relation between the normal and the pathological is the concept of normativity introduced by G. CANGUILHEM (1943). The possibility of simultaneously taking into account, hic et nunc, the illness, the patient and his environment constitutes an innovative approach to the solution of clinical problems. The shift in priority results from different aims more directly suited to the immediate needs of the patient. According to this view, hypotheses should be considered tentative and should be discarded whenever they fail to give results. They should be resorted to only to organise findings, to prevent oversimplification, to substantiate experience, for oversimplification and excessive generalisation are at the root of the notion that dementia is the unavoidable fate and natural state of the elderly.

III. A NEW CLINICAL APPROACH TO STATES OF DEMENTIFICATION

a. At present, clinical understanding of states of dementification is guided by the following principles :

1. medical aims are proportional to the value placed on human life and dignity;

2. physicians involved in the diagnosis and treatment of conditions for which there are as yet no known cures focus their attention on the patient, his environment and his care; this includes providing assistance where necessary. As it is not known when medicine will discover ethical cures, it is permissible to investigate morbid conditions in their own right;

3. clinical diagnosis is determined by treatment objectives. This means that diagnosis is subordinate to treatment. Its use should not be limited to the consolidation of scientific knowledge. Its prime purpose should be the well-being of the patient, his optimal adjustment to his condition. It should be essentially directed toward the enhancement and exercise of residual capacity. It should make adjustments for the bias introduced by clinicians, doctrines, theories and terminology. It demands not only the qualitative analysis of behaviour, but also its simultaneous interpretation according to both cross-sectional and longitudinal criteria, as well as evaluation of means of modifying it. It should disregard all but positive prognoses.

b. The structural analysis of behaviour constitutes a major step in the clinical evaluation of the dementias of later life. It provides a better understanding of the manner in which certain types of behaviour occur and of the functional significance of pathological behaviour. Developmental psychology, particularly that inspired by J. PIAGET, has led to a better understanding of clinical manifestations by calling attention to the adaptative aspect of operativity and instrumental performance. This has enabled clinicians to overcome the discrepancy between global intellectual impairment and instrumentality, that is to say between noeticians and anti-noeticians, which long hampered clinical progress with regard to states of dementification. It has opened up new avenues to the study of cognition in elderly patients with various degrees of dementification. Within this theoretical framework, thought is defined as an extension or internationalisation of action, while reasoning is seen as a mental experiment or an empirical internal groping which generates working hypotheses.

The developmental phases of J. PIAGET, which have been used to explain the organisation of behaviour associated with the dementification process, applies to periods during which various types of behaviour may be considered in a state of equilibrium. The state of equilibrium peculiar to a given developmental phase governs overall performance and behaviour. The transition from one developmental phase to another is not abrupt but rather all behavioural modifications remain consistent with the state of equilibrium regulating overall behaviour until a new state of equilibrium, incorporating the preceding, is fully established.

The developmental stages described by J. PIAGET have been observed in most of the operational fields in which the cognitive performance of the intellectually impaired patient has been tested (physical quantities, space, time, numbers, etc.). Within a given field the homogeneity of the operational level and the hierarchy of the developmental stages is maintained. In the intellectually impaired patient, however, we find relative homogeneity between the different operational fields and a specific reasoning process which results in low performance on temporospatial problems and logic in comparison th the so-called infra-logical capacities of the conservation of physical quantities. This can be explained by an alteration of anticipatory representation which is particularly evident in serial transformations and the implementation of inductive reasoning. As for praxias, there are organizational schemes which allow the coordination of spatial data independently of a sense of perspective, but which presuppose an intact ability to handle serial nesting.

By the same token the intellectually impaired may be able to control space through their bodies (ideomotor praxia) without being able to handle so called objective or euclidian space (constructive praxia), but must be able to handle practical space resulting from the temporospatial grouping of POINCARE and PIAGET (ideational praxia). It is in this manner that knowledge of the ratios between the various successive aspects of cognitive activity in the intellectually impaired elderly has made it possible to establish hypotheses about the origin and development of observed structural modifications.

c. Because any one type of behaviour may only be the uniform manifestation of various types of difficulties, the inferred mechanisms do not always furnish an accurate picture of the patient's optimal capacities. It has therefore been necessary to explain why the intellectually impaired prefer one kind of problem solving to another. It has also been necessary to investigate the laws governing the selection of actions announcing the appearance of a new type of problem-solving behaviour, for it became increasingly evident that this was the most relevant criteron for gauging the problems at hand. Nevertheless, it is certain that the range of possible problem-solving mechanisms, the ease with which they can be implemented and selected for a specific purpose remain dependent on the level of organisation of the cognitive processes, even when subjected to conative influences. In studying the sense of orientation of the intellectually impaired, the observer is struck less by difficulty in orienting correctly or by the different forms assumed by disorientation than by the patient's perseveration in a given approach to orientation and his failure to make use of mechanisms of orientation which he is known to retain intact.

To the extent that it adheres to the present objectives of medical action in geriatric psychiatry,this clinical concept of dementia, by drawing its inferences from an understanding of acquired behaviours offers a more functional approach. It is supported by the observation that the abilities of the dementified never appear absolutely stable, whatever the extent of organic lesions. It substantiates the postulate of B. INHELDER, according to which the structural analysis of a type of problem-solving behaviour must be confirmed by analysis of the choices the subject makes and uses effectively when he is confronted with a specific task to perform, i.e. choice of the processes of action.

IV. CONCLUSIONS

Geriatric psychiatry owes its identity as an independent specialty to the discovery and practical application of several basic rules which have resulted in recent advances in the clinical evaluation of mental impairments. These rules underscore the tenuousness of previous evaluative criteria. They reveal the flaws inherent in conventional views of behaviour and the inadequacies of the rating scales by which behaviour is currently gauged. They stress a clinical approach which is guided by therapeutic aims and revives the concept of dynamic medical action, particulary with a view to readjustment to a new level of residual capacity. In this manner, they show that problem-solving behaviour, previously considered the most reliable indicator of the extent of organicity, has been greatly overrated. Thus, for example, the induced grasping reflex, the oral reflex and resistance hypertonia occur later than previously, for the same degree of anatomically verified organic deterioration. The reestablishment of function, analysis of the structure and mechanisms of problem solving behaviour, a functional approach and the study of action processes are becoming the decisive criteria for the clinical management of mental impairment in the elderly and the springboard to future research and epidemiological investigations.

Acknowledgement

We wish to thank Dr. A. Hooton for translating from the original French.

VII. CLINICAL ASPECTS OF ALZHEIMER'S DISEASE: PART TWO

Presided by R.N. Butler (New York)

Senile Dementia: Outlook for the Future, pages 269–277

UNSOLVED CLINICAL PROBLEMS IN ADVANCED SENILE DEMENTIA

H.B.Stähelin, A.M.Hew-Winzeler, D.Behrens,
W.O.Seiler, J.Ulrich
Geriatric Clinics Kantonsspital and Felix Platter Spital and Institute of Pathology, University of Basle, 4031 Basle, Switzerland

INTRODUCTION

Senile dementia has undoubtly the greatest impact on the quality of life of the elderly population. Since ancient times clinical features are well known but only recently the disorder is recognized as a disease state rather than an effect of aging per se. The growing number of affected individuals and the consequences for our health-resources make it urgent to find ways and means to relieve the striken individual and the society at large.

Impressive advances were made in our knowledge about senile dementia. Several distinct forms, some of them amendable to improvement, were identified. Little or no progress however, occured in the therapy for senile dementia of the Alzheimer type (SDAT) which is alone or in combination with multiinfarction dementia (MID) responsible for the senile dementia in the majority of the affected subjects (11).

SDAT is from a clinical and practical point of view the most important affection. Since it is a disease of uncertain origin no prevention or treatment of the cause is available. Furthermore exact diagnosis during life time is difficult. These general remarks are well known and often cited. A corollary of these facts is, that therapy has to be at best symptomatic.

Patients with advanced stages of the dementia syndrome require extensive supportive care. Presently available therapy for clinical problems in advanced SDAT is in general not developed. Therapeutic measures are instituted according to symptoms in analogy to other distinct neurological or psychiatric diseases. It goes withaout saying that treatment which is effective in a different disease with similar symptoms may be without success in SDAT.

In analogy to research on atherosclerosis - a chronic disease of advancing age of multifactorial origin - one can take either an academic or a pragmatic view of senile dementia (2). The academic view looks for a complete understanding of the disease. Research will hopefully bring us one day toward a full understanding of SDAT and allow a cure or even better,prevention. The pragmatic view faces the fact that in the forseeable future neither cure nor prevention are likely to occur. Any improvement of the symptoms is welcome. The use of acetylcholine precursors or cholinergic compounds seems to be a first scientifically founded pragmatic approach. The cholinergic deficit-hypothesis is well founded on clinical pathological evidence (4). Until now however substitution with choline was not very successfull (6). Precursors, particularly lecithin are abundant in lipoproteins and one might wonder, whether the simple addition of choline or lecithin to the diet effectively increases the precursor concentration in the vicinity of the neurons or enhances the uptake of choline in the nerve terminal although it appears to be the case in animal studies (12). Nevertheless, drugs which improve cholinergic transmission and possibly prevent postsynaptic deterioration seem interesting and usefull.

Often an accurate diagnosis is not possible. Even brain biopsy or a specific biological marker will not enable us to decide in a patient with SDAT and MID often occuring together,which disease contributes more to the clinical condition.

RISK FACTORS IN SENILE DEMENTIA

We feel that prevention of MID should be more easily achievable if the risk factors for MID are diagnosed and treated carefully. In a small retrospective study we evaluated cardiovascular risk factors in SDAT and MID. According to necropsy data of our clinic, the neuropathologist identified 10 SDAT and 9 MID cases. The prevalence of diabetes, hypertension and coronary heart disease was compared as well as heart weight, serum lipid levels, body weight and brain weight. The significantly higher heart weight in MID and the high prevalence of hypertension identifies this condition as the most important risk factor especially if diabetes is also present (Tab.1). It may be noted that diabetes is much more frequently observed in MID but not absent in SDAT. Thus the hypothesis of hypoglycemia as causative factor in Alzheimer as put forward by Adolfsson is not corroborated in our experience (1).

Tab.1 Retrospective Comparison of SDAT and MID

		SDAT	MID
n		10	9
Age at Death		78,5 ± 6,6[1]	83,2 ± 6,4
Body Weight kg		53,8 ± 11,6	55,8 ± 8,5
Length cm		164,0 ± 11,5	165,0 ± 6,5
Hypertension	Yes	4	8
Coronary Heart Disease	Yes	3	6
Diabetes mellitus	Yes	1	4
Heart Weight g		378 ± 44	464 ± 114*
Brain Weight g		1210 ± 189	1194 ± 110
Cholesterol mmol/l		4,41 ± 0,72	3,77 ± 1,03
Triglycerides mmol/l		1,20 ± 0,45	1,26 ± 0,53

*) p 0,025
1) mean ± SD

Out of a group of 106 patients with organic brain syndrom who died between 1978 and 1980 19 were identified of suffering either from SDAT or MID.

The pragmatic lesson taught by these figures is that hypertension has to be treated most vigorously. Prevention of MID through hypertension control might improve the quality of life of a great number of our elderly citizens.

THE PROBLEM OF DEPRESSION IN SENILE DEMENTIA

In the differential diagnosis pseudodementia in depressive subjects has to be considered. We investigated, as a part of an ongoing multidisciplinary study of senile dementia, the suppression of cortisol by dexamethasone in 22 depressed senile dementia patients (Fig.1).

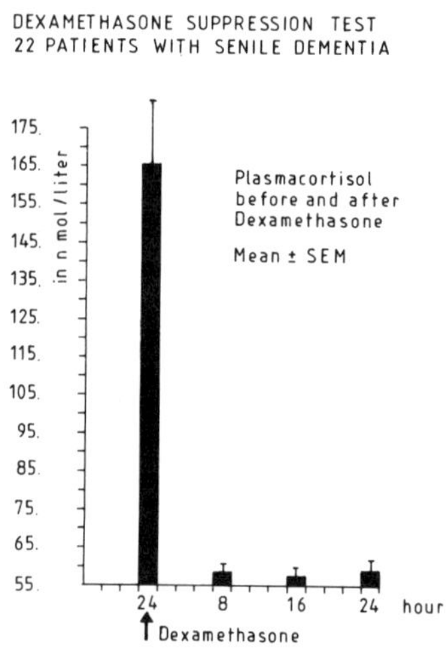

Fig. 1. In all but one subject dexamethasone suppressed the endogenous cortisol for 24 hours. The single exception showed no characteristic suppression as the 8 hours value but not the 24 hours value was above 165 nmol which is the upper limit suggested by Carroll (5).

The normal dexamethasone suppression test suggests that a further pathogenetic mechanism has to be invoked to explain the depressed state in senile dementia other than the one effective in depression. In keeping with this observation is the well known fact that antidepressant drug therapy has to be administred in low dosages in the elderly. The response is often unsatisfactory and the high prevalence of anticholinergic side effects and toxicity is well known.

The pragmatic conclusion therefore is: In senile dementia there exists a demand for more specific drugs to improve symptoms of depression. The large number of affected subjects would certainly warrant specific research directed at this goal.

EXTRAPYRAMIDAL SYMPTOMS IN SENILE DEMENTIA

In advanced cases of SD, Apraxia, incontinence and extrapyramidal symptoms (EPS) become increasingly prominent. In these patients a therapeutic dilemma exists. Treatment by anticholinergic drugs might in theory aggravate the underlying disease. EPS might also result from treatment with neuroleptic drugs. The extrapyramidal disorders of Alzheimer disease are well recognized since the work of Pearce (9). The relation between Parkinson disease and dementia is also well documented. Lieberman et al. found moderate to marked dementia in 32% of 520 patients with idiopathic Parkinsonism (8). Boller et al. observed a similar prevalence of SD in patients with Parkinsonism (3). The latter found a good correlation between dementia and extent of Alzheimer changes. From a theoretical point of view dopa could also aggravate SDAT by inhibition of the remaining cholinergic system. Certainly anticholinergic drugs seem unfavorable in SDAT. It appears that drug induced hallucinations are more likely to occur in patients with Parkinson disease and concomitant SDAT. In contrast to idiopathic Parkinsonism, abnormalities of the dopaminergic system have not been a consistent finding in primary degenerative dementia.

These ideas prompted us to investigate the clinical symptoms, drug therapy, and histopathological findings in senile dementia. 78 patients of the geriatric clinic (43 males, 35 females) were thoroughly documented during 1980-1982. Until now 40 patients died. A complete clinical and neuropathological workup was possible in 37 patients. (One patient died too early after enrollement, another had a massive intracerebral hemorrhage and in a third brain autopsy was not possible).

Of 37 patients 28 had histological signs of SDAT (Fig.2). MID was observed in 17 patients, 14 of whom had simultaneously SDAT. Signs of Parkinsons disease were found in 6 patients, 3 in combination with SDAT, one in combination with MID. 3 subjects had almost normal brain histology, in one a Steele-Richardson, in an other a Wernicke Korsakow syndrome were found.

PROSPECTIVE STUDY ON SENILE DEMENTIA

Necropsy Findings SDAT	MID	PAR	n	m/f	AGE (MEAN±SD)
■	□	□	11	6/5	83.5 ± 6.8
■	■	□	14	7/7	85.7 ± 6.2
■	□	■	2	1/1	81
■	■	■	1	0/1	75
□	■	□	1	1/0	86
□	■	■	1	1/0	78
□	□	■	2	2/0	67.5
□	□	□	5	4/1	75.2 ± 5.9

Symptoms of Parkinsonism were observed in 50% of our patients with SDAT (group 1 and 2, Tab.2). Pomara and co-workers (10) reported in 40%,moderate to pronounced EPS in SDAT. They found a significant correlation between EPS and cognitive impairment. This indicates that in advanced disease stages EPS become more predominant. Of our patients 1/4 were in such an advanced stage that cognitive tests (e.g. the Mini Mental Status of Folstein) were no longer applicable. In our group 2 (SDAT + MID) the severity of EPS seemed to be probably sligthly lower than in group 1 (SDAT). The pathological changes in substantia nigra and locus coeruleus were however comparable (Tab.2). In the SDAT + MID group basal ganglia were affected more severely. In this group tardive dyskinesia was more frequent.

Tab.2 Extrapyramidal Symptoms and Neuropathological Findings in Senile Dementia

Clinical and Pathological Findings	SDAT n = 11	SDAT + MID n = 14
Parkinson Symptoms	5 (45%)	7 (50%)
Average EPS-Score[1]	1.4	1.3
Tardive Dyskinesia	3 (27%)	6 (43%)
Substantia Nigra[2]	1.3	1.54
Locus Coeruleus	1.1	1.2
Basal Ganglia	0.7	1.2

1) Tremor, Cogwheel sign, and walk were scored and averaged.
2) Pathological changes were graded from 0-3 and averaged.

Griffiths et al. (8) among others already pointed out that arteriosclerosis might possibly contribute to the production of senile Parkinsonism, but clinical symptoms did not allow a distinction between SDAT or MID in our study.

Dopaminergic therapy was given in 1/2 of all cases, anticholinergic therapy over 1/3 (Tab.3). Possibly, the higher EPS score in SDAT reflects only the fact that approximately 90% of SDAT patients received neuroleptic treatment. In the SDAT + MID group the percentage was lower (around 60%).

Tab.3 CNS-Drugs[1] in Patients with Advanced Senile Dementia

Drugs	SDAT n = 11	SDAT + MID n = 14
Neuroleptics	9 (82)*	9 (64)
Antidepressant	6 (55)	8 (57)
Anticholinergic	3 (27)	4 (29)
Dopa etc.	5 (45)	5 (36)

1) During hospital stay *Percentage

IN CONCLUSION

Therapy of EPS in our group was probably too pragmatic. In SDAT, neuroleptic therapy may be dangerous if it coexists with idiopathic Parkinsonism. On the other hand anticholinergic and dopaminergic drugs are of doubtfull theoretical value in the treatment of EPS in SDAT. The clinical impression, however, is that these drugs do not aggravate the dementia in an obvious way. This certainly casts some doubt on the importance of the choline-deficit model in advanced SDAT. A better understanding of advanced stages of primary degenerative dementia is needed in order to cope more effectively with this often prolonged, expensive and distressing period of the illness. Besides the search for a cure and prevention of SDAT more effort and more research has to go into the study of the more advanced stages of the disease. I am well aware of the obstacles, difficulties and complexities of such an endeavour. But the attempt to influence symptoms of SDAT by therapies derived solely by analogy from other neurological and psychiatric diseases is too simplistic and unsatisfactory.

REFERENCES

1) Adolfsson R, Bucht G, Lithner F, Winblad B (1980). Hypoglycemia in Alzheimer's disease. Acta Med Scand 208: 387.
2) Blackburn H (1975). Contrasting professional views on atherosclerosis and coronary disease. N Engl J Med 292: 105.
3) Boller F, Mizutani T, Roessmann U, Gambetti P (1980). Parkinson disease, dementia and Alzheimer disease: clinicopathological correlations. Ann Neurol 7: 329.
4) Bowen DM, Sims NR, Benton S, Haan EA, Smith CCT, Neary D, Thomas DJ, Davison AN (1982). Biochemical changes in cortical brain biopsies from demented patients in relation to morphological findings and pathogenesis. Aging 19: 1.
5) Carroll BJ, Curtis GC, Mendels J (1976). Neuroendocrine regulation in depression, II, discrimination of depressed from non depressed patients. Arch Gen Psychiat 33: 1051.
6) Ferris SH, Sathananthan G, Reisberg B, Gershon S (1979). Long-term choline treatment of memory-impaired elderly

patients. Science 205: 1039.
7) Griffiths RA, Dalziel JA, Sinclair KGA, Dennis PD, Good WR (1979). Tremor and senile Parkinsonism. J Gerontol 36: 170.
8) Lieberman A, Dziatolowski M, Kupersmith M, Serby M, Goodgold A, Korein J, Goldstein M (1979). Dementia in Parkinson disease. Ann Neurol 6: 355.
9) Pearce J (1974). The extrapyramidal disorder of Alzheimer's disease. Europ Neurol 12: 94.
10) Pomara N, Reisberg B, Albers S, Ferris S, Gershon S (1981) Extrapyramidal symptoms in patients with primary degenerative dementia. J Clin Psychopharmacol 1: 398.
11) Tomlinson BE (1970). Observations on brains of demented old people. J Neur Sci 11: 205.
12) Wurtman RJ, Zeisel SH (1982). Brain choline: its sources and effects on the synthesis and release of acetylcholine. Aging 19: 303.

Senile Dementia: Outlook for the Future, pages 279–282

APHASIA AS A FIRST SIGN OF DEMENTIA

Assal G., Favre C., Regli F.

Centre de Neuro-Psychologie et pathologie
du langage - CHUV
1011 Lausanne - Suisse

Aphasia is quite common in the evolution of degenerative dementia (Alzheimer's disease, Pick's dementia, senile dementia). It frequently starts with a difficulty in finding words often developping into the syndrome of isolation speech area(transcortical sensory aphasia). Articulatory and syntax disorders are absent but the semantic function is deeply disorganized. (Whitaker 1976, Assal et al. 1981, Appel et al. 1982). As a rule aphasia is not one of the first signs of dementia although such a case was reported by Wechsler (1977).

Slowly progressive aphasia which severity contrasts with preserved mental aptitudes during a long period of time was discussed lately by Mesulam (1982). We report here the observation of a patient whose evolution has some similarities with Mesulam's cases.

Case report

M. C. is a 64 years old right handed female who presented 4 years ago depressive manifestations followed by elocution difficulties. Neurological examination and computerized tomography (CT) scan were normal at the time. Almost four years after onset the patient's behavior is still adapted: she lives alone, does her housework and works part-time. Neurological examination is again normal. CT scan shows a cortico-sub-cortical atrophy with a widening of both sylvian fissures without asymmetry. In the meantime language disorders have much worsened and spontaneous language is now limited to badly articulated utterances. The rare intelligible sequences are agrammatic. Repetition and denomination are almost impossible. Auditory verbal comprehension is impaired even for simple commands. There is a dissociation between good understanding of semantics and severe difficulties in understanding syntax and grammar. As for written language, oralization of reading is similar to oral language, that is unintelligible. Understanding of reading follows the same pattern as understanding of oral language (a dissociation between semantic and syntax/grammar). Graphism is good in writing, copying is correct (not slavish), spontaneous writing is agrammatic but well spelled. Dictation of letters is possible. Concerning words, there is a dissociation between good preservation of concrete words and strong impairement in the writing of functors. Written denomination is much better than the oral one. The patient has no difficulty in written calculation but is unable to calculate orally. Constructive and ideomotor praxias are but slightly impaired; there is an important buccofacial apraxia. Somatognosia is not impaired. Visual recognition is good. Memorization of Rey's 15 words is successful if presentation and reponses are written. Evocation of the Complex figure of Rey is sufficient. Cognitive functions are lowered but still normal (Performance scale of WAIS : 90.Progressive Matrix : C 25).

Three months later a neuropsychological control shows a general deterioration of language functions but behavior and practo-gnosia remain unchanged.

Discussion

Our observation shows a severe and progressive global aphasia still worsening at the present time with mild associate desorders. In the case of a degenerative dementia such a severe aphasia would accompany a global deterioration of non verbal functions. In our patient global deterioration is on the contrary progressing very slowly and remains minimal. The CT scan findings show a light cortico-sub-cortical atrophy with widening of both sylvian fissures without asymmetry. No focalized lesion is present. Atrophy seems to be progressive but it is difficult to be positive about it since the CT scans were obtained with different techniques.

This symptomatology suggests a focalized cerebral degeneration as seen in Mesulam's observations. This author recently reported six case stories with language disorders beginning in the presenium (except a 17 years old patient). At onset patients have difficulty in finding words (except the patient cited who has a pure word deafness), then language deficits slowly worsen ; but no global aphasia is described. Neurological examination remain normal or lightly impaired and non verbal intellectual aptitudes are often unchanged for a long period of evolution. Neuroradiological findings suggest a left hemispheric perisylvian lesion. No case was anatomically investigated allowing for a precise etiological diagnosis. A cerebral biopsy made for one of the patients fails to show any modification specific of degenerating dementia.

It seems that Mesulam's findings and our own observation draw the attention on a still little known syndrome which neuropathological basis are not yet verified.

References

Appel J, Kertesz A, Fisman M (1982). A study of language functioning in Alzheimer patients. Brain and language 17 : 73-91.

Assal G, Delaloye A, Regli F (1981). Troubles du langage lors des démences séniles. Extraits du compte rendu du congrès de psychiatrie et de neurologie de langue française. 79ème session, p.331-336.

Mesulam M.M (1982). Slowly progressive aphasia without generalized dementia. Annals of neurology II : 592-598.

Wechsler A.F (1977). Presenile dementia presenting as aphasia. J. of neurol, neurosurg. and psychiatry 40 : 303-305.

Whitaker H (1976). A case of the isolation of the language functions. Studies in neurolinguistics 2 Academic Press, p 1-57.

Senile Dementia: Outlook for the Future, pages 283–289

THE PHILOTHERMAL RESPONSE: DIAGNOSTIC TEST FOR ALZHEIMER DISEASE?

Lissy F. Jarvik, M.D., Ph.D., and Steven S. Matsuyama, Ph.D.

Psychogeriatric Unit, West Los Angeles Veterans Administration Medical Center, Brentwood Division, Los Angeles, California 90073
and
Department of Psychiatry and Biobehavioral Sciences, UCLA, Los Angeles, California 90024

Supported in part by the National Institute of Mental Health Grant #MH 36205, West Los Angeles Veterans Administration Medical Center, Brentwood Division.

THE VIEWS EXPRESSED ARE NOT THOSE OF THE V.A.

Despite modern advances in medical technology (e.g., CT scan), the clinical diagnosis of dementia of the Alzheimer type (DAT) is difficult to make and remains a diagnosis of exclusion. Thus, there is, at the moment, no single laboratory test or combination of tests specific for DAT. An intensive search is underway for biological markers not only to aid in diagnosis, but also to shed light on etiology and pathogenesis, so that rational treatment may be developed and preventive measures taken.

In our laboratory we are evaluating the philothermal response as a potential biological marker for DAT. Philothermal response is the term we use to designate the tendency of cells to migrate along a temperature gradient toward the warmer temperature. The experimental technique to assess the philothermal response developed in our laboratory (Kessler et. al., 1979; Fu et. al., 1982), is designed to allow application of the temperature gradient by eliminating thermal convection. The basic methodology is as follows: We draw a sample of venous blood and prepare a polymorphonuclear leukocyte (PMN) cell suspension which we then add to hollow flat glass microslides that are partially filled with an agarose gel solution (0.75%). The preparation is then exposed to a temperature gradient for three hours (1.4 °C/mm).

The philothermal response is a function of the cell concentration and temperature gradient. Moreover, there are day-to-day variations. To assess these variations, we examined the total number of migrating cells in cell suspensions made daily from blood samples of two nominally healthy volunteers during a five-day period with isolated repeat determinations during the next two months. Despite the variability, there was no overlap between the two individuals (Fu et. al., 1982).

Initially, we investigated the philothermal response in relation to aging (Kessler et. al., 1979) since it is well known among physicians, but unfortunately not well documented, that with advancing age there is a reduced febrile response to infection and also a slight lowering of normal basal body temperature. When no significant age-related abnormalities were detected, we expanded our studies to include patients with DAT since there are theoretical grounds for expecting an abnormal philothermal response in these patients. Thus, an intact microtubular system is required for cell orientation and directed, unlike random, cell migration (Malech et. al., 1977). And, a microtubular defect has been postulated in DAT (Heston, 1976). Microtubules also play an important role in chromosome separation, and a microtubular abnormality may underlie the increased frequency of aneuploidy reported in DAT (Jarvik et. al., 1971; Matsuyama, in press). The defective cell migration reported in individuals with chromosomal abnormalities, most notably Down syndrome (Khan et. al., 1975; Seger et. al., 1976), supports the postulated relationship. Finally, there is the possibility that the philothermal response constitutes a new host defense mechanism and that the poor resistance to infection so often seen in patients with DAT may be the result of a defect in this host defense system. It is against this background that we investigated the philothermal response of cells obtained from patients with a clinical diagnosis of DAT.

The present report extends our previous publication

(Jarvik et. al., 1982) and concerns the findings derived from 18 patients with DAT, 10 men and 8 women, ranging from 55 to 90 years (mean = 74.8 $\pm$ 10.2 years). The clinical diagnosis of DAT was made in accord with the DSM III criteria for primary degenerative dementia after psychiatric, medical, and neurological examinations as well as clinical laboratory studies (including T4, folic acid, and serology). Fifteen of the patients (83%) had had CT scans and 13 (72%) EEGs; the results were consistent with the diagnosis of DAT. For comparison, we assess 18 relatively healthy individuals without mental disorder, matched by sex and age (ranging from 57 to 89 years, mean 72.9 $\pm$ 7.6 years) as closely as possible to the patients.*

The total number of cells (N) which had migrated in response to the temperature gradient was only slightly and insignificantly higher for the DAT patients than for the mentally normal individuals (271 $\pm$ 140 vs. 258 $\pm$ 97, respectively). However, these two groups did differ significantly in terms of the distance covered by the five cells furthest from the cell suspension source. This leading front parameter, D, was significantly shorter for the DAT patients (mean 808 $\pm$ 160 micrometers) than the mentally normal individuals (mean 998 $\pm$ 126 micrometers).

Another statistical parameter of the philothermal response, and one we believe may be the most meaningful clinically, is the value R, which is the ratio of the number of proximal cells (cells within the interval from 210 to 420 micrometers) to the number of distal cells (700 micrometers and beyond). A high R value indicates relatively few distal cells. The R values for the 18 DAT patients ranged from 4.8 to infinity; 15, however, had an R value greater than 11. By contrast, only one of the 18 mentally normal individuals had an R value greater than 11 (69-year-old man with R of 12.8). The remaining 17 had R values ranging from a low of 4.4 to a high of 10.2.

Clearly, it is important to have some estimate of the replicability of the R value. So far, we have accumulated data from seven individuals who had determinations at intervals ranging from one day to two years. Even though

*The current report adds seven patients with DAT and seven controls to those previously published (Jarvik et. al., 1982).

there was considerable variability, the R ratios which had all been below 11 at first examination, remained below 11 upon repeat examination.

Based on the above results, the philothermal response as quantified by the R value, appears to differentiate at least a subgroup of DAT patients from mentally normal individuals; 83% of the former, but only 5.6% of the latter, had an R of 11 or more. To date, none in the comparison group, but four of the 18 DAT patients have died, all with R values over 11, and we were able to obtain autopsies on three of them. In each case, the neuropathological examination confirmed the clinical diagnosis of DAT. However, the differentiation is not equivalent to diagnostic specificity.

To begin to answer the question of specificity, we evaluated the philothermal response of patients with clinically diagnosed multi-infarct dementia (MID) and with major depressive disorder unipolar type (DSM-III criteria). The three MID patients (two women and one man, ages 66-74 years) whose duration of illness ranged from four to 10 years, all had low R values (3.0, 4.2 and 4.3). All but one of the seven depressed patients (four women and three men, ranging in age from 50-70 years), also had R values below 11. The single exception was a 63-year-old man with an R of 11.2.

Collectively, these data suggest that the nonspecific accompaniments of dementing illness, as well as the symptoms of depression often seen in patients with DAT, are not responsible for the impaired cellular migration as quantified by R values over 11. Clearly, there is a need to evaluate a larger sample of patients with DAT, as well as patients with other dementing (e.g., MID, Huntington disease, and Parkinson dementia) and physical illnesses (e.g., rheumatoid arthritis, multiple sclerosis). The defect in cell migration (R greater than 11) was not a function of age, sex, or duration of illness. Nor was it related to specific medical problems; patients with hypertension, generalized arteriosclerosis and osteoarthritis having R values above as well as below 11. Individuals without diagnosed physical illness had among the lowest (4.4) as well as the highest (infinity) R values. Most of the patients were taking medications (diuretics, phenothiazines, and tricyclic antidepressants being the most common), but the few who were not, also had R values over 11. Many in the comparison group were not taking any medications, including the one with the elevated R (12.8). Others were taking diuretics, thyroid or aspirin and still had R values below 11. Five of the seven depressed patients were taking tricyclic antidepressants (imipramine or doxepin) at the time the blood sample was drawn, and yet, four of them had R values below 11, while the fifth had an R value of 11.2. The MID patients also received medications (including phenothiazine) and all had low R values. Thus, no single disease or drug was implicated in high R values.

As of now, we lack information on the mechanisms responsible for the reduced numbers of distally migrated cells which result in elevated R values. The numerous possibilities include a deficit of a fast moving subpopulation of cells, a slower average speed of individual cells, or a declining speed of cellular locomotion over time. In situ observations revealed the frequent occurence of cell collisions in the migration space which could well impair effective locomotion. Finally, and perhaps most importantly, less effective directed migration related to a microtubular defect could also result in apparent slowing of cell motion. These as well as other possible mechanisms await elucidation. Meanwhile, our studies suggest that the cellular response to a temperature gradient is compromised in a subgroup of DAT patients.

The question also arises whether or not exogenous factors present in the sera of patients with DAT are capable of modulating the philothermal response of normal cells. To answer this question, we assessed the effects of sera obtained from patients with a clinical diagnosis of DAT on the cells derived from healthy normal adults, and compared them to the effects of sera from young and elderly mentally healthy individuals (Matsuyama and Fu, in press). Serum samples were obtained from 12 individuals as follows: four patients with DAT, two men (61 and 83 years old) and two women (73 and 85 years old) with a mean age of 75.5 years; four relatively healthy normal individuals matched for age and sex to the DAT patients, two men (61 and 87 years old), and two women (69 and 84 years old) with a mean age of 75.3 years; and four healthy young adults, two men (24 and 36 years), and two women (28 and 33 years old), with a mean age of 30.3 years.

Polymorphonuclear leukocytes were obtained from three healthy non-demented individuals, one woman (28 years old), and two men (36 and 87 years old). The individual cell suspensions were aliquotted and serum was added to each for a final concentration of 10% (The serum samples were all coded by an individual who was not directly involved in the experiment). The microslide tubes were filled with these cells suspensions which were then exposed to the temperature gradient for three hours.

The results were strikingly different for the sera from patients with DAT and all others. In the presence of serum from normal adults a large number of cells (137-352) migrated from the cell suspension source, while in the presence of serum from DAT patients, very few cells (12-20) migrated beyond the meniscus. Overall, there was a significant serum effect (df: 3 and 8, $F=17.4$, $P<0.001$) and the response to DAT serum differed significantly from that to normal elderly serum ($P<0.001$).

We wondered whether the serum from the DAT patients acted as a chemoattractant and thereby prevented the cells from exhibiting the normal philothermal response. We investigated this possibility and found only one of the four DAT sera exhibiting any chemoattractant activity at all. Thus, chemoattraction cannot explain the consistent inhibitory effect of the serum samples from each of the four DAT patients. Clearly, a factor (or factors) in the serum of these four DAT patients was (were) capable of inhibiting the philothermal response. It remains to be established whether the sera of patients with DAT contain inhibitory factors or lack migration stimulating factors. The nature of the factor(s) remains to be explored, initially by traditional biochemical procedures. While the serum factor(s) may represent a biological marker(s) for DAT, there is also the possibility that it (they) may signal subclinical infection.

In summary, our preliminary findings of abnormal philothermal response in patients with DAT--as well as humoral factors in their serum capable of significantly affecting that response--are promising. Further investigations are needed to assess the usefulness of the philothermal response as a biological aid in the diagnosis of DAT. Aside from increasing our sample sizes as well as investigating individuals with other dementias and physical illnesses, every attempt will be made to obtain neuropathological confirmation of the clinically diagnosed DAT patients and the mentally normal elderly adults with normal as well as elevated R values. As in any scientific inquiry, confirmation of findings by independent laboratories is essential, and we eagerly await the results of attempts at replication.

Fu TK, Kessler JO, Jarvik LF, Matsuyama SS (1982). Philothermal and chemotactic locomotion of leukocytes: Methods and results. Cell Biophys 4:77.

Heston LL (1976). Alzheimer's disease, trisomy 21, and myeloproliferative disorders: Associations suggesting a genetic diathesis. Science 196:322.

Jarvik LF, Altshuler KZ, Kato T, Blumner B (1971). Organic brain syndrome and chromosome loss in aged twins. Dis Nerv Syst 32:159.

Jarvik LF, Matsuyama SS, Kessler JO, Fu TK, Tsai SY, Clark EO (1982). Philothermal response of polymorphonuclear leukocytes in dementia of the Alzheimer's type. Neurobiol of Aging 3:93.

Kessler JO, Jarvik LF, Fu TK, Matsuyama SS (1979). Thermotaxis, chemotaxis and age. Age 2:5.

Khan AJ, Evans HE, Glass L, Shin YH, Almonte D (1975). Defective neutrophil chemotaxis in patients with Down's Syndrome. J Pediatr 87:87.

Malech HL, Root RK, Gallin JI (1977). Structural analysis of human neutrophil migration: Centriole, microtubule, and microfilament orientation and function during chemotaxis. J Cell Biol 75:666.

Matsuyama SS (in press). Genetic factors and chromosomal abnormalities in dementia of the Alzheimer type. In Reisberg B (ed): "Alzheimer's Disease and Senile Dementia," New York: The Free Press.

Matsuyama SS, Fu TK (in press). Inhibition of normal polymorphonuclear philothermal response by serum from dementia of the Alzheimer type patients. Age.

Seger D, Wildfever A, Bushinger G, Roman W, Catty D, Dybus L, Haferkamp O, Stroder J (1976). Defects in granulocyte function in various chromosome abnormalities. Klin Wochenschr 54:177.

Senile Dementia: Outlook for the Future, pages 291–303

MECHANISM OF ELECTROENCEPHALOGRAPHIC SHARP WAVE DISCHARGES IN DEMENTING ILLNESSES

Roger D. Traub, M.D.[1,2]
W. Douglas Knowles, Ph.D.[1]
Timothy A. Pedley, M.D.[2]

[1]IBM T.J. Watson Research Center,
Yorktown Heights, N.Y. 10598, U.S.A.

[2]Neurological Institute
New York, N.Y. 10032, U.S.A.

The electroencephalogram (EEG) of patients with Creutzfeldt-Jakob disease (CJD) often exhibits generalized sharp wave discharges, occurring with regular periods of 0.5 to 2.0 seconds (Burger et al., 1972). The EEG of patients with Alzheimer disease (AD) uncommonly contains generalized sharp waves (Watson, 1979; Faden and Townsend, 1976; Ehle and Johnson, 1977), and when present these waves do not show the typical periodicity of CJD (Gloor, 1980). Myoclonus, while reported in both diseases, is the rule in CJD (Traub et al., 1977), and the exception in AD (Jacob, 1970; Mayeux et al., 1980). There is an increased incidence of generalized seizures in both conditions (Traub et al., 1977), but in neither are they common. These observations must derive fundamentally from the different ways in which these disease processes affect the function of individual neurons and the interactions between neurons.

Two possibly distinct electrophysiological processes require explanation: (1) the mechanism whereby cellular activities become synchronized to produce EEG sharp waves (and also perhaps myoclonic jerks); and (2) the mechanism whereby cellular activities become periodic in CJD. Recent basic research in the context of epileptogenesis has provided insight into both of these processes, and suggests hypotheses that may explain the electrophysiological differences in these two diseases.

In 1981, we developed a theory to explain the periodic synchronized EEG events seen in CJD patients (Traub and Pedley, 1981). We proposed that these transients were analogous to interictal spikes, which have been shown in several experimental models of epilepsy to result from the synchronized bursting of a population of neurons. We further suggested that synchronization of neuronal bursting might occur in CJD because of viral-induced cell fusions, that result in de novo electrotonic junctions. We noted that high amplitude periodic EEGs could be seen in other infectious encephalitides (herpes simplex, SSPE) whose causative viruses could also induce cell fusion, at least in vitro. Our hypothesis assumes wider interest in view of the EEG sharp waves sometimes noted in AD patients. Spongiform changes may at times be seen in AD brains (Flament-Durand and Couck, 1979), and familial AD brain has as much in vitro cell-fusing activity as does CJD brain (Moreau-Dubois, Brown et al., 1981).

In the last few years, considerable progress has been made in understanding cellular mechanisms of epileptogenesis. In particular, the dominant role of chemical synaptic connections, as opposed to electrotonic junctions, has been established for the synchronized bursting during penicillin-induced "interictal spikes" in vitro (Schwartzkroin and Prince, 1978; Wong and Traub, 1983; Traub and Wong, 1983b). In this paper, we shall review two models of epileptogenesis as they relate to dementing illness: the hippocampal slice perfused with convulsant agents, and generalized penicillin epilepsy. In the slice, chemical synaptic connections mediate both synchronization itself and certain high frequency (10-20 Hz) oscillations analogous to tonic seizures. Periodic behavior of long periods (>4 seconds), on the other hand, probably results from intrinsic refractory intervals of individual cells in the population. Electrotonic junctions are likely to have modulatory effects. The cellular basis of generalized penicillin epilepsy is not known in as much detail, but this epilepsy model (originally developed to provide insight into absence seizures) is also highly relevant to the CJD problem: in generalized penicillin epilepsy, periodic EEG spikes having a wide cortical distribution also occur.

Epilepsy in the hippocampal slice: The hippocampal slice is able to manifest epileptiform activity analogous to an interictal spike: synchronized population cellular bursts with associated field potential transients. The relevant cellular mechanisms involve both intrinsic neuronal properties and the synaptic connections between neurons.

The principal neurons in the hippocampus are the pyramidal cells. Their soma-dendritic membranes contain a number of different voltage-sensitive ionic channels: Na^+, K^+, Ca^{2+}, "slow" Ca^{2+}-mediated K^+ channels, and perhaps other channels as well. Under the influence of synaptic inputs, these channels interact with one another to produce different modes of electrogenesis: isolated action potentials, trains of action potentials, and so-called intrinsic bursts. The latter can be generated by brief stimuli and also occur spontaneously. They consist of a train of 3 or more action potentials riding on an increasing slow depolarizing wave, followed by one or more "slow spikes" and then sometimes by one or more fast spikes, lasting 30-50 ms in all (Wong and Prince, 1981; Wong, Prince and Basbaum, 1979; Traub, 1982). Bursting is followed by a long duration, intrinsically-mediated afterhyperpolarization (AHP) caused at least in part by a K^+ current (Alger and Nicoll, 1980; Hotson and Prince, 1980).

Excitatory synaptic mechanisms within the hippocampal slice: Cells within CA3 have mutual excitatory synaptic interconnections (MacVicar and Dudek, 1980a). These interconnections are apparently sparse, since these authors observed one cell exciting another in only 5 out of 88 simultaneous pair recordings. The anatomical substrate of these mutual excitatory connections is unknown.

Action of convulsant agents in the slice: Epileptiform activity may be induced in the hippocampal slice by several different means. 1) Perfusion with penicillin or bicuculline produces blockade of synaptic inhibition (Wong and Prince, 1979; Dingledine and Gjerstad,1980; Schwartzkroin and Prince, 1980). 2) Lowering extracellular Cl^- also diminishes IPSPs (Ogata, 1978). 3) Kainic acid increases excitatory mechanisms (either synaptic or intrinsic membrane) (Lothman et al., 1981). 4) Raising extracellular $[K^+]$ increases cellular excitability (Hablitz and Lundervold, 1981; Prince and Schwartzkroin, 1978). Pencillin and bicuculline, in blocking synaptic inhibition, transform the effects one cell has on other cells, so that an output which normally elicits EPSP-IPSP sequences in other cells will instead elicit an EPSP alone. The stage is therefore set for signal amplification through a recurrently interconnected population.

Epileptiform activity in the hippocampal slice: Experimental epileptiform activity in the slice consists of synchronized cellular depolarizing bursts. These occur spontaneously and rhythmically, with a period of several seconds, and can be evoked by localized stimuli (Schwartzkroin and Prince, 1977, 1978; Wong and Traub, 1983; Traub and Wong, 1983a). During such an event an extracellular electrode records a so-called "ringing field potential" lasting 50-120 ms. Between events the field potential is flat. The intracellular manifestation of the population event consists of a depolarizing burst which can be recorded in any pyramidal cell in the slice. This burst occurs synchronously with the ringing field potential. A sustained AHP follows the epileptiform burst in each cell. Depolarization of a small number of CA2-CA3 cells with very small local applications of KCl can evoke a population event (Wong and Traub, 1983),save and intracellular stimulation of a single CA3 cell can at times evoke the complete event (Miles and Wong, 1982). The fact that these in vitro synchronized events seem to grow from activities beginning in very small subpopulations may serve to distinguish them from the generalized synchronized EEG phenomena of CJD.

The generation of synchronized bursts requires chemical synaptic transmission. If chemical transmission is blocked in a low-Ca^{2+} high-Mg^{2+} medium, then synchronized population discharges do not occur (Schwartzkroin and Prince, 1978; Oliver, Hoffer and Wyatt, 1978). In addition, if a cell is hyperpolarized by an injected current during the population event, one observes a depolarizing wave that is apparently an EPSP (Johnston and Brown, 1981; Wong and Traub, 1983). Thus, the depolarizing burst in each cell seems to arise from excitatory inputs impinging on it from other cells. These inputs trigger bursts in follower cells in the relative absence of synaptic inhibition. When a synchronized burst is triggered by a local stimulus, there is a latent period of about 100 ms during which the field potential and most intracellular potentials remain flat (i.e. at their respective resting potentials).

Synchronization model: Penicillin-induced epileptiform synchronized bursts have been reproduced with a simulation model based on known physiological principles: intrinsic bursting, chemical excitatory synaptic connections within CA3, and synaptic disinhibition (Traub and Wong, 1982). To model each individual cell, a CA3 cell simulation program was used (Traub, 1982). In a network of 100 model neurons, cells were interconnected randomly with a 5% probability that one cell directly excites any other. Synaptic connections were strong enough that bursting in one cell would evoke bursting in its followers. In this way, a localized stimulus (e.g. to 4 cells in the published example) would cause a set of "initiating" cells to burst. The initiating cells excite other cells to burst, and they in turn excite still others. This sequential excitation process is what produces the long latency to the population event. The simulated epileptiform synchronized discharge is terminated as the individual bursts are shut off by intrinsic membrane processes.

Periodicity of synchronized events: As mentioned above, epileptiform events occur periodically in the disinhibited hippocampal slice, as they do in in vivo acute epileptogenic foci, and less regularly in some human cases of focal epilepsy. Even in the resting slice, that is, one not treated with a convulsant agent, CA3 pyramidal neurons burst spontaneously, but asynchronously, with a period of about 1 second. If we assume that some cells continue to burst at 1 Hz in the disinhibited slice, computer simulations show that for suitable strengths of the excitatory synapses the population will exhibit periodic synchronized discharges at 0.5 Hz (Traub and Wong, 1983a). Period doubling occurs for the following reason: during alternate pacemaker cell bursts, almost all of the cells are still sufficiently hyperpolarized from the preceding population discharge, so that a new population event cannot be generated. This same model also reproduces the experimental observation that an interpolated population event resets the rhythm of succeeding periodic synchronized discharges (Traub and Wong, 1983a). This model does not yet explain why periods of 10 or more seconds can occur between epileptiform events. It is possible that the intrinsic bursting periods of individual cells are slowed in the presence of convulsant agents.

Electrotonic junctions: effects on synchronization: Electrotonic junctions have been seen in different regions of the hippocampal slice (Taylor and Dudek, 1982; MacVicar and Dudek, 1980b, 1981, 1982; Miles and Wong, 1982). Dye-coupling has also been observed between hippocampal neurons in vivo (MacVicar, Ropert et al., 1982) and between neocortical neurons in vitro (Gutnick and Prince, 1981). There is ultrastructural evidence for gap junctions in neocortex (Sloper, 1972). Electrotonically coupled cells occur in small clumps, rather than forming a syncytium that includes a significant population. Thus, it is unlikely that a stimulus to a few cells could spread solely through electrotonic junctions to cause synchronized bursting involving a significant region of the hippocampus. However, at least some pairs of neurons are electrotonically coupled with sufficient tightness so that intrinsic bursting evoked in one cell can in turn cause bursting in the other cell (Miles and Wong, 1982). We wish to know how electrotonic junctions modulate the synchronization process, given an underlying network of excitatory chemical synapses. A recent simulation study (Traub and Wong, 1983b) indicates that electrotonic junctions can have important, but sometimes surprising, effects. The effects a given set of electrotonic junctions have on the synchronization process depend on the behavior of the chemical synapses (Traub and Wong, 1983b). For example, with one set of parameters, they may serve to prevent synchronization, but with different parameters they may enhance synchronization. Determination of these relevant electrophysiological parameters (chemical and electrotonic interconnections and intrinsic membrane properties) in CJD and AD brain would be of great interest.

Generalized penicillin epilepsy: This experimental epilepsy model has been compared with human absence seizures because of the similarity of electrographic (Fisher and Prince, 1977a, 1977b; Gloor, 1979) and behavioral (Gloor, 1979) manifestations. Generalized penicillin epilepsy arises because of the interaction of a normal thalamus with a pharmaologically altered cortex. There are a number of excitatory thalamo-cortical projections systems, stimulation of which can produce characteristic cortical evoked responses. During barbiturate anesthesia in animals, 12-16 Hz rhythmic EEG waves (spindles) can occur in spontaneous runs. The waves in any given cortical region are apparently evoked by activity in specifically related regions of the ventrobasal thalamus (Andersen and Andersson, 1974).

After systemic administration of penicillin to an animal, 3-5 Hz rhythmic spike-wave patterns are seen in runs in the EEG. These occur synchronously between the two hemispheres, and the corpus callosum is required for this synchrony (Musgrave and Gloor, 1980). They are caused by the action of the drug on the cortex itself rather than on the thalamus: application of the drug in dilute solutions to the cortex elicits the phenomenon, while application to the thalamus does not (Gloor, Quesney and Zumstein, 1977). The thalamus must, however, be connected to the penicillin-treated cortex for the 3-5 Hz spike-wave to occur. Penicillin-treated isolated cortex displays a different and disorganized epileptiform activity (Pellegrini, Musgrave and Gloor, 1979). Intracellular recordings indicate that many (but not all) cortical neurons increase their firing rate or burst during the "spike", and most are hyperpolarized during the "wave" (Fisher and Prince, 1977b). The hyperpolarization appears to be an IPSP rather than an intrinsic membrane event since 1) it is decreased following increases in intracellular $[Cl^-]$, and 2) it appears even in the absence of a preceding cellular burst (Fisher and Prince, 1977b).

This model of epilepsy resembles CJD in that generalized periodic EEG events occur in both, albeit with different frequencies. It is not known if the thalamus is also required in CJD to trigger the EEG events in a pathologically altered cortex (Rayport, 1963; Nelson, 1968).

There are three further types of data which may indirectly shed light on epileptogenic mechanisms in the dementias. First, it is known in AD that there is a loss of cholinergic terminals in neocortex and hippocampus. There is now considerable intracellular information on the effects of acetylcholine (ACh) on hippocampal neurons (Benardo and Prince, 1981, 1982a, 1982b). Iontophoresed ACh often depolarizes neurons, in association with an increase in input resistance; these effects have been attributed to a decrease in a K^+ current. However, ACh also can hyperpolarize pyramidal cells, an effect perhaps secondary to ACh-induced stimulation of inhibitory interneurons. It is therefore not possible to predict the effects of ACh on tissue as a whole, since the response is a summation of effects on different cell types. Likewise, we can not predict the physiological effects of a chronic deficiency of ACh. It is interesting, however, that pharmacologic blockade of cholinergic transmission in cats leads to EEG delta waves (Schaul et al., 1978). This may be relevant to the slowing of background EEG rhythms in AD (Gordon and Sim, 1967).

Second, there is simplification of dendrites in AD and loss of dendritic spines in AD and CJD (Buell and Coleman, 1979; Scheibel, 1979; Landis et al., 1981). Schwartzkroin and Wyler (1980) have indicated that, other things being equal, this would promote the electrical coupling between dendrites and soma, and might increase excitability.

Finally, there are interesting data on the aging rat hippocampus suggesting that synapses onto granule cells are lost with senescence. Physiological compensation occurs, however, in that the effective strength of the remaining synapses is increased, perhaps by lowering the firing threshold of the granule cells (Barnes and McNaughton, 1980).

In conclusion, basic studies of epileptogenesis have lead to important insights concerning synchronization and rhythmicity of cellular activities. To apply these directly to the dementias, we need cellular electrophysiological data from this group of diseases. Intracellular recordings from human brain specimens studied in vitro have proved useful in investigating epilepsy (Prince and Wong, 1981; Schwartzkroin et al., 1983). A potential practical problem is the transmissible nature of CJD (Gajdusek et al. 1977). However, the existence of a cheap and easily constructed slice recording chamber (i.e. one that might be reusable after virus decontamination) (Nicoll and Alger, 1981) suggests that electrophysiological recordings may indeed be feasible from human diagnostic brain biopsy specimens or from brain specimens from animals with experimental CJD. Should this kind of experimentation be possible, we are likely to gain more direct understanding of the electrophysiological abnormalities occurring in human dementias.

Experiments in this direction can be guided by three hypotheses, not mutually exclusive: (1) EEG synchronization is enhanced by neuronal fusion, the latter being common in CJD and unusual in AD. (2) Intrinsic neuronal inhibitory mechanisms (e.g. slow K^+ conductances) remain relatively intact in CJD and AD, explaining why generalized seizures do not occur universally, despite the epileptiform EEG. (3) In those patients who do have seizures, there may be selective loss or dysfunction of inhibitory interneurons.

References

Alger BE, Nicoll RA (1980). Epileptiform burst afterhyperpolarization: calcium-dependent potassium potential in hippocampal CA1 pyramidal cells. Science (USA) 210:1122.

Andersen P, Andersson SA (1974). Thalamic origin of cortical rhythmic activity. In Creutzfeldt O (ed): "Handbook of Electroencephalography and Clinical Neurophysiology, Vol. 2-C", Amsterdam: Elsevier, p 2C-90.

Ball MJ (1980). Features of Creutzfeldt-Jakob disease in brains of patients with familial dementia of Alzheimer type. Can J Neurol Sci 7:51.

Barnes CA, McNaughton BL (1980). Physiological compensation for loss of afferent synapses in rat hippocampal granule cells during senescence. J Physiol 309:473.

Benardo LS, Prince DA (1981). Acetylcholine induced modulation of hippocampal pyramidal neurons. Brain Res 211:227.

Benardo LS, Prince DA (1982). Cholinergic excitation of mammalian hippocampal pyramidal cells. Brain Res 249:315.

Benardo LS, Prince DA (1982). Ionic mechanisms of cholinergic excitation in mammalian hippocampal pyramidal cells. Brain Res 249:333.

Buell SJ, Coleman PD (1979). Dendritic growth in the aged human brain and failure of growth in senile dementia. Science 206:854.

Burger LJ, Rowan AJ, Goldensohn ES (1972). Creutzfeldt-Jakob disease: an electroencephalographic study. Arch Neurol 26:428.

Coyle JT, Price DL, DeLong MR (1983). Alzheimer's disease: a disorder of cortical cholinergic innervation. Science 219:1184.

Dingledine R, Gjerstad L (1980). Reduced inhibition during epileptiform activity in the in vitro hippocampal slice, J Physiol (Lond) 305:297.

Ehle AL, Johnson PC (1977). Rapidly evolving EEG changes in a case of Alzheimer disease. Ann Neurol 1:593.

Faden AI, Townsend JJ (1976). Myoclonus in Alzheimer disease. Arch Neurol 33:278.

Fisher RS, Prince DA (1977a). Spike-wave rhythms in cat cortex induced by parenteral penicillin. I. Electroencephalographic features. Electroenceph Clin Neurophysiol 42:608.
Fisher RS, Prince DA (1977b). Spike-wave rhythms in cat cortex induced by parenteral penicillin. II. Cellular features. Electroenceph Clin Neurophysiol 42:625.
Flament-Durand J, Couck AM (1979). Spongiform alterations in brain biopsies of presenile dementia. Acta Neuropathol (Berl) 46:159.
Gajdusek DC, Gibbs CJ, Jr, Asher DM, Brown P, Diwan A, Hoffman P, Nemo G, Rohwer R, White L (1977). Precautions in medical care of, and in handling materials from, patients with transmissible virus dementia (Creutzfeldt-Jakob disease). New Eng J Med 297:1253.
Gloor P (1979). Generalized epilepsy with spike-and-wave discharge: a reinterpretation of its electrographic and clinical manifestations. Epilepsia 20:571.
Gloor P (1980). EEG characteristics in Creutzfeldt-Jakob disease. Ann Neurol 8:341.
Gloor P, Quesney LF, Zumstein H (1977). Pathophysiology of generalized penicillin epilepsy in the cat: the role of cortical and subcortical structures. II. Topical application of penicillin to the cerebral cortex and to subcortical structures. Electroenceph Clin Neurophysiol 43:79.
Gordon EB, Sim M (1967). The E.E.G. in presenile dementia. J Neurol Neurosurg Psychiat 30:285.
Gutnick MJ, Prince DA (1981). Dye coupling and possible electrotonic coupling in the guinea pig neocortical slice. Science USA 211:67.
Hablitz JJ, Lundervold A (1981). Hippocampal excitability and changes in extracellular potassium. Exper Neurol 71:410.
Hotson J, Prince DA (1980). A calcium-activated hyperpolarization follows repetitive firing in hippocampal neurons. J Neurophysiol 43:409.
Jacob H (1970). Muscular twitchings in Alzheimer's disease. In Wolstenholme GEW, O'Connor M (eds): "Alzheimer's Disease and Related Conditions", London: Churchill, p 75.
Johnston D, Brown TH (1981). Giant synaptic potential hypothesis for epileptiform activity. Science USA 211:294.
Landis DMD, Williams RS, Masters CL (1981). Golgi and electron-microscopic studies of spongiform encephalopathy. Neurology 31:538.

Lothman EW, Collins RC, Ferrendelli JA (1981). Kainic acid-induced limbic seizures: electrophysiologic studies. Neurology 31:806.

MacVicar BA, Dudek FE (1980a). Local synaptic circuits in rat hippocampus interactions between pyramidal cells. Brain Res 184:220.

MacVicar BA, Dudek FE (1980b). Dye-coupling between CA3 pyramidal cells in slices of rat hippocampus. Brain Res 196:494.

MacVicar BA, Dudek FE (1981). Electrotonic coupling between pyramidal cells: a direct demonstration in rat hippocampal slices. Science USA 213:782.

MacVicar BA, Dudek FE (1982). Electrotonic coupling between granule cells of the rat dentate gyrus: physiological and anatomical evidence. J Neurophysiol 47:579.

MacVicar BA, Ropert N, Krnjevic K (1982). Dye-coupling between pyramidal cells of rat hippocampus in vivo. Brain Res 238:239.

Mayeux R, Hunter S, Fahn S (1980). More on myoclonus in Alzheimer disease. Ann Neurol 8:200.

Miles R, Wong RKS (1982). The origins of primary and secondary synchronized bursts in disinhibited hippocampal slices. Soc Neurosci Abstr 8:910.

Moreau-Dubois M-C, Brown P, Goudsmit J, Cathala F, Gajdusek DC (1981). Biologic distinction between sporadic and familial Alzheimer disease by an in vitro cell fusion test. Neurology 31:323.

Musgrave J, Gloor P (1980). The role of the corpus callosum in bilateral interhemispheric synchrony of spike and wave discharge in feline generalized penicillin epilepsy. Epilepsia 21:369.

Nelson J (1968) On the origin of diffuse spikes in Jakob-Creutzfeldt's disease. Electroenceph clin Neurophysiol 24:395.

Nicoll RA, Alger BE (1981). A simple chamber for recording from submerged brain slices. J Neurosci Methods 4:153.

Ogata N (1978). Possible explanation for interictal-ictal transition: Evolution of epileptiform activity in hippocampal slice by chloride depletion. Experientia 34:1035.

Oliver AP, Hoffer BJ, Wyatt RJ (1978). Interaction of potassium and calcium in penicillin-induced interictal spike discharge in the hippocampal slice. Exper Neurol 62:510.

Pellegrini A, Musgrave J, Gloor P (1979). Role of afferent input of subcortical origin in the genesis of bilaterally synchronous epileptic discharges of feline generalized penicillin epilepsy. Exper Neurol 64:155.

Prince DA, Schwartzkroin PA (1978). Nonsynaptic mechanisms in epileptogenesis. In Chalazonitis M, Boisson M (eds): "Abnormal Neuronal Discharges", New York: Raven Press, p 1.

Prince DA, Wong RKS (1981). Human epileptic neurons studied _in vitro._ Brain Res 210:323.

Rayport M (1963). Electroencephalographic, corticographic and intracerebral potentials in two anatomically verified cases of Creutzfeldt-Jakob disease. Electroenceph clin Neurophysiol 15:922

Schaul N, Gloor P, Ball G, Gotman J (1978). The electromicrophysiology of delta waves induced by systemic atropine. Brain Res 143:475.

Scheibel AB (1979). The hippocampus: organizational patterns in health and senescence. Mech Ageing Dev 9:89.

Schwartzkroin PA, Prince DA (1977). Penicillin-induced epileptiform activity in the hippocampal _in vitro_ preparation. Ann Neurol 1:463.

Schwartzkroin PA, Prince DA (1978). Cellular and field potential properties of epileptogenic hippocampal slices. Brain Res 147:117.

Schwartzkroin PA, Prince DA (1980). Changes in excitatory and inhibitory synaptic potentials leading to epileptogenic activity. Brain Res 183:61.

Schwartzkroin PA, Turner DA, Knowles WD, Wyler AR (1983). Studies of human and monkey "epileptic" neocortex in the in vitro slice preparation. Ann Neurol 13:249.

Schwartzkroin PA, Wyler AR (1980). Mechanisms underlying epileptiform burst discharge. Ann Neurol 7:95.

Sloper JJ (1972). Gap junctions between dendrites in the primate neocortex. Brain Res 44:641.

Taylor CP, Dudek FE (1982). Physiological evidence for electrotonic coupling between CA1 pyramidal cells in rat hippocampal slices. Brain Res 235:351.

Traub RD (1982). Simulation of intrinsic bursting in CA3 hippocampal neurons. Neuroscience 7:1233.

Traub RD, Gajdusek DC, Gibbs CJ Jr (1977). Transmissible virus dementia: the relation of transmissible spongiform encephalopathy to Creutzfeldt-Jakob disease. In Smith WL, Kinsbourne M (eds): "Aging and Dementia", New York: Spectrum, p 91.

Traub RD, Pedley TA (1981). Virus-induced electrotonic coupling: hypothesis on the mechanism of periodic EEG discharges in Creutzfeldt-Jakob disease. Ann Neurol 10:405.

Traub RD, Wong RKS (1982). Cellular mechanism of neuronal synchronization in epilepsy. Science USA 216:745.

Traub RD, Wong RKS (1983a). Synchronized burst discharge in disinhibited hippocampal slice. II. Model of cellular mechanism. J Neurophysiol 49:459.

Traub RD, Wong RKS (1983b). Synaptic mechanisms underlying interictal spike initiation in a hippocampal network. Neurology 33:257.

Watson CP (1979). Clinical similarity of Alzheimer and Creutzfeldt-Jakob disease. Ann Neurol 6:368.

Whitehouse PJ, Price DL, Clark AW, Coyle JT, DeLong MR (1981). Alzheimer disease: evidence for selective loss of cholinergic neurons in the nucleus basalis. Ann Neurol 10:122.

Wong RKS, Prince DA (1979). Dendritic mechanisms underlying penicillin-induced epileptiform activity. Science USA 204:1228.

Wong RKS, Prince DA (1981). Afterpotential generation in hippocampal pyramidal cells. J Neurophysiol 45:86.

Wong RKS, Prince DA, Basbaum AI (1979). Intradendritic recordings from hippocampal neurons. Proc Nat Acad Sci USA 76:986.

Wong RKS, Traub RD (1983). Synchronized burst discharge in the disinhibited hippocampal slice. I. Initiation in the CA2-CA3 region. J Neurophysiol 49:442.

Senile Dementia: Outlook for the Future, pages 305–316

EVOKED POTENTIALS IN THE STUDY OF NORMAL AND PATHOLOGICAL AGING

Solomon Laurian, MD

Psychiatric University Clinic
of Lausanne (Dir.: Prof. C. Müller)
CH-1008 Prilly-Lausanne

The recording and analysis of electrical brain potentials obtained from scalp electrodes constitute a non-invasive, harmless and quite accessible method for evaluation of cerebral functions.

Brain spontaneous and evoked potentials were discovered by Caton in 1875, in the rabbit. About half a century later, Berger recorded the spontaneous activity in man, using scalp electrodes. By the beginning of the sixties, the advent of averagers permitted the recording of sensory evoked potentials (EPs), also from scalp electrodes. Since then, this technique aroused increased interest not only for neurophysiologists, who thought they had an instrument potentially able to measure the specific function of a definite brain area, but also for clinical physicians in search of non-invasive methods for the routine examination of CNS integrity.

The EPs are generally not observable in EEG recordings, being greatly attenuated at the surface of the scalp and submerged by the ongoing spontaneous electrical activity of the brain. The commonest method for extracting the evoked responses from the background activity is by averaging most conveniently done by using digital techniques of computation. The result of this computation is the average evoked response, a complex curve containing a series of positive and negative waves beginning about 1 msec after the stimulus and continuing for 300-500 msec or more; these components are defined by their polarity and latency or position (fig. 1).

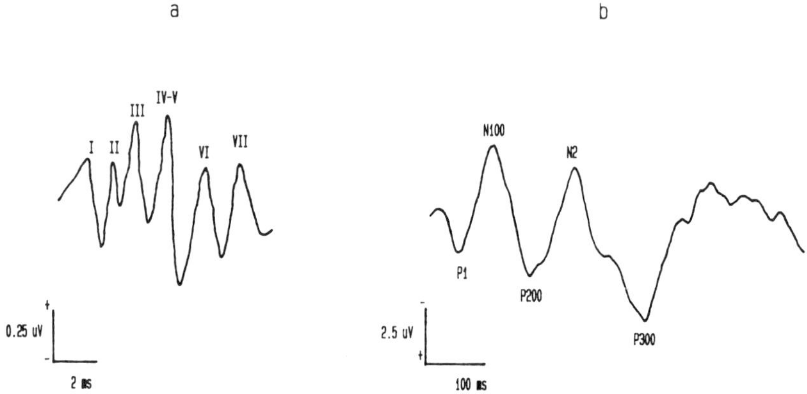

Fig. 1. Evoked potentials induced by auditory stimuli. a) Brain stem evoked responses to monoaural clicks at 65 dB HL; components are designated by roman numerals.
b) Cortical evoked responses to binaural tones at 70 db HL; components are designated by polarity (N,P) and a number indicating the position (1, 2, etc.) or the modal latency of the peak in msec (100, 200, etc.)
Note that different time bases and calibration signal were used in a) and b).

The earlier waves, lasting for 100 to 200 msec, depend upon the stimulus modality and are primarily determined by the physical characteristics of the stimulus (exogenous components, Donchin, 1975), whereas the later ones, having very clear and important psychological correlations, depend rather on the state of the subject and the experimental context (endogenous components). The anatomical sources of some waves are now well established, but the origin of others is unknown; some components seem to have multiple sources.

EPs and Normal Aging

Many studies have been performed in elderly persons, using evoked potentials to seek a better understanding of the mechanisms of normal and pathological aging. Extensive investigations on the life-span changes in EPs were performed by Beck and Dustman (1975), Beck et al. (1975), Dustman et al. (1977). There has emerged a consistent picture of age changes in cortical sensory evoked potentials. The auditory evoked responses (AERs) undergo only insignificant changes in the elderly. In contrast, visual (VERs) and somatosensory (SERs) evoked responses show stable latencies and increased amplitudes in some components up to 100 msec and increased latencies and decreased amplitudes in the waves extending from 100 to 200 msec. Celesia and Daly (1977) studied the effects of aging on VERs to pattern-reversal stimulation and reported a significative increase of latencies of the first major negative and of the first major positive deflection with advancing age. Goodin et al. (1978) reported some systematic changes with age also for AERs consisting in an increase of P2 latency at a rate of 0.7 msec/year and a decrease of the N1-P2 amplitude at a rate of 0.2 μV/year. Besides, they observed a more nearly equipotential distribution of N1-P2 amplitude with age. Likewise, Liberson (1976) mentioned scalp distribution changes of EPs as a function of age, namely a progressive shift of localization of SERs of maximal amplitude from the centro-frontal to the posterior parietal regions.

As regards brainstem responses (BSRs) to auditory stimuli, Rowe (1978) reported longer peak latencies in the elderly, whereas Beagley and Sheldrake (1978) found that the amplitude of wave V tends to decrease with age. Otto and McCandless (1982) and Maurizi et al (1982) observed that the BSRs waveforms were disorganized and less easily identifiable in senescence. Data presented by Harkins and Lenhardt (1980) suggest that most changes in these waves in healthy elderly persons can be accounted for by presbycusis.

A number of studies have attempted to investigate some more functional aspects of the age-related changes in sensory evoked potentials. Ford et al (1979) studied the abilities to attenuate irrelevant stimuli and to detect target stimuli in elderly subjects, in order to test different hypotheses on the origin of their difficulties in performing tasks requiring high levels of attention. They used an experimental paradigm allowing evaluation of N1(latency about 100 msec)and P3 (latency 300-500 msec) EPs components. The former was shown to be sensitive to the level of attention, whereas the latter is related both to the subject's expectancy and the length of time necessary to make a decision. The results showed that the amplitudes of N1 were not significantly different between the young and old subjects, suggesting a similar level of general attention to auditory stimuli during the task in both groups. Whereas the P3 amplitude did not discriminate between the old and young subjects, the P3 latency was significantly later in the elderly, suggesting that they take longer to decide whether an event is relevant or not. Goodin et al (1979) reported that the latency of the P3 component increased systematically, at a rate of 1.64 msec/year, with increasing age. It is possible that some effects of age on cognitive functions can be accounted for by influences of such latency prolongations on information processing.

Dustman and Snyder (1982) tested the hypothesis of cortical inhibitory deficits in old subjects through an investigation of the augmenting-reducing phenomena related to the intensity of visual stimuli. As expected, oldsters demonstrated greater amplitude enhancement to increased flash intensity than young adults, probably related to a reduced turnover of inhibitory neurotransmitters as well as to structural deficiencies in the elderly.

The concept of performance decrements in the elderly was studied by Marsh and Thompson in a CNV (contingent negative variation) experimental paradigm. The CNV is a slow negative wave occurring when a conditioning stimulus is followed a few seconds later by an imperative stimulus demanding a response. Subjects had to judge whether the second of a pair of tones was higher, lower or the same in pitch as the first tone of the pair. Surprisingly, the older subjects demonstrated an ability to make a sensory discrimination which a group of younger ones did not accomplish. Such findings raise serious questions regarding age decrements in perceptual function in healthy elderly subjects.

Recently, Porjesz et al (1980) used a P3 paradigm in a study of VERs to visuo-spatial stimuli in order to assess similarities in brain functioning between alcoholics and old people. Previous neuropsychological studies indicated that alcoholics may exhibit behavioral deficits similar to those of the elderly. The results of this study indicated that the N1-P2 and N2-P3 components are significantly decreased in amplitude in the chronic alcoholics. In contrast, these components are of normal amplitude in the elderly subjects, but occur significantly later. It was concluded that, despite behavioral similarities between alcohol-related deficits and those of the aging process, the nature of brain dysfunction is quite different in the two groups.

EPs and Pathological Aging

An area of EP research, which has been particularly successful is represented by studies on geriatric patients presenting signs of mental deterioration. In comparison with healthy old subjects, the psychogeriatric patients show quantitative as well as specific alterations in the amplitude, latency, morphology, topographic distribution, hemispheric symmetry.

Several studies showed prolonged latencies of some components of sensory evoked potentials. Straumanis et al (1964) reported longer latencies of VERs components occurring later than 100 msec after the light flash. Visser et al (1976) investigated the VERs in senile and presenile dementia patients. When compared to normal subjects, the results indicated that patients had longer latencies for all peaks, except for an early component around 70 msec. Hendrickson et al (1979) recorded AERs in elderly depressives, dements, patients with a combination of depression and dementia and normal elderly controls. The latencies were significantly longer in dements than in controls; depressives had intermediate latencies. Although the AER is of value in distinguishing the experimental groups, it does not appear to be a good indicator of the severity of dementia. Laurian et al (1977) investigated AERs in two groups of demented patients suffering from Alzheimer's disease or simple senile dementia and a group of nondemented aged controls. The latencies of the N1 and P2 components were longer in both groups of patients than in controls.

Goodin et al (1978) found that of the various evoked potential components elicited by tones, the P3 component is the most sensitive both in normal and pathological aging. They demonstrated that impaired mental functioning in dementia, regardless of the etiology, is highly correlated with changes in the latency and amplitude of the P3 component of the AER. The magnitude of the P3 latency in particular reliably distinguished the patients with dementia from neurological patients with normal mental function. Thus, if a P3 latency which exceeds normal by two standard deviations is adopted as the criterion for defining dementia electrophysiologically, 80 percent of demented patients would be correctly classified. Interestingly, patients with functional rather than organic disorders rarely had P3 latencies exceeding the normal range. Using the same P3 latency criterion in combination with the Mini-Mental State scores, Brown et al (in press) correctly separated the majority of the demented from the non-demented patients. The misclassifications were entirely false negative with respect to dementia. Snydulko et al (1982) studied the AERs in a group of 12 patients presenting moderate progressive dementia of unknown etiology and a group of age-matched normal controls. The most striking difference in waveform between groups was for the P3 component, their results supporting its potential diagnostic utility.

A few investigations approached some aspects

of the topographic distribution of EPs in senile psychoses. Gerson et al (1976) studied the AERs and the VERs in 17 geriatric patients presenting senescent cognitive impairment and 27 normal controls matched for age. Subjects were tested in 5 different experimental conditions. Consistent differences were obtained between the two groups with respect to the symmetry of the EPs between corresponding regions of the two hemispheres, systematically greater in normals. Moreover, imposition of an information-processing activity caused a marked increase in EPs symmetry in the normals and a decrease in the seniles. Presumably, the two hemispheres of the brain of the seniles are less well coordinated than in normal aged persons and this incoordination is further accentuated by imposing an information-processing load. In the authors' opinion, the diminished concordance between the two hemispheres could constitute the primary cause of the cognitive disorders in senile dementia.

An interesting peculiarity in topographic distribution of EPs in senile dementia was reported by Laurian et al (1977, 1982). The VERs to flashes were recorded at vertex and occipital electrodes in 10 patients suffering from simple senile dementia, 7 patients presenting Alzheimer's disease and 5 old nondemented controls. Whereas the waveforms in the occipital region were quite similar for the three groups, at the vertex the responses in Alzheimer patients differed strikingly from those recorded in the two other groups (fig. 2).

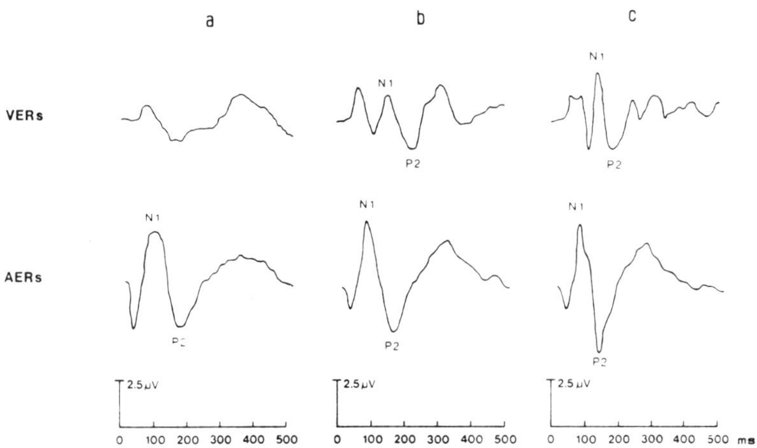

Fig. 2 Visual and auditory evoked responses (grand mean waveforms) in three groups of old persons : a) = patients suffering from dementia of Alzheimer's type (n = 7); b) = patients presenting simple senile dementia (n = 10); c) = controls (n = 5). Each wave represents the average of all responses of all subjects.

In these last two groups, the VERs presented the usual configuration with a N1-P2 component always identifiable; in the Alzheimer group, in contrast, the N1-P2 component was almost not discernible or completely missing. These data confirm the assumption that the vertex and occipital VERs probably represent different neurophysiological phenomena and it may be inferred that the structures responsible for the genesis of the vertex VER are severely impaired in Alzheimer patients. The lack or an alteration of the vertex VER are very probably linked with a deep organic and/or functional brain disorder which may serve as a diagnostic criterion in psychogeriatry. On the other hand, the AERs wave form was quite similar in these groups.

Diagnostically interesting changes in VERs have also been observed in the later stages of Jakob-Creutzfeld disease (Lee and Blair, 1973). Serial VERs were investigated in one patient who showed an exagerated response to visual stimuli. Initially, the responses were markedly enlarged; as the disease progressed, there was an increase in latency and decrease in amplitude of early components and a reversal of polarity in the late part of the response. It is suggested that many of these changes might reflect a loss of normal inhibitory influences on the cortex.

Conclusion

One of the most striking trends in the investigations on EPs has been their application to the study of normal and pathologic aging. From these studies one could infer that the EPs to sensory stimulation exhibit systematic modifications with increasing age. At present, these changes cannot be correlated with specific deteriorations of central or peripheral mechanisms, but they strongly suggest anatomical and functional alterations in the involved neuronal structures. Biochemical changes in aging, represented by decreases in inhibitory and excitatory neurotransmitters and their associated enzymes, as well as neuropathological modifications consisting of loss of cells and dendrites have been described.

The longer latencies observed in the elderly are compatible with a decrease in normal conduction time as a consequence of an alteration in myelination. The increase in amplitude of some early components might be the result of a decrease in normal inhibitory influences on the cortex, whereas the diminished amplitude in later peaks presumably reflects a lower efficiency of the activatory reticular system.

The use of the endogenous components made it possible to evaluate various aspects of cognitive function and to demonstrate a slowing of cognitive processing with increasing age. Smith et al (1980) reviewed the EP research that has focused on aging process and proposed some conceptual models to explain the age-associated differences observed.

On the other hand, some measures of EPs, such as the P3 latency, appear to constitute a worthwhile diagnostic tool in senile dementia. Recently, John (1977) proposed a new approach, called "neurometrics", based upon quantitative measurements of salient features extracted from spontaneous and evoked brain electrical activity data, which reflect various aspects of brain function related to sensory, perceptual and cognitive processes as well as to structural and functional integrity of different neuroanatomical systems. Neurometric data obtained from 60 normal elderly persons and 60 senile demented patients were subjected to a cluster analysis that permitted correct classification of 85 % of them.

Undoubtedly, the evoked potential technique offers a unique approach for assessing the level of brain function and constitutes a valuable instrument not only for studies on aging, but also one of clinical usefulness in psychogeriatry.

References

Beagley HA, Sheldrake JB (1978). Differences on brainstem response latency with age and sex. Brit J Audiol 12 : 69.

Beck EC, Dustman RE (1975). Changes in evoked responses during maturation and aging in man and macaque. In Burch N, Altshuler HL (eds) "Behavior and brain electrical activity", New York : Plenum Press, p 431.

Beck EC, Dustman RE, Schenkenberg T (1975). Life span changes in the electrical activity of the human brain as reflected in the cerebral evoked response. In Ordy JM, Brizzee KR (eds) "Neurobiology of aging", New York, Plenum Press, p 175.

Berger H (1969). Hans Berger on the electroencephalogram of man (english translation by P. Gloor) Electroenceph Clin Neurophysiol Suppl 28 : 75.

Brown WS, Marsh JT, LaRue A (in press). Event-related potentials in psychiatry : differentiating depression and dementia in the elderly. Bull Los Angeles Neurol Soc.

Caton R (1875). The electrical currents of the brain. Brit Med J 2 : 278.

Celesia GG, Daly RF (1977). Effects of aging on visual evoked responses. Arch Neurol 34 : 403

Donchin E (1979). Event-related brain potentials : a tool in the study of human information processing. In Begleiter H (ed) "Evoked brain potentials and behavior", New York : Plenum Press, p 13.

Dustman RE, Schenkenberg EG, Lewis EG, Beck EC (1977). In Desmedt JE (ed) "Visual evoked potentials in man : new developments", Oxford : Clarendon Press, p 363.

Dustman RE, Snyder EW (1981). Life-span changes in visually evoked potentials at central scalp. Neurobiology in aging 2 : 303.

Ford JM, Hink RF, Hopkins WF, Roth WT, Pfefferbaum A, Kopell BS (1979). Age effects on event-related potentials in a selective attention task. J Geront 34 : 388
Gershon IM, John ER (1976). Average evoked response (AER) in the electroencephalographic diagnosis on the normally aging brain : a practical application. Clinical Electroenceph 7 : 77.
Goodin DS, Squires KC, Henderson BH, Starr A (1978a). Age-related variations in evoked potentials to auditory stimuli in normal human subjects. Electroenceph Clin Neurophysiol 44: 447.
Goodin DS, Squires KC, Starr A (1978b). Long latency event-related components of the auditory evoked potential in dementia. Brain 101 : 635.
Harkins SW, Lenhardt M (1980). Brainstem auditory evoked potentials in the elderly. In Poon LW (ed) "Aging in the 1980's", Washington : American Physiological Association, p 101.
Hendrickson E, Levy R, Post F (1979). Averaged evoked responses in relation to cognitive and affective state of elderly psychiatric patients. Brit J Psychiat 134: 494.
Laurian S, Lobrinus A, Wertheimer J, Gaillard JM (1977). Evozierte Potentiale bei seniler Demenz. In Lauter H (Hrsg) "Gerontopsychiatrie 6. Janssen Symposien", Düsseldorf, p 57.
Laurian S, Gaillard JM, Wertheimer J (1982). Evoked potentials in assessment of brain function in senile dementia. In Courjon J, Mauguière F, Revol M (eds) "Clinical applications of evoked potentials in neurology", New York : Raven Press, p 287.
Lee RG, Blair RDG (1973). Evolution of EEG and visual evoked response changes in Jakob-Creutzfeldt disease. Electroenceph Clin Neurophysiol 35 : 133.
Liberson WT (1976). Scalp distribution of somatosensory evoked potentials and aging. Electromyogr Clin Neurophysiol 16 : 221.
Marsh GR, Thompson LW (1973). Effects of age on the contingent negative variation in a pitch discrimination task. J Geront 28: 56.
Maurizi M,Altissimi G, Ottaviani F, Paludetti G, Bambini M (1982). Auditory brainstem responses (ABR) in the aged. Scand Audiol 11: 213.

Otto WC, McCandless GA (1982). Aging and the auditory brain stem response. Audiology 21: 466.
Porjesz B, Begleiter H, Samuelly I (1980). Cognitive deficits in chronic alcoholics and elderly subjects assessed by evoked brain potentials. Acta Psychiat Scand Suppl 286: 15.
Rowe MJ (1978). Normal variability of the brain stem auditory evoked response in young and old adult subjects. Electroenceph Clin Neurophysiol 44: 459.
Smith DBD, Thompson LW, Michalewski HJ (1980). Averaged evoked potential research in adult aging - status and prospects. In Poon LW (ed) "Aging in the 1980's", Washington : American Physiological Association, p 135.
Straumanis JJ, Shagass C, Schwartz M (1965). Visually evoked cerebral response changes associated with chronic brain syndromes and aging. J Geront 20: 498.
Syndulko K, Hansch EC, Cohen SN, Pearce JW, Goldberg Z, Montan B, Tourtellotte WW, Potvin AR (1982). Long-latency event-related potentials in normal aging and dementia. In Courjon J, Mauguière F, Revol M (eds) "Clinical applications of evoked potentials in neurology", New York : Raven Press, p 279.
Visser SL, Stam FC, van Tilburg W, Op den Velde W, Bloom JL, de Rijke W (1976). Visual evoked response in senile and presenile dementia. Electroenceph Clin Neurophysiol 40: 385.

Senile Dementia: Outlook for the Future, pages 317–323

VALIDATION WITH THE POSITRON EMISSION TOMOGRAPHY OF A CLINICAL BATTERY FOR THE DIFFERENTIAL DIAGNOSIS OF DEMENTIAS : PRELIMINARY COMMUNICATION

Theodore Hovaguimian, M.D., Philippe Magistretti, M.D., Ebba Mahler, M.D. and Jean-Pierre Junod, M.D.

Geriatric Institutions and Department of Radiology, University of Geneva, Geneva, Switzerland

INTRODUCTION

This paper introduces a research project on senile dementia which the Geriatric Institutions and the Nuclear Medicine Department of the University of Geneva are about to develop in collaboration with the World Health Organization and the Swiss National Fund for Scientific Research.

The main objective will be to improve the clinical diagnostic criteria for organic dementias in order, particularly, to allow a better distinction between the senile dementias of Alzheimer type and the vascular dementia, for there are grounds to expect that, in the near future, these two morbid entities will become the object of specific therapeutic interventions, the success of which will depend on the adequate selection of the patients liable to benefit of them.

A refinement of the differential diagnosis of organic dementias has now become possible in view of the parallel development of two methodologies:

The first methodology results from the increased observation of individual symptoms of dementia and a systematic study in epidemiological investigations which brought a better definition of the cognitive, behavioral, psychosocial, neurological or physical disorders accompanying this condition and produced reliable instruments to detect and measure these disorders in a standardized way.

The other methodology is linked to the development of a second generation of brain scanners, namely those using the Positron Emission Tomography that opens the field to functional dynamic studies of the cerebral blood flow topography, the glucose metabolism and an ever increasing number of other metabolic activities of the brain.

While it was only possible, so far, to establish a delayed correlation between clinical and laboratory findings, i.e. between the symptoms observed in the course of the dementing illness and their causal diagnosis established at autopsy, we are able today to establish instant correlations between clinical profiles of impairment of various functions measured with standardized methods and an imaging of the brain technique liable to give precise information on the etiology of dementia.

BRIEF REVIEW OF THE KNOWLEDGE IN THE FIELDS OF CLINICAL DIAGNOSIS OF DEMENTIA AND ITS INVESTIGATION WITH THE POSITRON EMISSION TOMOGRAPHY

Among the first attempts to systematize operational clinical criteria for differential diagnosis of organic dementias is the work of Mayer-Gross, Slater and Roth (Mayer-Gross 1954) who reported the respective psychiatric manifestations of senile dementia and cerebral arteriosclerosis. Birkett studied the validity of psychiatric criteria for distinguishing between senile and arteriopathic brain disease in a report where he compared mental symptoms of two groups of demented patients classified on basis of necropsy and confirmed the usefulness of some characteristics, such as the more acute onset, the better preservation of personality and insight and a greater mood lability to identify the multi-infarct group.

Hatchinsky and his colleagues (Hatchinsky 1975) developed a summary of statements about these features in a rating scale they called the ischemic score. These authors published data on the measurement of cerebral blood flow of demented patients; those who were classified as vascular on the basis of the ischemic score seemed to actually belong to a specific subgroup in which blood flow and oxygen consumption were lower than in the other demented patients.

In the particular field of cognitive functions, the work of Ajuriaguerra, Tissot and Richard in Geneva (Tissot 1980) includes a very complete attempt to analyse the semeology of intellectual defects of dementia in search of a differential aetiological classification.

In short, the studies of this school take as a paradigm that, when dementia results from progressive and diffuse lesions, as it is the case with senile dementia of Alzmeimer type, the disintegration of intelligence will follow the reverse pathway of the steps of its development described in the child by Piaget (Piaget 1970); while, in a dementia with more focalized lesions, be it degenerative (such as Pick's dementia) or vascular (multi-infarct dementia), the impairments of the various cognitive functions can be considered, according to these authors, as mere local defects added one to another, and no longer as the global performance of a system with an organization characteristic of an operatory level of intelligence.

A validation study of this model was carried out by Todorov, Constantinidis and Elston (Todorov 1975) who found an agreement between clinical diagnosis and anatomo-pathological findings varying between 19% and 78%, depending on the clinical diagnostic sub-group; the highest correlation belongs to the pre-senile sub-groups.

Beside this model of genetic psychology, the concept of homogeneous and non-homogeneous intellectual impairments is also found in several clinical observations that established a consensus on an empirical notion that diffuse cerebral atrophy leads to a global and generalized deterioration, while impairment remains multi-focal in arteriopathic dementia.

This clinical observation proves, however, to be difficult to ascertain by psychometric tests, which are not unanimously recognized to be useful for differential diagnosis. Thus, while, for instance, Perez et al. (Perez 1975), who used sub-tests of the W.A.I.S., reported a high level of discrimination between vascular and non-vascular, others, like Miller (Miller 1980), expressed their doubts about the possibility to expect from the psychometric approach more than presumptions concerning some clinical forms of dementia.

The last two decades have witnessed a large increase in clinical assessment tools for the diagnosis of dementia, which borrowed from one another to a large extent. The Mental Health Division of the World Health Organization inventorized, in a manual to be published shortly, more than 100 instruments, published on an international level, and aiming at the measurement of various aspects of mental aptitudes and adaptation capacities of the aged.

Over the last years, however, there has been a shift of emphasis from the tests measuring specific functions to multi-dimensional batteries; these are instruments designed to allow the measurement of a variety of more or less independent functions, such as physical status, intellectual capacity, social performance, mood and behavior, etc.; thus, a multi-dimensional battery provides for a subject profiles of impairment of several functions.

In parallel to the development of this assessment methodology, new insights are being brought concerning the physiopathology of dementia through the development of the Positron Emission Tomography (P.E.T.).

In this technique, a radionuclide, i.e., a labelled pharmaceutical or biological agent, is administered to the subject. When reaching the target organ, e.g. the brain, the product is captured by the neurones and starts emitting positrons; the positrons will travel in the matter of the organ over a short distance before entering into contact with a electron. Positrons and electrons form a complex that annihilates itself and emits two Gamma rays in opposite directions.

The image is obtained with external detectors that operate in coincidence, i.e., that reckon an event only when the opposite detector is stimulated; thus, the location of the contact point between positrons and electrons is determined precisely.

A tomographic reconstruction of the image, which is made out of millions of events detected in that way, uses the same algorythmes as the Computerized Axial Tomography.

An inherent advantage of the P.E.T., in comparison with previous scintigraphic methods, such as the Xenon method, is its capacity to provide a topographic representation in slices of the blood flow and metabolism. Thus, with a radionuclide such as the fluoro-deoxy-glucose, the P.E.T. can measure, in each tomographic slice of the brain, the tissular concentration of this glucose analogue, and reflects the energy consumption at that level. Thereby, a mapping of cortical and sub-cortical metabolism is obtained.

A small number of research teams are currently exploring the brain with the P.E.T. The literature on the results of this investigation in dementia is scarce. Lenzi and Jones (Lenzi 1980) reported a significant decrease of frontal and central activity of the brain in the demented. Kuhl, in a more recent publication (Kuhl 1983), noted the contrasts between the uniform distribution of the glucose metabolism in normal subjects,and the patchy image observed in patients with vascular dementia.

SUMMARY OF THE PROPOSED PROJECT

The study will first pool the dimensions inventorized in the most relevant instruments for the assessment of mental, social and physical disorders of dementia in a comprehensive multi-dimensional pilot battery.

Then, the signs and symptoms included will be examined with regard to their frequency and patterns of occurrence in correlation with objective indications about the type of dementia obtained with the P.E.T. technique.

Regarding the technical aspects of the P.E.T., the Division of Nuclear Medicine at the University Hospital of Geneva has, in collaboration with the CERN (European Organization for Nuclear Research), brought some new developments to the positron camera detectors, which are now providing images of a better quality with an enhanced power of resolution.

It is being anticipated that, with these latest developments, the P.E.T. technique will allow a precise discrimination of possible metabolism differences between various relevant functional areas of the brain.

Then, in mapping the brain activity of a series of demented patients, it is expected to identify a group with their uniformly reduced metabolism, to which the patients with senile dementia of Alzheimer type will probably belong, and another with a patchy distribution of activity, in which the multi-infarct patients will fall.

An appropriate statistical treatment of the data gathered with the pilot battery, which will be administered to the same series of patients, will finally determine the specificity and the sensitivity of each clinical element and the discriminatory power of their combinations with regard to the diagnostic category.

REFERENCES

Hachinsky VC et al. (1975). Cerebral blood flow in dementia. Arch Neurol 32:632.

Kuhl DE (1983). Mapping cerebral glucose metabolism in stroke, degenerative disease and epilepsy. In Magistretti P (ed.): "Functional radionuclide imaging of the brain," Raven Press, New York.

Lenzi GL, Jones T (1980). Cerebral metabolism-to-blood flow relationships with respect to aging and dementia. In Amaducci L et al. (eds.): "Aging of the brain and dementia. Aging," New York: Raven Press, vol.13, 99-102.

Mayer-Gross W, Slater E, Roth M (1954). "Clinical Psychiatry." London and Baltimore.

Miller E (1980). Cognitive assessment of the older adult. In Birren JE, Sloan RB (eds.): "Handbook of mental health and Ageing," Englewoods Cliffs, New Jersey: Prentice-Hall. 520-536.

Perez FI, Rivera VM, Meyer JS, Gay JRA, Taylor RL, Matthew NT (1975). J Neurol Neurosurg Psychiat 38:533

Piaget J (1970). "L'Epistémologie génétique." Paris.

Tissot R (1980). "Etats déficitaires cérébraux liés à l'âge." Genève: Georg.
Todorov AB, Go RCP, Constantinidis J, Elston RC (1975). Specificity of the clinical diagnosis of dementia. Journal of the neurological Sciences 26:81.

VIII. THERAPEUTIC POSSIBILITIES

Presided by D.D. Orlovskaya (Moscow)

Senile Dementia: Outlook for the Future, pages 327–337

COMPARISONS OF THE CARE OF THE DEMENTED ELDERLY IN NEW YORK AND LONDON

Barry J. Gurland*
Peter S. Cross*
A.H. Mann**
Alastair Macdonald***

*Center for Geriatrics & Gerontology
Columbia University and the New York State Office of Mental Health
100 Haven Avenue
New York, New York 10032
**Royal Free Hospital, London
***Institute of Psychiatry, London

INTRODUCTION

Over the past decade, the United States-United Kingdom Cross-National Project has carried out a series of comparisons of the care of the elderly (65 years +) in New York and London (Gurland et al., 1983; Cross et al., 1983; Cross et al., In Press; Mann et al., In Press; Copeland et al., 1975). These studies are listed in Table 1. Here we will attempt to draw from these studies some general conclusions about the care of the elderly with dementia that bear upon health and social service policy and planning for the next two decades.

In both the community and institutional studies, randomly drawn samples were studied. In the institutional studies the numbers in the samples of cases of dementia are substantial but in the community studies, these numbers are small; however, the latter cases do have the merit of being part of large represenative samples of the community elderly.

In the results that follow the term 'pervasive dementia' is used to refer to cases identified as having an organic brain syndrome of a clinical level of severity and following new and explicit criteria (Gurland et al., 1982).

Table 1. Sequence of US-UK cross-national studies

Study 1.	Geriatric Hospital Study: Examination of 50 consecutive geropsychiatric admissions in New York and 50 in London. Three month follow-up.
Study 2.	Geriatric Community Study: Examination of a resentative sample of 445 elderly subjects living in the community in New York and 396 in London. One year follow-up. Services received and family support also studied.
Study 3.	Geriatric Institutional Study: Examination of 162 and 159 geriatric residents randomly selected from all long term care facilities in respectively New York and in London. Organization and costs of institutions also studied.
Study 4.	Geriatric Alternatives to Institutions Study: Examination of quality, costs, and outcome of care given to matched groups of frail elderly in institutional and community based settings in New York and London.

RESULTS

Our key findings in this respect are as follows:

Prevalence rates of pervasive dementia do vary between populations but are between 3-5% of the elderly (65 years and older) residing in the community and about 50% of the 4 to 5% of elderly population in long-term care facilities. Thus, the point prevalence of dementia in the total elderly population is about 5-7%.

Almost all these pervasive dementias are to some degree rendered disabled and dependent on others because of their condition. A majority of the pervasive dementias in the community (in New York 19 out of 22 cases; in London 5 out of 9) are dependent on others to a degree that would require nursing home care were they not being looked after at home. Conversely, dementia accounts for about 20-50% of the severly dependent elderly in the community.

The pervasive dementias reside for relatively lengthy periods in the community; at a one year follow-up of the community resident pervasive dementias only a very few (in New York 2 out of 21 with 1 unknown; in London 1 out of 9) had been admitted to long term care institutions and most were still alive (16 of 21 in New York with 1 unknown; 8 out of 9 in London). At least as many pervasive dementias live outside long-term care facilities as in them (in New York about twice as many) (Gurland et al., In Press).

Figure 1. Formal home care services for the dependent elderly in New York and London as a proportion of total providers.

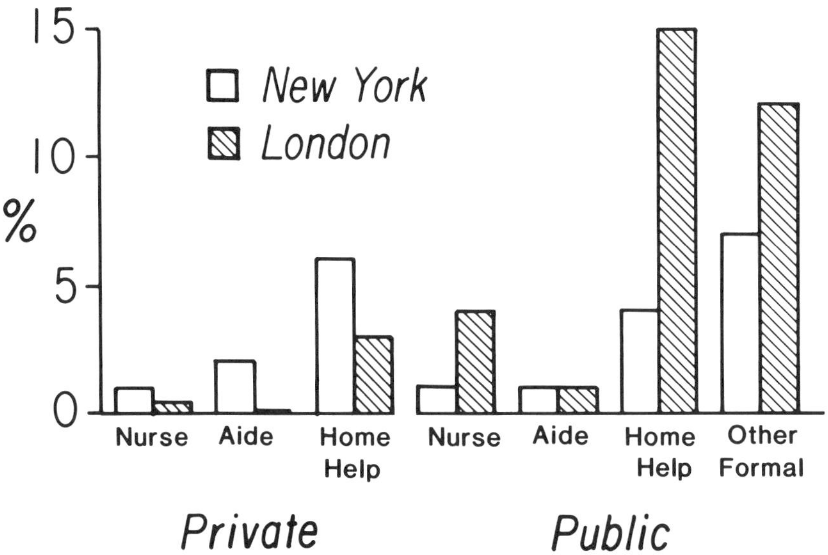

Note: Number of dependent elderly: 132 in New York, 124 in London. Number of total providers (private and public): 234 in New York, 209 in London.

Given a basic modicum of home care services, the proportion of dementias prevented from entering institutions may not be predictably increased by merely increasing the activity of home care services or the numbers of alternatives to institutional care (such as day care centers or day hospitals). The US-UK data show a higher proportion of the elderly population with pervasive dementia in New York than in London; although the latter city has a greater activity in community based formal services (see Figure 1). This point is also supported with respect to the elderly (N=132 in New York and 124 in London) who are dependent from any cause and require to be assisted to remain in the community these are found in about equal proportions (around 30%) of the New York and London elderly populations.

The greatest influence on keeping dementias out of institutions is probably the family. Few pervasive dementias live alone (4 out of 21 in New York and 1 out of 9 in London).

Despite the greater number of dementias in the community as compared to institutions, medical services are organized to serve the needs of cases of dementia in institutions rather than in the community. In London, 3 of the 9 community resident dements had not been seen by a doctor in over a year. In New York, medical services were received more often but house-calls were virtually non-existent. Yet because of their extreme old age (about half or more are 80 years or older) these community based dementias require good medical as well as social care. The correlation between the score on a dementia scale and on a scale of immobility for the community elderly was .33 and .30 in New York and London respectively.

In institutions, active medical care is not necessarily the same as good care. Figure 2 shows that dementias in New York receive phenothiazines significantly more often than do dementias in London (43% vs. 20% respectively). Yet such behavior problems as wandering, being noisy at night or inappropriate behavior were equally frequent in the two cities among the dements in institutions (Mann et al., In Press). The cross-national differences in use of phenothiazines is probably related to corresponding differences in the long term care systems. The distribution of cases of dementia (those with Mental Status Questionnaire scores of 8 or more) in long term care facilities shows that the vast majority (90%) of cases in New York are in skilled nursing facilities; in London, the majority (51%) are in homes not intended for provision of skilled nursing care (Local Authority Part III accomodation or voluntary and private residential homes). It appears that increased tranquillization is associated with a 'medical-nursing model' of care without corresponding benefits in reduction of behavior disorder.

Figure 2. Percentage of residents receiving phenothiazines in long term care facilities.

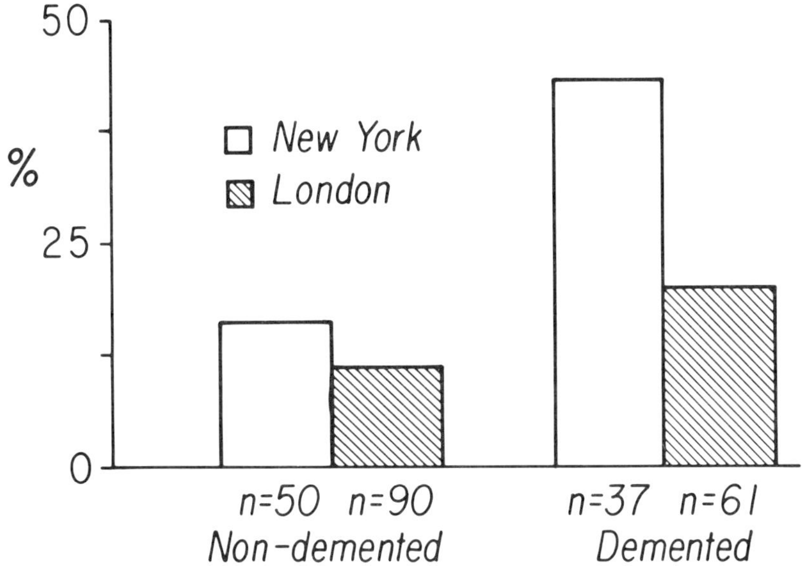

DISCUSSION

One may expect the prevalence of dementia to increase over the next 20 years because the very old (80+ years) segment of the population will grow in absolute numbers and as a proportion of the population; and because better health care and palliative pharmacological treatments will be developed to prolong the lives of the elderly in general and the dementias in particular. This rise in prevalence of dementias will probably be tempered but not prevented by improved recognition and treatment of remediable dementias.

The response of the health and social care system to the growing demands for care of the dementias shows cross-national differences in emphasis on social versus medical-nursing models; institutional versus community services; and formal versus informal approaches. Such differences are analogous to the shifts in emphasis that can be seen over time in a given care system. These cross-national results suggest that such shifts should not be a redirection but a balancing of resources.

Neither an institutional nor a community orientation to care can stand, one without the other. Despite cross-national differences in these emphases a substantial proportion of dementias are admitted to institutions in both New York and London. A certain proportion of dementias warrant instititional care even where active home care services have been established. Moreover, as the community-based enterprise expands it may begin to serve cases that are not imminently destined for institutional admission and may set limits of tolerance for demands by these cases on service time which leads to accelerated pressures for institutional admission. It is notable that the London formal home care services are more active than those in New York in supporting the dependent elderly but that there are relatively fewer severe cases of dependency supported in London than in New York. Furthermore, about a third of the dementias in New York were receiving full-time or daily services (16 hours or more per week) from formal sources whereas no dementias were receiving this much formal service in London.

Similarily, neither social, nursing, nor medical models of care suffice alone. Dementia (as can be seen by its correlations with a range of problems) is a disorder requiring multidisciplinary efforts. With social problem scales the dementia scale correlated as follows (New York data first, London second; underscoring indicates that the correlation is statistically significant at $p \leq .05$): Inadequate activities, .28 and .25; Isolation, .13 and .09; Environmental disadvantage .09 and .01; and Financial disadvantage .18 and .03. Furthermore, the optimization of health, and control of acute confusional states in the homebound dementias tends to be neglected; on the other hand, we have seen that the medical care of dementias in institutions may be overzealous.

The social emphasis given to institutional care in London while providing the semblance of a more comfortable quality of life than is seen in the New York facilities does not seem to improve the morale of patients. Scores on a scale of depression-demoralization were found to be higher among those elderly (who could report their symptoms) in London than in New York institutions (55% vs. 39%); with the greatest cross-national discrepancy being among the most severely disabled (71% vs. 30% in London and New York respectively) (Mann, et al., In Press); perhaps because attention to rehabilitation is inadequate in the institutions run on a social model.

These cross-national results underline the necessity for a model of care which balances social, nursing and medical aspects. However, the system of care required for dementia needs to be not only balanced but flexible. Some of the demands on service in the next twenty years are unpredictable. Partly this is caused by unexpected (and often unwanted) effects of new interventions. A possible displacement of family support of the demented by formal home care services might be inferred from the cross-national data. The lesser activity of formal home care services in New York compared with London appears to be compensated by greater activity of informal services (see Figure 3).

Figure 3. Reciprocal relationship of services from formal and informal home care sources.

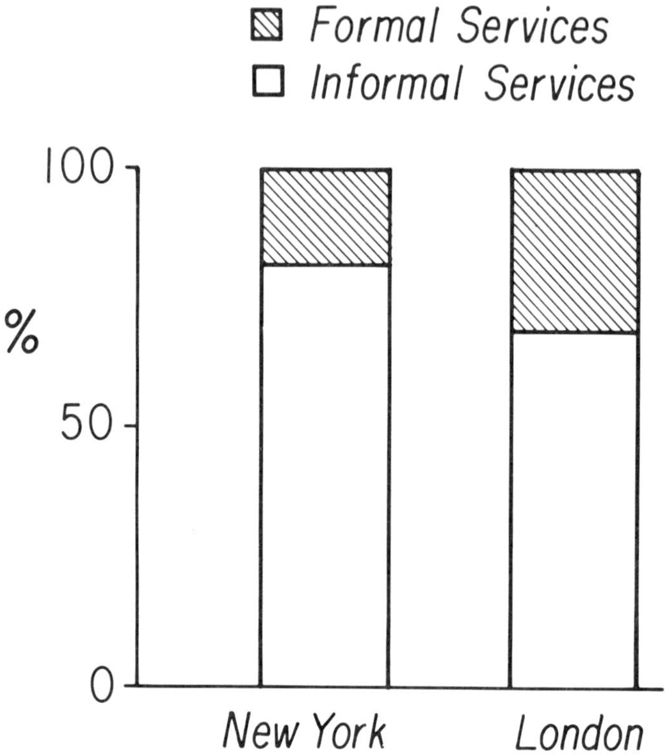

Note: In New York 30% (of 445 subjects) were dependent; In London 31% of 396 subjects. Figure includes only the primary provider.

There is also unpredictability in shifts in the politics of funding the various components of continuum of care that constitutes the long term care system.

By and large, the health and social care system needs to maintain elastic capacity and vigour in all components while recognizing the realities of limits on overall costs.

Finally, it is important that the planning

of health care services is carried out on a more discrete level of specificity in matching services to a typology of clinical problems and contexts relating to dementia. For example, different services are called for in rapidly progressive dementias than in the slowly advancing dementias (the usual form in the old-old); in those with and without behavior problems; and in those with strong or with weak social supports. In the cross-national study it appears that community based services have major impact in reducing (though not eliminating) institutional admission rates among the dependent elderly with weak (not absent) social supports; whereas, where supports are strong these services may have little success in reducing the need for institutional beds.

CONCLUSION

Advances in therapeutic interventions and support for the elderly with dementia should be viewed in the context of the health care system in which the new model of care will be imbedded. Without this perspective, there is a risk that the attractions of an innovative approach to care will be overwhelming and imbalance the system to the detriment of the patients or family. The cross-national comparisons of the US-UK Project show different emphases in the long term care systems of New York and London but do not disclose a clearcut advantage to either side. Rather, these studies suggest the need to make both systems as balanced and flexible as possible.

REFERENCES

Copeland JRM, Kelleher MJ, Kellett JM, Fountain-Gourlay AJ, Cowan DW, Barron G, DeGruchy J (UK) with Gurland BJ, Sharpe L, Simon RJ, Kuriansky J, Stiller P (US) (1975). Cross-national study of diagnosis of the mental disorders: A comparison of the diagnoses of elderly psychiatric patients admitted to mental hospitals serving Queens County New York and the former borough of Camberwell, London. British Journal of Psychiatry 126:11-20.

Cross P, Gurland BJ, Mann AH (In Press). A comparison of the frail elderly in day treatment and long-term care in New York City and London. Acta Psychiatrica Scandinavica Supplement.

Cross PS, Gurland BJ, Mann AH (1983). Long-term institutional care of demented elderly people in New York City and London. Bulletin of the New York Academy of Medicine 59:267-275.

Godlove C, Richard L, Graham R (1982). "Time for Action: An Observation Study of Elderly People in Four Different 'Care Environments'." Sheffield: University of Sheffield, 1982.

Gurland B, Bennett R, Wilder D (1981). Reevaluating the place of evaluation in planning for alternatives to institutional care for the elderly. Journal of Social Issues 37 (3): 51-68.

Gurland B, Copeland J, Kelleher M, Kuriansky J, Sharpe L, Dean L (1983). "The Mind and Mood of Aging: The Mental Health Problems of the Community Elderly in New York and London." New York: Haworth Press.

Gurland BJ, Dean LL, Copeland J, Gurland R, Golden R (1982). Criteria for the diagnosis of dementia in the community elderly. Gerontologist 22:180-186.

Gurland BJ, Wilder DE, Cross P (In Press). Public health aspects of Alzheimer's and related dementias. In Kelly E (ed): "Alzheimer's Disease and Related Dementias." Springfield, Illinois: Charles C Thomas.

Mann AH, Gurland BJ, Cross P (Submitted for publication). A comparison of the prescriptions received by the elderly in long-term care institutions in New York and London.

Mann AH, Gurland BJ, Cross P (1982). A comparison of the long-term care of the elderly in New York and London and implications of the differences. Paper presented at the meeting of the epidemiology section of the World Psychiatric Association at Johns Hopkins University May 16, 1982.

ACKNOWLEDGEMENTS

The studies discussed in this paper were supported in part by grants from the National Institute of Mental Health (5R13MH09191) and the Adminstration on Aging (90-A-1649; 90AT-2155; 93-P-57467).

Senile Dementia: Outlook for the Future, pages 339–352

Mutual-Help Groups for Caregivers in the Management of Senile Dementia: A Research Agenda

George L. Maddox, Ph. D.

Duke University

Durham, North Carolina 27710

Medical research and therapeutic maneuvers typically focus on individuals and the diseases that plague them. These characteristic preferences are only slightly modified by interest in the sociocultural context of disease etiology, course, and treatment illustrated by epidemiology and social medicine. The basic and clinical research agenda for Senile Dementia of the Alzheimer's Type (SDAT) and its treatment typically encountered in the United States confirms expectations (see e.g., White House Conference on Aging, 1981).

This paper proposes a complementary, corrective research agenda. We propose that, in the immediate future, systematic psychosocial research on caregiving and on informal mutual-help groups for non-professional, non-institutional caregivers should be given a priority equal to that given to SDAT and to the SDAT patient. My reasons are straightforward.

First, for all the public emphasis on the current and future demand SDAT patients will place on the formal care system, most of the care provided for most SDAT patients is now and in the foreseeable future will be provided informally by kith and kin. While systematic research has not established this conclusion for the management of SDAT, research on the care provided for other seriously impaired older persons does (Laurie, 1977). We have not been but should be curious about the effectiveness of informal caregiving. But we should be equally curious about whether caregiving has the possibility if not the probability of turning a caregiver into a patient and, if not, why not. Systematic research on the effects of informal caregiving is scarce, particularly in the United States. A recent study of informal residental caregiving for older adults documents high levels of demand on and stress among caregivers (Noelke and Poulshock, 1982). While the study did not focus on SDAT, it did focus on stress-producing factors of particular relevance for the SDAT caregiver--personal care dependency, cognitive impairment, and disruptive behavior. It is noteworthy that 80% of the caregivers were 50 years of age or older and, on average, have been providing care for over six years. The documented negative impact of caring on caregivers' health and well-being was substantial.

Participation by caregivers in mutual-help groups, we argue, probably does or could play an important role in insuring that informal caregiving is therapeutically beneficial for the SDAT patient and protective for caregivers. This is intuitively believable and often asserted but undemonstrated.

Second, the best possible investment of societal resources in health care is in basic research promising an understanding of disease etiology and feasible strategies of prevention. We commend basic biomedical research on SDAT. But, if experience with other complex major diseases is relevant, we are at this time multiple millions of dollars and decades away from preventing or controlling the effects of SDAT. This is not a counsel of dispair. It is a realistic appraisal and it is the basis for concentrating on psychosocial research regarding what can be done in the meantime for patients through caregivers, particularly a meantime that is likely to span a decade or two.

In the meantime, therefore, we suggest a major initiative in basic and applied psychosocial research on mutual-help groups for SDAT caregivers. The emphasis on research is important. Many clinicians and biomedical research investigators indicate they believe mutual-help groups for caregivers can be useful in therapeutic and other ways (see, e.g., Mace and Rabins, 1981). Their support of basic behavioral and social scientific research on such groups is less obvious.

Third, beyond any therapeutic potential mutual-help groups for caregivers may have for SDAT patients and caregivers, we propose that basic research on such groups promises useful incidental benefits of considerable importance both for society and for biomedical research investigators. We argue that available evidence on mutual-help groups indicates they not only may assist caregivers in coping with the stress of caring for a seriously impaired individual but also 1) may increase the effectiveness of patient care; 2) may provide a mechanism for the practical education of professionals who have minimum interest in and experience with SDAT; 3) may enhance social advocacy to reduce established barriers to formal care (e.g. lack of care, access to available care, insurance coverage exclusions); and 4) may provide a political base for support of public funding of basic and applied biomedical research. Further, we believe enthusiastic support for basic and applied research on SDAT mutual-help groups by the biomedical research community would contribute significantly and usefully to the application of the perspective of social medicine in which biomedical, behavioral and social factors interact directly and beneficially in the case of caregivers and indirectly in the case of the SDAT patient. In turn, the application of the perspective of social medicine to SDAT promises to benefit patients, caregivers, the total research community, and society.

REVIEW OF THE LITERATURE

In the absence of systematic research, there is very little definitive information on the role and effect of mutual-help on informal caregivers managing SDAT patients in community settings. A research agenda to explore the therapeutic potential of mutual-help groups is needed to replace the speculation characteristically encountered in the literature on caring for the non-institutionalized SDAT patient. However, a great deal of information is now available on mutual-help groups as a generic type of social support network. Fortunately this voluminous literature is surveyed with reasonable comprehensiveness in five sources (Caplan and Killilea, 1976; Lieberman and Borman, 1979; Hamburg and Killilea, 1979; Katz, 1981; and Wan, 1982). These sources provide the basis for summary generalizations which follow about the conceptualization, origins, growth and development, functions and outcomes of mutual-help groups. These summary generalizations, in turn, constitute the background for our subsequent proposal of a research agenda to explore the actual and potential therapeutic significance of such groups for the SDAT patient and caregiver. We will comment on mutual-help groups generated specifically in response to SDAT insofar as limited current experience permits.

Conceptual and Definitional Issues. The social and emotional bonding of individuals into social networks of individuals who perceive a shared fate and affirm mutual responsibilites for one another is a basic building block of all stable social groups. Kinship groups are prototypic mutual-help groups. In complex, socially differentiated societies, kinship-like social networks also appear in large numbers and great variety apparently to compensate for the attenuation of kinship ties, the limited capacity of kin groups to provide needed social support, or both. While specialized mutual-help groups are extraordinarily common in the United States, which is known for its proliferation of specialized organizational froms, similar developments have been documented, for example, in the United Kingdom, Holland, Poland, Yugoslavia and Latin America. While specialized support groupings take many forms (e.g., as alternatives to professional care, as adjuncts to professional care, as contexts for alternative lifestyles, or as political action groups), mutual-help denotes a particular type of socially bonded exchange relationship focused primarily, at least initially, on assistance in adapting to some stressful events or circumstances. Events or circumstances related to illness--one's own or other's--are particularly likely to generate mutual-help groups. As a case in point, almost every major category of disease in the International Classification of Diseases has generated in the United States some type of mutual-help group.

In psychosocial terms, the essence of mutual-help groups is the provision of a reliable exchange network in which participants believe they are loved, are cared for, and are the certain beneficiaries of a network of mutual obligations. Mutual-help groups typically function to provide 1) models of emotional mastery in responding to traumatic events and circumstances; 2) guidance in the cognitive interpretation of and response to these events and circumstances; 3) consensual validation for self-esteem or for the re-invention of the self in the face of significant loss; and 4) instrumental, palpable, practical help in securing needed resources.

This characterization of mutual-help groups makes it reasonably clear that such groups are not relevant for SDAT patients themselves in a way similar to the role played for the alcoholic by Alcoholics Anonymous, the prototypic mutual-help group for patients with an alcohol abuse problem. Therefore, the proper analogy for our purposes is Al-Anon, the counterpart group for the spouses of the patient with this problem (Ablom, 1974).

Origins--The fundamental importance of group solidarity and of the bonding of group members in exchange relationships is a very old idea well-documented in both ethological and social scientific research. Isolation from groups and the disorganization of established exchange relationships demonstrably produce aberrant behavior and increase the risk of morbidity and mortality.

Mutual-help groups in human populations tend to be insured at least minimally for most individuals by the bonds of kinship. Naturally occurring kinship groups tend to be supplemented by the creation of special support groups in complex societies in which kinship bonds are attenuated or missing and in which relatively novel problems affect large numbers of individuals, as in the case of SDAT.

Initiative in constructing mutual-help groups typically is taken initially by laypersons rather than professionals or by professionals with atypical attitudes toward therapy. This initiative is most likely to occur in response to events or circumstances for which consensual definitions of the cause, course, and means of control are unknown or ambiguous, again as in the case of SDAT. When professionals are involved in initiating mutual-help groups, they tend to have distinctive, non-traditional perspectives and to serve as facilitators of group development rather than as formal leaders.

In December, 1979, for example, the National Institute on Aging of the (U.S.) National Institutes of Health facilitated a meeting of existing lay and professional leadership from "family support groups" for caregivers maintaining a SDAT patient at home. By January, 1981, a national organization--the Alzheimer's Disease and Related Disorders Association (ADRDA)--was created. At Duke University in 1979 a social worker with experience in community organization facilitated a meeting of caregivers interested in creating a local mutual-help group. The leadership of the group that emerged in Durham, North Carolina, was composed totally of laypersons; as a matter of principle, professionals served only as advisors and facilitators. This local group was the nucleus subsequently of other local groups in 23 communities geographically spread throughout the state involving over 2,000 families. The North Carolina groups subsequently affiliated collectively with the national organization (Gwyther, 1982).

It is relevant to note that mutual-help groups sometimes appear to emerge in response to perceived professional ineffectiveness and indifference or hostility toward the kinds of problems most likely to generate social support groups. While this is surely one incentive for group formation, it should not be exaggerated. Observed mutual-help groups typically involve professionals at least in a support role, a majority of group participants typically have received professional care, and a substantial minority maintain an active personal relationship with a professional.

Growth and Development--Authoritative current assessments of the number and rate of growth of various mutual-help groups do not exist. In the past decade, however, such groups are known to be numerous in both the United States and Europe. A current estimate for all types of mutual-help groups in the United States is that over 500,000 groups involving several million persons exist. In the health field alone ten national organizations involving over 2.5 million persons exist; a single mutual-help organization, Alcoholics Anonymous, has over 27,000 local chapters. Informed observers have documented analogous developments in some European countries.

No reliable basis for estimating expected growth rates for mutual-help organizations exists. This is understandable since informal organizations have difficulty in identifying members whose involvement varies over time; in any case, for such organizations documenting participation is not a primary concern. Apparent growth, however, can be dramatic. National ADRDA in the United States, which emerged in January, 1981, reported one year later 40 local chapters and 200 family support groups. In North Carolina, one support group in 1981 involving a small number of family members had evolved two years later into mutual-help family support groups in 23 communities involving over 2,000 family members.

Published research suggests at least two questions of practical as well as theoretical importance in the growth and development of mutual-help groups. The first deals with the dynamics of self-selection among participants and the natural course of their participation. As we will note later, these dynamics are complicated and not only warrant research but also constitute a significant problem for designing research on the impact of group participation. The second deals with the observed tendency over time for informal groups which emphasize charismatic leadership initially to become bureaucratized as they become part of a formal, national organization. The effect of this organizational transformation on group objectives and on the experience of participants, while expected to be significant, is not well documented.

Participant Needs and Group Functions--Mutual-help groups that are, as in the case of those responsive to caregivers of SDAT patients, focused on coping and adaptation to the stresses of caregiving, typically have four primary functions matched implicitly or explicitly with recognized needs: 1) cognitive definition and re-definition of stressful and possibly stigmatizing experiences; 2) containment of powerful and potentially immobilizing emotion; 3) practical exchange of goods and services; and 4) models for reorganizing, re-integrating, and re-inventing the self in the face of the significant loss.

This specification of personal needs and related group functions observed in mutual-help groups generally are recognizable and intuitively plausible to clinicians and investigators of group dynamics. This specification is also consonant with our personal experience with participants in a large number of mutual-help groups for SDAT caregivers (Gwyther, 1982). Both published research and our observations indicate the importance of understanding the timing, salience and elaboration of individual needs and related group functions over the course of participation. The natural evolution of needs in terms of their salience and elaboration appears to proceed typically in this order: cognitive clarification; exploring ways both to express and contain emotion; testing of "reliable availability" of others and their capacity and willingness to provide or help in securing required services; and, finally, new conceptions of the self, particularly when relief from the overwhelming burden of caregiving implied by the phrase "the 36-hour day" is an urgent concern.

The need for cognitive definition of SDAT underlies a profound interest in reliable, authoritative information about the etiology of the disease, about its heritability and about the expectable course of the illness. Concern among caregivers about the etiology of SDAT warrants a special comment. SDAT is currently and correctly classified as a "non-specific" disease; that is, a disease which, like many types of mental illness or drug abuse, lacks a definitive etiology, definitive natural course, and definitive intervention. The associated ambiguity insures that the caregiver will have difficulty in interpreting for self and others the unusual behavior of an otherwise apparently normal person; caregivers characteristically feel stigmatized. They want to know "what kind of disease is this?" and they worry about whether the disease is a form of mental illness to which they contributed. The prospect that the disease might be organic in origin, possibly genetic, is only partly reassuring. Siblings and children of the SDAT patient, e.g., are obviously frightened by the implications of genetic heritability. The need to define SDAT as a medical rather than a psychiatric disorder or mental health problem, the caregiver quickly learns, has important implications for health insurance coverage and access to health facilities. Analogous practical concerns were appreciated 35 years ago by E. M. Jellinek, the effective advocate for alcoholics who managed to get the American Medical Association House of Delegates to declare that "alcoholism is a disease." His explicit goal was to reduce the experienced rejection of the alcoholic by hospitals and insurance companies.

Mutual-help groups for SDAT caregivers clearly function as a context for observing models of emotional expression and containment of profound feelings of loss, sorrow, and anger. Feelings of shame are frequently expressed and group meetings provide an occasion for "coming out of the closet, of going public" with a socially stigmatized problem.

The exchange of actual goods in SDAT caregiver groups appears to be limited. Members do offer each other, however, some rather important services, including, e.g., information about the disease, "reliable availability" should there be a need, practical advice on problem management, and insights into how the existing formal services work or can be made to work more effectively. Group meetings provide a plausible, legitimate reason to take leave briefly from caregiving responsibilities and to ask kith and kin to provide respite services.

The fact that more experienced caregivers meet in the same group with less experienced ones insures the probability that models of cognitive restructuring, of emotional containment, and of practical exchange of advice will be available for the novice. Concomitantly, the experienced participant has the opportunity to experience the satisfaction of being a helper. Experience in Alcoholics Anonymous and Al-Anon suggests that a small number of persons become a quasi-professional cadre in mutual-help groups who find personal satisfaction through helping. But the process by which this happens is not altogether clear. We know it is not a highly probable outcome for most participants.

Relatively late in the experience of group participants the reorganization and re-invention of the self become salient. Observers of Al-Anon for the spouses (typically the wife) of alcoholics note that experienced participants focus on themselves and <u>their</u> problems almost to the exclusion of "the patient" (Ablom, 1974). This re-assertion and possible re-invention of the self may be facilitated by the death of, separation from, or disidentification with "the patient"; and at this point the caregiver is eligible to and may "graduate" from the group. Apart from a large number of factors that might explain marginal or temporary participation in mutual-help groups, "graduation" is a type of potentially successful outcome that naturally insures turnover in membership.

At relatively advanced stages of group process, mutual-help groups--or at least their leadership--may become involved in professional and public education, in political advocacy, and in fundraising. Such activities tend to be the primary concerns of the national bureaucratic superstructures which are grafted onto the base of popular support implicit in local mutual-help groups. There is no question that, if the experience of the United States is generalizable, bureaucratic leadership can and does use local groups effectively to illustrate need for societal resources to attack some neglected problem and to provide evidence of widespread support for legislation and the allocation of public resources for research, training, and services.

Outcomes. There is currently no systematic evidence from research that mutual-help groups generally and for caregivers of the SDAT patient in particular have predictably beneficial outcomes for participants or the patients they serve. The basic sources cited at the beginning of this paper document in a compelling way that access to and participation in supportive social exchange networks appear to be beneficial. An extensive body of research on coping and adaptation has argued that perceived and actual integration into a reliable social exchange network probably work through known connections between behavior and what are called by biomedical scientists "three great organic systems"--the central nervous system, the endocrine, and the immunological system. Most of the research on beneficial effects of social support systems has concentrated on patient's themselves. To extrapolate these findings to an associated person, in our case a caregiver, would be reasonable but would remain an extrapolation (see, e.g., White House Conference on Aging, 1982).

The difficulties for research investigators attempting to assess the effects of mutual-help groups directly on SDAT caregivers and indirectly on patients are formidable. First, one would have to decide what to measure. The problem has at least two components. Is one concerned with the indirect effects on the SDAT patient, the direct effects on the caregiver, or both? Further, would the outcomes of interest be symptom relief or greater competence in functioning or personal integration (i.e., the professional therapist's primary interest) or all three?

Second, when to measure? The fluid dynamics of group participation, coupled with different stages in the conditions of the patient to which the caregiver responds, suggest why one would expect differential effects of participation among individuals at a point in time and for the same individual over time. Symptom relief, competence in functioning, and personal integration might occur not at all, selectively, or in complex combinations for individuals over time.

Third, the fluid dynamics of group participation and the

probable differential timing of outcomes present especially challenging problems of sample design.

We proceed to our next section on a research agenda fully aware of these challenges but confident that the high stakes involved make the challenges worth accepting. We expect biomedical scientists, acutely aware of their own challenges in understanding SDAT, to be sympathetic and supportive.

A RESEARCH AGENDA

Our suggested agenda includes four broad categories of research on mutual-help groups for SDAT caregivers:

1. The dynamics of group formation and maintenance;

2. The outcomes of participation directly for participants and indirectly for patients;

3. Principles and decision rules for professionals in the support and therapeutic use of mutual-help groups; and

4. The broader societal implications of mutual-help groups and related national associations of such groups.

In brief, we would benefit from the kind of systematic attention to SDAT caregiver groups provided in the case studies of other mutual-help conveniently illustrated in the Lieberman and Borman (1979) monograph. Further, we recommend the research design outlined by Pearlin *et al* (1981) to investigate the role of support groups in the mediation of stress as a prime model to use as a point of departure in developing the scientific information needed.

The Dynamics of Group Formation and Maintenance. We know that effective mutual-help groups occur naturally, with kinship grouping as the prototype (Noelke and Poulshock, 1982). Naturally occuring groups available to an SDAT caregiver may be able to supply models of emotional containment in the face of traumatic experience and to supply an exchange of essential support services. Two factors argue, however, for reliable knowledge about the construction of supplemental support groups. First, for a minority of caregivers, viable kinship groups are literally not available or accessible. Second, for the majority it is improbable that existing kin groupings have the information necessary for useful cognitive definition of SDAT that would assist in dealing with probable concomitant stigma; in providing models of emotional control in the face of a socially stigmatized condition; in providing cognitive mapping of relevant professional and non-professional services and their effective use; and in offering models of role redefinition for caregivers.

Further, reliable information is needed on how the essentially charismatic leadership of mutual-support groups can be mobilized and maintained in the face of tendencies toward professional dominance and bureaucratization. Both professionalism and bureaucratization are potentially countervailing forces in the maintenance, and possibly the therapeutic effectiveness, of mutual-help groups for SDAT caregivers.

The Dynamics of Effective Group Participation--While we know intuitively that participation in constructed mutual-help groups is self-selective, no definitive research exists on the process of selection, on the degree of involvement, or on termination of participation. This is true of all mutual-help groups, not just SDAT groups. We know from observation that SDAT mutual-help groups have a mix of participants with varying degrees of sophistication and experience; this fact is essential to understanding why the experienced members are able to assist novice members. However, we know very little about the optimum mix of experience and inexperience that affects the efficacy of therapeutic outcomes; and we know little about the forces that predict normal "graduation" from the group in contrast to drop-out and about the maintenance of a cadre of experienced helpers. Further, systematic evidence about how the effects of group experience on SDAT caregivers translates into their sense of well-being, their functioning, and their use of health care for themselves and for the SDAT patient is not available.

We now know enough, however, about how to conceptualize group processes and outcomes, about the measurement of outcomes and about research design and sampling problems to undertake the necessary systematic research.

Appropriate Professional Utilization of Groups--Professionals who include care of SDAT caregivers in their purview as an integral part of care for the SDAT patient are currently working within the proverbial "black box." Intuitively they suspect that mutual-help groups are possibly if not probably useful but they do not know for whom or under what circumstances. Professionals, in brief, lack principles to guide their support of mutual-help groups and they lack decision rules regarding the utilization and limits of mutual-support groups as adjuntive therapy and about what their relationship to such groups should be. The development of appropriate decision rules presupposes the existence of reliable information about groups and their dynamics which does not exist currently for professionals in practice or in training.

The Societal Implications of Groups--In the United States, the national organization of SDAT mutual-help groups, ADRDA, issued a proclamation in March, 1982, entitled "A Disease of the Century." The hyperbole of the title has some basis in fact. The prevalence of SDAT in increasingly aging populations is high and the estimated personal and societal costs of the disease are impressive. The stated mission of ADRDA includes not only family support but also public and professional education, advocacy and research. Significantly, among the types of education and research offered to illustrate the societal bnefits of ADRDA, education and research on SDAT mutual-help groups is not featured.

To end as we began, this paper is not intended to persuade that basic or clinical research on the biomedical aspects of SDAT is unimportant. Quite the contrary, basic biomedical research which promises prevention or amelioration of SDAT is a premier investment. Rather this paper intends to persuade that basic psychosocial research on how, under what circumstances and for whom SDAT mutual-help groups are beneficial is also important. Further we argue that both whether and how, in addition to therapeutic benefits, such groups are integral to public and professional education, and support of research warrant careful documentation.

In our view, it is important to establish how and under what circumstances the potentially therapeutic benefits of mutual-help groups can be acheived at the same time broader societal goals are pursued. Further, it is important to establish whether and how mutual-help groups have a beneficial impact on the way societal health care resources, legislation, and allocation of research resources are affected by social processes as elemental and as mobilizable as the basic social forces that promote and insure social solidarity.

Ablom J (1974). Al-Anon family groups. Am J Psychotherapy 28:1:30-45.
Caplan G, Killilea M (eds) (1976). "Supportive Systems and Mental Health." New York: Grune & Stratton.
Gwyther L (1982). Caring for caregivers: A statewide family support program mobilizes mutual help. Durham, NC: Duke University Center Report on Advances in Research 6:4 (whole issue).
Hamburg B, Killilea M (1979). Relation of social support, stress, illness, and the use of health services. In Surgeon General of the United States, "Healthy People: Background Papers." Washington, DC: Department of Health, Education and Welfare.
Katz A (1981). Self-help and mutual-aid: An emerging social movement? Ann Rev Sociol 7:129-155.
Laurie W F (1978). Employing the Duke OARS methodology in cost comparisons: Home services and institutionlization. Durham, NC: Duke University Center Report Report on Advances in Research 2:2 (whole issue).
Lieberman M, Borman L (1979). "Self-help Groups for Coping with Crisis." San Francisco: Jossey-Bass.
Mace N, Rabins P (1981). "The 36-Hour Day." Baltimore: The Johns Hopkins Press.
Noelke L, Poulshock S (1982). "The Effects of Caring for Impaired Elderly in Residence." Cleveland, Ohio: Benjamin Rose Institute.
Pearlin L, Lieberman M, Menagham E, Mullen J (1981). The stress process. J Health Social Behav 22:337-356.
Wan T (1982). "Stressful Life Events, Social Support Networks, and Gerontological Health." Lexington, MA: Lexington Books.
White House Conference on Aging (1981). Report of the Mini-Conference on Alzheimer's Disease. Washington, DC.

Senile Dementia: Outlook for the Future, pages 353–364

SENILE DEMENTIA - REFLECTIONS ON REHABILITATION PROCEDURES

Margaret Zinder

Psychologie
Hôpital de Psycho-Gériatrie
Prilly, 1008 - Suisse

We propose in this paper to describe a research orientation on the rehabilitation of subjects suffering from senile dementia, to clarify the theoretical course to follow and analyze the main landmarks along this route. A number of problems will be proposed for consideration, even though we are aware that they may assume different forms or even become irrelevant as the theory is put to the test of practice. A review of the work upon which ours has been based, and of work having different objectives, will supply a brief survey of the various psychological approaches to senile dementia. We shall conclude with an illustration of our general approach by two practical applications.

By rehabilitation, we refer to all the various means aimed to maintain or recuperate for the senile dement an optimal degree of autonomy, taking into consideration his mental deterioration, in day to day activities. We shall revert in greater detail below to this concept of optimal autonomy, which implies a certain mastery by the subject of his environment. If the action of the subject is regarded as the basis for construction of the internal and external world of the individual, it will also constitute the basis of all rehabilitation activity in the demented subject.

The elaboration of a system of aids tending toward the autonomy of the subject, toward his capacity to carry out everyday tasks without passive dependence on his social circle, implies making the concept of autonomy operational. Between the subject and a task to be carried out or a goal to be achieved, there is a relationship of adjustment or reciprocal adaptation, the quality of which determines the degree of autonomy with regard to the task in question. This dynamic interplay between subject and object has been taken by Piaget(1967;1974)to express the idea of adaptation or adequation, whose motor mechanism he studied, as well as the successive forms or structures of the genesis of intelligence. Piaget (1976)situated the motor for adaptation at the level of behavior itself, while considering subject-environment adequation as the product of an active construction. He treated intelligence as the specific organ of the most stable and also the most mobile adaptation, the one most compensatory for perturbation. The regulatory mechanism of equilibrations constituting the dynamic of behavior is therefore the functional constant of all the successive forms of adaptation, from the instinctive to the intellectual forms. At every ontogenetic level, subject and milieu are reciprocally adapted to one another through an assimilation of external objects to the structures of the subject and an accomodation of these structures to external reality. These are the functional characteristics of the Piaget system on which we focus in attempting to evaluate the dynamic relationship between the dement and his immediate environment.

From the structural point of view, the successive forms or structures upon which the cognitive elements pattern themselves, from the earliest habits acquired by the infant to the hypothetical-deductive operations of the young adult, define the potentialities of the individual, that is, his level of competence or his cognitive baggage. These forms succeed one another according to a necessary sequence of integration and each of them summarizes or subsumes the tools of knowledge thus far acquired in the course of ontogenesis. This theoretical Piagetian model served as the basis for the Geneva team of Ajuriaguerra and Richard (1972), who supported the hypothesis that in senile dementia the deterioration of cognitive functions follows a course opposite to that of their construction.

Marianne Boehme (1973) has relativized this hypothesis, maintaining the impossibility of perceiving any one of these evolutive stages in its entirety during the process of dementification, since it is the operativity itself which defines these structures which would be disturbed in the pathological process of dementia. The problems involved in this study, dealing with orientation in space, relate directly to the active adequation of the knowing subject to reality.

It is nevertheless necessary to recall that Piaget considered adaptation in its evolution and knowledge in its genesis. From the structural point of view, the Piagetian subject understands reality without any effective or successful participation in it. For our part, we are interested in the actual adaptation of the senile dement and in his activity, not only reflexive but practical and finalized. These divergences question the theoretical model on two main points :

1. The control by the adult subject of his cognitive instruments, already acquired and structured.
2. The programming or planning of the action, subject to representation of the purpose aimed at.

The control of instruments is the special subject of the study by P. Vermersch (1978) of work psychology, which seeks to understand the functioning of an adult operator in a situation of training or work. In summing up this author's work, we may say that on the basis of Piaget's theory he arrives at a hypothetical model of cognitive adult functioning, related to stages in their genesis and their qualities of equilibration. Depending on the situation, the operator uses one or another of the planning registers, to which other registers are subordinated, which succeed one another or act in combination in the course of the task. Various factors of choice have to be reckoned with, such as the instruments which the work demands or what its representation induces, and a more or less voluntary control, inhibiting the tendency to assimilate the object before organizing and processing the data concerning it.

The question of programming itself is the subject of work by B. Inhelder et al (1978; 1980) of the Geneva school. These authors, studying what they call the procedures of discovery, aim at the reconstitution of a psychological model of the subject in the course of resolving a finally completed task.

Such a model would function according to two alternating orders of procedure:

- A descending control or teleonomic order, consisting for the subject, on the basis of representations of the task to be carried out or a goal to be reached, of evoking and applying these familiar schemata, pursuant to a plan of action.
- An ascending control or productive order which consists of performing a series of appropriate actions on the basis of the significance accorded to the indices of the situation.

To illustrate the practical application of these ideas, we present some observations of a woman patient, disoriented in the space of the ground-floor of the hospital where she spent her daytime hours. It was considered important for the autonomy of this patient, that she should be able to go to the toilet alone. Our approach to the situation consisted of several stages:

1. The spontaneous movements of the patient are observed. These observations show that she only starts in the right direction after an initial visual exploration of the space. She continues in the direction chosen until she comes to the first unmarked door, which opens into the dining room. Then she either explores this room visually or enters it, which takes her away from her objective. Taken back into the corridor, she finds the toilet by reading the signs on the doors.

2. The visuo-spatial configuration of the initial space is modified by removing a picture and shifting a plant symmetrically from left to right. The patient, indecisive at first, goes to the side where the plant is now located, she appears confused and returns to her starting point.

3. When we cover up the sign on the toilet door, the patient looks attentively at the cover, hesitates, and then opens the door to identify the room behind it. When the sign for the toilet is moved to the preceding door, she takes this to be the door to the toilet.

The general procedure for accomplishing the task consists in the coordination of perceptions and movements, without coordination of the whole pattern, subordinated to the objective. This objective is construed by the patient to be a simple extension of her actions. She set her course step by step, correcting her errors after making them. Her reactions when the plant is displaced showed that she had used it as an index for the direction to follow. This index was associated with the sensory-motor schema of turning to the left, which itself was constructed of the repetition of walking in that direction. The conflict between this schema and the perceptive-motor information registered by the patient when the plant was moved disturbed her behaviour. Once the direction was chosen, the places were recognized by signs; if not, exploring them diverted the patient from her objective.

In the light of these results, it is apparent that the autonomy of the patient in her movements depends on two conditions :

1. Conservation of the sensory-motor schema of turning to the left. In order to assure this conservation, it is important on the one hand that the patient be motivated to go to the toilet alone and, on the other hand, that we do not modify the visuo-spatial configuration integrated in her schema.

2. Maintenance of the conduct of searching for the objective. We should make sure that the patient is not obliged to go through a place physically in order to identify it. It would suffice to keep her from losing track of her objective for all the doors on the corridor to be marked, since she only enters rooms which are not identifiable from the outside.

As we can see, observation of the spontaneous perambulations of the subject and intervention on the conditions under which she carries them out enables us to deduce the type of procedure adopted and also the instruments used at different stages. In the case described, the patient did not resort to representation, which in fact had proved to be very perturbed in specific tests designed to develop this function. On the other hand, she was able to read and to deal with a variety of visuo-spatial data.

The problematic in the second study we shall present deals with social interaction between subjects suffering from senile dementia. Why do we speak of social interaction in this connection ?

The hospital, inherently, is a place which brings together persons from all possible origins. While cohabitation is an essential condition, encounters between individuals are nevertheless relatively uncertain at times, and these encounters have not been the subject of systematic observation. It is true of course that we do have occasional and often fragmentary information about interactions between hospitalized patients. These usually consist however of subjective impressions of developments which are difficult to quantify. In addition, the situations have the major disadvantage that it is difficult to repeat and systematize them for experimental purposes. We wanted to determine therefore if observations of this kind can be repeated, developed and systematized in the framework of an ergotherapy workshop. Our initial interest is in attempting to understand to what extent the interaction between subjects confronted by the same task may serve as a factor contributing to rehabilitation. While our medium term purpose is to work with our patients on activities which bear a relation to the tasks of everyday life, we decided in an initial phase to base our experimentation on Piaget's operational tasks. These tasks present the advantage that they not only make possible quantitative measurement of a performance but also enable us to make a qualitative evaluation of development. We are therefore concerned with studying both the modalities and the effects of interactions and in so doing to determine whether cooperation, in the sense of an operation carried out jointly, between two subjects, can be a source of individual progress for the partners.

What importance does Piaget (1965)attribute to social interactions in the genesis of cognitive structures ?

He demonstrates that alongside of maturation of the role exercised by action on reality and of equilibration, another fundamental factor intervenes, that of social interaction and transmission. Although Piaget refers to the importance of this factor on cognitive evolution in his theoretical work, he did very little to verify this experimentally. The studies carried out by Perret-Clermont (1979)and by Doise and Mugny (1981)provided us with both a theoretical and experimental basis for our own work. In her studies with children, Perret-Clermont demonstrated that they benefit from interaction with partners of a genetic level which is inferior, equal or superior to their own if two conditions are fulfilled. The first condition, of course, is the capacity to communicate with others; the second is to perceive the conflict of centration between one's own point of view and that of the other child.

The proposed model illustrates the constructivist and interactionist point of view of the Geneva school. To theories of the "modeling effect", the authors oppose the Piagetian vision of the genesis of cognitive structures. This does not result from passive appropriation by the child of behavior or knowledge but from a structuralizing action on reality which is carried out especially well through inter-individual coordination. The interaction does not merely supply an ingredient to assimilate into the schema of the subject but engenders an act of accomodation which in turn generates progress, inasmuch as the performance of a model at a higher level than that of the subject cannot, of course, be directly assimilated by the subject. Such models correspond to levels of structuration different and more complex than his own, which implies that any progress can only be the result of an act of accomodation, permitting reorganization of the cognitive structures of the subject.

Accordingly, any difference between points of view is conflictual, generates perturbations only to the extent that it is merely perceived, without being directly assimilated into an overall structure. We may say then that the sociocognitive conflict causes disequilibriums which necessitate the elaboration of new forms and hence the construction of new operations (Piaget 1975)

Following this outline of the theoretical and methodological basis of our work, we shall briefly summarize our experiment.

Our experimental procedure includes four stages:

- a preliminary test
- a phase of interaction
- 2 follow-up tests

The preliminary and follow-up tests are given only to the individual subjects, while the phase of interaction calls for two subjects to cooperate in supplying a common response to the problem presented.

The task given is one of Piaget's (1948)which we have adopted in a simplified form, the relating of points of view. This task utilizes a model consisting of a house, a tower and a pine tree on a square base, measuring 50 cm on each side. After the subject has identified and named each object on the model, the experimenter shows him four pictures of the same landscape as seen from different points of view. The subject is asked to designate, successively, the picture which represents his own point of view and the one showing the opposite point of view. He then localizes the point of view corresponding to one of the pictures.

During the phase of interaction, a similar problem is presented, based on the furniture in the office. The role of the experimenter, in the tests given individually, consists of offering counter suggestions and helpful indices to the subject and of recalling the instructions. During the interaction phase, the experimenter intervenes to reinforce cooperation between the subjects, to recall the reciprocal arguments and on occasion, to emphasize the difference in the points of view of the subjects.

The population examined is composed of three groups :

- an experimental group of patients at the Psychogeriatric Hospital at Prilly
- two control groups.

One of the control groups consists of subjects suffering from senile dementia who attend a day hospital; the other of aged people with no particular pathology.

This research procedure permits consideration of several poles of centration. The first is of course to examine the effect of interaction. We shall attempt to determine whether cooperation between patients improves performance and also, by the follow-up tests, to ascertain the stability of this effect. Secondly, we shall try to differentiate between the effect attributable to the interaction and that induced by the intervention of the experimenter. We hope, through the use of the two control groups to find out if there are significant differences in the behavior of the subjects based on whether or not they participate in the interaction phase. Thirdly, our study will be concerned with the interaction itself, that is, the communication between the subjects and its modalities. Accordingly, we shall :

- examine as a whole all the verbal and non verbal conduct of the patients, their use of codes and conventional signs;
- verify the existence of rules of communication, implicit or explicit;
- try to identify elements which may be specific to communication between demented subjects.

In conclusion, the two studies presented have a double objective : to elaborate a theoretical model of the functioning of the senile dement and to develop a method of rehabilitation.

The encounter this represents between ergotherapy and genetic psychology is an expression of our general approach, consisting of a reciprocal adjustment between theory and practice.

REFERENCES

Ajuriaguerra J.de et al (1972). De l'application des méthodes de la psychologie génétique à l'étude des fonctions cognitives dans l'âge avancé.

Rev. franç. géront. p 17.
Boehme M (1973). La détérioration dans la démence sénile. Démence sénile simple-sénescence.Delachaux et Niestlé (ed). Neuchâtel. p 216.
Boula JG et al (1979). Les niveaux d'intervention ergothérapeutique en psychogériatrie. Jassen pharmaceutica p. 223.
Doise W et al (1981). Le développement social de l' intelligence. Inter Editions.
Gut AM et al. Les déments séniles interagissent-ils. unpublished.
Inhelder B (1978). De l'approche structurale à l' approche procédurale: introduction à l'étude des stratégies. Actes XXIe Congrès intern.de psychologie.PUF. p 99.
Inhelder B et al (1980). Procédures et significations dans la résolution d'un problème concret. Bull. psychol no 345. T XXXIII. p 645.
Perret-Clairmont AN (1979). La construction de l' intelligence dans l'interaction sociale. Peter Lang.
Pierrehumbert B et al (1978). Activité et réhabilitation dans les démences de la vieillesse. Archives suisses de neurologie, neurochirurgie et de psychiatrie. Vol 122. Fascicule 2 p 315.
Piaget J (1948). La représentation de l'espace chez l'enfant. PUF.
Piaget J (1965). Etudes sociologiques. Librairie Droz-Genève.
Piaget J (1967). Biologie et connaissance. Paris: Gallimard.
Piaget J (1974). Adaptation vitale et psychologie de l'intelligence. Paris: Hermann.
Piaget J (1975). L'équilibration des structures cognitives. Etudes d'épistémologie génétique. Vol XXXIII. PUF. Paris.
Piaget J (1976). Le comportement moteur de l'évolution. Paris: Gallimard.
Vermersch P (1978). Une problématique théorique en psychologie du travail: Essais d'application des théories de J.Piaget à l'analyse du fonctionnement cognitif de l'adulte. Le Travail humain. T 41. no 2. p 265

Zinder M, Brull J, Wertheimer J (1982). Pour une compréhension des fonctions cognitives du dément sénile dans une perspective de réhabilitation. Revue suisse de psychologie pure et appliquée. No 4. p 265.

Senile Dementia: Outlook for the Future, pages 365–379

PHARMACOLOGICAL RATIONALE FOR A TREATMENT OF SENILE DEMENTIA WITH CO-DERGOCRINE MESYLATE

Marco Ermini, Ph.D. and Rudolf Markstein, Ph.D.

Sandoz Ltd., Pharmaceutical Division

4002 Basel, Switzerland

Introduction

Senile Dementia of the Alzheimer Type (SDAT) is characterized by various morphological and neurochemical changes.

While it is obvious that the current knowledge is limited to only a few of the neuronal systems possibly involved in the pathogenesis and consequences of the disease, it may provide us with a - preliminary - basis for the development of a rationale for drug treatment.

Basically, there are two aspects to be considered for any pharmacotherapeutic approach.

On the one hand, an attempt could be made to causal treatment that would eventually result in an actual cure or even prevention of the disease.

On the other hand, on a secondary level, a more symptomatic approach may be envisaged, which will not "cure" the patient but at least alleviate some of the more deleterious impairments, such as loss of memory function, over a certain time.

While the causes responsible for the development of the disease are still under dispute (viral, genetic, toxic, dietetic?) one attempt could be directed towards preventing the neurons and neuronal processes to be lost. In particular neuronal systems innervating the cerebral cortex and the hippocampus, with their origin in deeper subcortical structures such as the nucleus basalis of Meynert or the Locus coeruleus appear to be important (for review see Bowen et al., 1979, De Boni and Crapper, 1980, Mann, 1983). Alternately, regeneration of the destroyed neuronal processes could also be considered.

Furthermore, it could be attempted to prevent or reverse the structural abnormalities found in cortical and hippocampal neurons, particularly the formation of neurofibrillary tangles and plaques, although it is not known, whether these elements are the cause or merely the consequence of metabolic disturbances of the affected cells.

However, up to now, no reasonable pharmacotherapeutic approach to such structural alterations has emerged so far (e.g. provoking sprouting of new dendrites). More feasible appears to be the attempt to keep the remaining neuronal systems functional either by enhancing neuronal activity presynaptically (e.g. synthesising and release of the respective neurotransmitter substances) or postsynaptically (e.g. by providing stimulatory input).

Currently, much emphasis is put on the cholinergic neurons of the frontal and temporal cortex, as well as of the hippocampus, which were found to show substantial decrease in the activity of choline acetyltransferase (CAT), as well as of acetylcholinesterase (AChE) (for review see: Bartus et al., 1982, Coyle et al., 1983). This finding is brought into relation to the loss of cognitive function, especially of memory formation and retrieval, as one of the most conspicuous and debilitating symptoms of SDAT (Perry et al. 1975, Rossor 1982).

However, despite the fact that pharmacological manipulation of memory function in amimals and man by anticholinergic agents and their reversal by drugs potentiating central cholinergic function (Davis et al., 1978, Drachman, 1978, Sitaram et al., 1978) point to the validity of using such drugs in the case of SDAT-dependent memory impairment, the outcome of such trials in SDAT patients has been rather inconclusive up to now (Corkin, 1981, Marchbanks, 1982, Thal et al., 1981).

On the other hand, besides the cholinergic systems, also monoaminergic systems were found to be affected in SDAT. In particular, the noradrenergic systems originating in the Locus coeruleus, the nigrostriatal dopaminergic pathway, and the serotoninergic projections of the Raphe nuclei to various brain regions, including the hippocampus and cerebral cortex, appear to be involved (Adolfsson et al., 1979, Gottfries, 1982, Mann et al., 1982, Rossor 1982, Rossor 1981).

The involvement of monoaminergic systems in SDAT appears to be less unequivocal than that of the cholinergic ones and the existence of subtypes of SDAT was suggested as a possible explanation for the inconsistent findings (Bartus et al., 1982, Carlsson et al., 1980, Coyle et al., 1983). It may also be one indication for a difference in etiology between Alzheimer´s disease and SDAT. Recently, the L. coeruleus and its projection to the fore-brain and its cholinergic structures has drawn considerable interest, since nerve cell degeneration has been found there more consistently than in other monoaminergic systems (Bondareff et al., 1982, Mann, 1983, Mann et al. 1982).

A therapeutic attempt of enhancing L. coeruleus neuronal function as well as of the other monoaminergic systems may, at least symptomatically, be of some benefit for the SDAT patient. Besides direct effects due to L. coeruleus stimulation, activation e.g. of the limbic dopaminergic and serotoninergic systems may result in an improvement, if not necessarily of the memory function per se, but of attention, mood and motivation, which in turn may facilitate cognitive and memory function (Coyle et al., 1983, Gottfries, 1980, Rossor, 1981). On the other hand, direct support of monoaminergic subcortical structures, even if affected only secondarily, may be desirable for the same reasons.

Co-dergocrine (Hydergine): An example for a drug modulating monoaminergic systems

Co-dergocrine mesylate (Hydergine, Sandoz) has been found to exert beneficial effects on geriatric patients with mild to moderate stages of SDAT (for review see Exton-Smith et al., 1983, Fanchamps, 1983, Loew and Weil, 1982). In view of the possible role of monoaminergic systems in SDAT, the treatment of SDAT patients with co-dergocrine may be based on a pharmacological rationale involving the specific pharmacological characteristics of this drug.

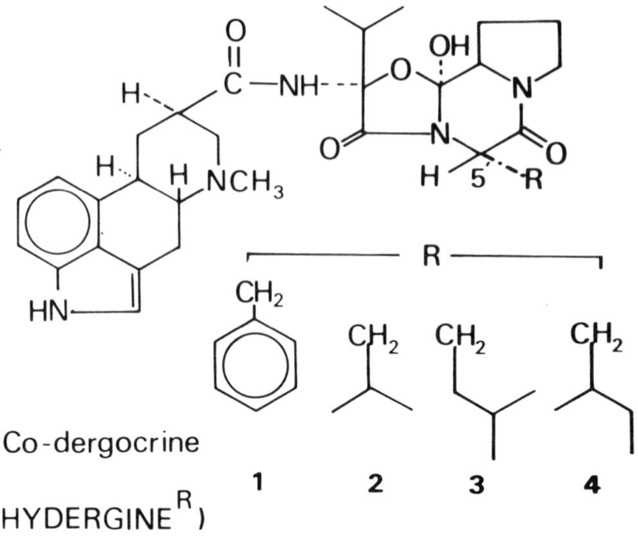

Figure 1

Chemical structures of the components of co-dergocrine (Hydergine, Sandoz).

1 = dihydroergocristine, 2 = dihydroergocornine, 3 = dihydro-alpha-ergokryptine, 4 = dihydro-beta-ergokryptine. The mesylates of 1, 2, 3 and 4 are present in the ratio 3:2:2:1, respectively.

Like most of the ergots but in a wider range, co-dergocrine interacts with central monoaminergic systems.

In particular, it was found to exhibit mixed agonist-antagonist activity both in dopaminergic and serotoninergic, and antagonist activity in noradrenergic central systems.

Studies including the induction of contralateral turns in rats with unilateral striatal lesions (Ungerstedt model) (Loew et al., 1980), the analgesic effect of morphine in rabbits (Deporteere et al., 1975), the induction of emesis in dogs (Papp et al., 1966, Wang and Glaviano, 1954), the counteraction on hypoxia-induced amnesia in rats (Jäggi et al., 1976), the effects on selfstimulation in rats

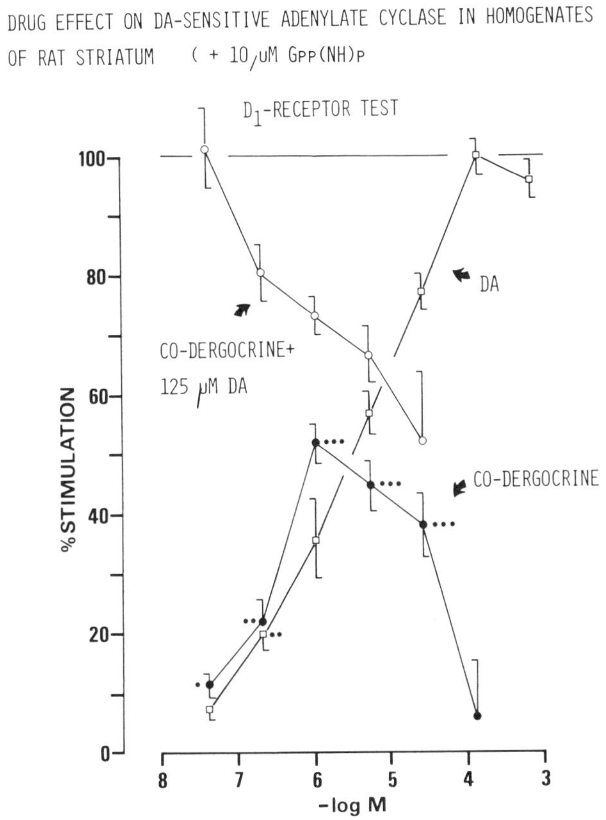

Figure 2

Mixed agonist-antagonist effects of co-dergocrine (Hydergine) at D1 receptors. Effect of various concentrations of dopamine (DA) (□) and co-dergocrine alone (●), and co-dergocrine in combination with 1.25×10^{-6}M DA (O) on cyclic AMP formation in homogenates of rat striatum. Results are expressed as percentage of the maximal stimulation elicited by 1.25×10^{-6}M dopamine. Basal cyclic AMP production was 113.3±4.3(n=8) pmoles cyclic AMP/mg protein/min., rising to 206.0±2.2 (n=8) pmoles cyclic AMP/mg protein/min.in the presence of 1.25×10^{-6}M DA. Values in the figure are means of ± S.E.M. of three experiments. Significant differences from controls: *2P < 0.05, **2P < 0.01, ***2P< 0.001 (student`s t-test). (Markstein, 1983). Co-dergocrine alone acted as an agonist at concentrations up to 10^{-6}M, and as an antagonist at concentrations above. In the presence of 1.25×10^{-6}M dopamine, co-dergocrine acted as an antagonist aleady at concentrations of 10^{-7}M and above.

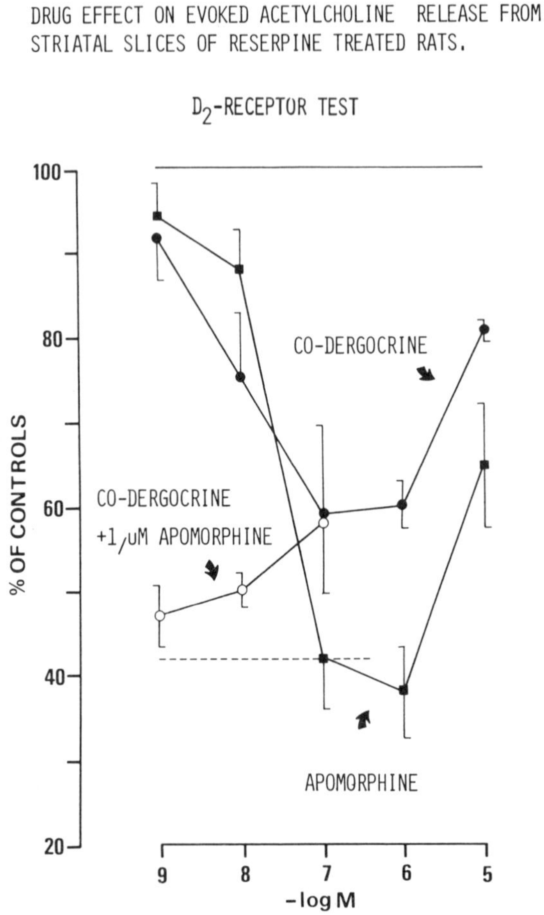

Figure 3

Mixed agonist-antagonist effects of co-dergocrine (Hydergine) at D2 receptors. Effects of various concentrations of apomorphine (■) and co-dergocrine (●) alone, and of co-dergocrine in combination with 10^{-7}M apomorphine (O) on electrically evoked tritium overflow from rat striatal slices preincubated with [^{3}H] choline (rats pretreated with reserpine). After preincubation, the slices were superfused and stimulated twice for 2 min. each at 2Hz (S_1, S_2). Drugs were added 30 min. before S_2. Drug effects are expressed as percentage of control ratios (Markstein, 1983). The mean of control ratios was 0.86 $\pm$ 0.015 (n=24). Values in the figure are means $\pm$ S.E.M. of two to six experiments. Co-dergocrine alone acted as an agonist at concentrations up to 10^{-7}M, and as an antagonist at concentrations above. In the presence of 10^{-6}M apomorphine, co-dergocrine acted as an antagonist at concentrations of 10^{-9}M and above.

(Copeland et al., 1981, Poschel and Ninteman, 1981), and the lowering of serum prolactin in rats and man (Flückiger and Del Pozo, 1980, Hofmann et al., 1979) point to dopamine-agonistic activity of co-dergocrine in vivo.

In vitro studies served to further differentiate these effects. Co-dergocrine was found to be a mixed agonist-antagonist both at D1 and D2 receptor subtypes of rat striatal preparations with an affinity higher than dopamine.

At low concentrations of dopamine, co-dergocrine enhanced dopaminergic function, at high dopamine concentrations, it counteracted excessive stimulation. (Markstein, 1983).

Regarding serotoninergic systems co-dergocrine appears also to be effective in in vivo on functions that are believed to be related to serotonin agonistic action such as its influence on the sleep-wakefulness cycle of rats and cats (increase of wake phase and decrease of R.E.M. phase (Carruthers-Jones et al., 1978, Loew et al., 1976, Loew and Spiegel, 1976, Susic and Masirevic, 1981), and the suppression of P.G.O. spikes in reserpinized cats (Deporteere et al., 1975, Züger et al., 1978).

Similar to the effects on dopaminergic systems, co-dergocrine was observed to exert partial agonistic action in serotonin systems in vitro. Again on adenylate cyclase-linked serotonin receptors a partial effect was found.

It was also observed to act as an agonist on serotonin receptor subtypes pharmacologically distinct from the adenylate cyclase-linked receptors (Ermini and Markstein, 1982).

In noradrenergic systems the antagonistic effects of co-dergocrine on alpha-adrenoceptors are known, at least in part, ever since the drug has been produced and described pharmacologically more than 30 years ago, when its "sympathicolytic" properties were discovered (Kühns, 1949).More recently, central effects of co-dergocrine on alpha-adrenoceptors were investigated in a more differentiated way. In vivo it was found that chronic administration of the drug to rats over periods of several weeks up to two years resulted in a lowering of cortical and cerebellar cyclic AMP concentration, as well as in reduced sensitivity of cortical slices to noradrenaline-stimulated cyclic AMP formation (Markstein and Wagner, 1978). In addition, the firing rate

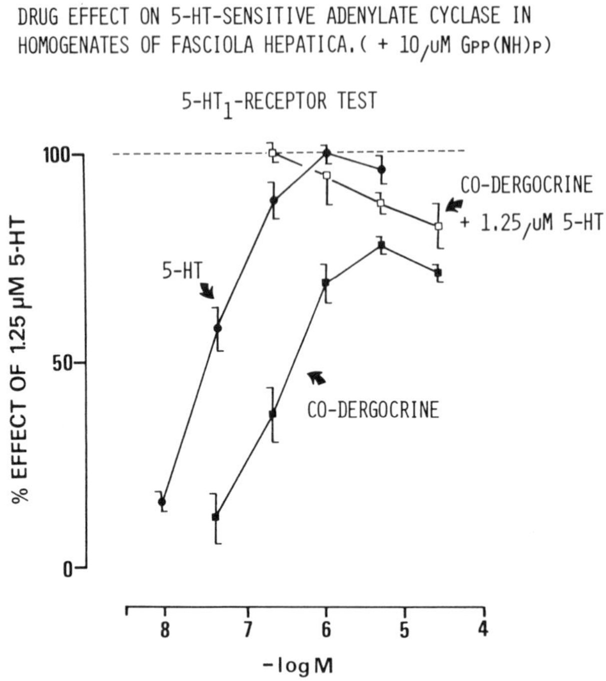

Figure 4
Mixed agonist-antagonist effects of co-dergocrine (Hydergine) at 5-HT-1 receptors. Effects of various concentrations of serotonin (5-HT) (●), and co-dergocrine alone (■), and of co-dergocrine in combination with 1.25×10^{-6}M 5-HT (□) on cyclic AMP formation in homogenates of the liver fluke Fasciola hepatica. Results are expressed as a percentage of maximal stimulation elicited by 10^{-6}M 5-HT. Basal cyclic AMP production was 205±9.5 pmoles cyclic AMP/mg protein/min. rising to 1280±17 pmoles cyclic AMP/mg protein/min. in the presence of 10^{-6}M 5-HT. All values are means ± S.E.M. of triplicate experiments (Ermini and Markstein, 1982). Co-dergocrine alone acted as an agonist at concentrations up to 10^{-5}M, and as an antagonist at concentrations above. In the presence of 1.25×10^{-6}M 5-HT, co-dergocrine acted as an antagonist at concentrations of 10^{-6}M and above.

of rat L. coeruleus neurons was increased upon administration of co-dergocrine at doses between 0.1 - 1.0 mg/i.p., which was interpreted as being suggestive for alpha-2 receptor blockade (Olpe and Steinmann, 1981).

In vitro it was found that co-dergocrine exerted non-competitive blockade of alpha-1 adrenoceptors involved in stimulation of cAMP formation in rat cerebral cortex slices.

It counteracted also clonidine-induced inhibition of noradrenaline release from rat occipital cortex slices, suggesting antagonist properties at presynaptic alpha-2 adrenoceptors (Ermini and Markstein, 1982, Markstein et al., 1983).

The stronger antagonistic potency on presynaptic alpha-adrenoceptors than on postsynaptic alpha-adrenoceptors may be interpreted such that in the case of an up-regulated noradrenergic function down-regulation is inflicted and, in the case of a down-regulated situation, compensatory up-regulation could occur (Ermini and Markstein, 1982).

In conclusion, the behavioral effects and the biochemical investigations have shown that co-dergocrine has multiple effects on dopaminergic and serotoninergic systems. It acts there as a mixed agonist-antagonist, and might, therefore, be able to compensate for a transmitter deficit in one brain structure and, at the same time, counteract an overactivity of the respective transmitter system in other brain regions. The noradrenergic system may be affected in a similar way, however, by a different mechanism of action. In this system, co-dergocrine increases stimulation-evoked noradrenaline release by blocking inhibitory presynaptic autoreceptors but at the same time restricts the postsynaptic effects. Co-dergocrine appears, therefore, to restore balance in the functional interplay between the different monoaminergic transmitter systems.

The effect of co-dergocrine in the different monoaminergic synapses could be compared with the action of a chemical buffer system and, consequently, co-dergocrine was called a synaptic buffer substance (Ermini and Markstein, 1982).

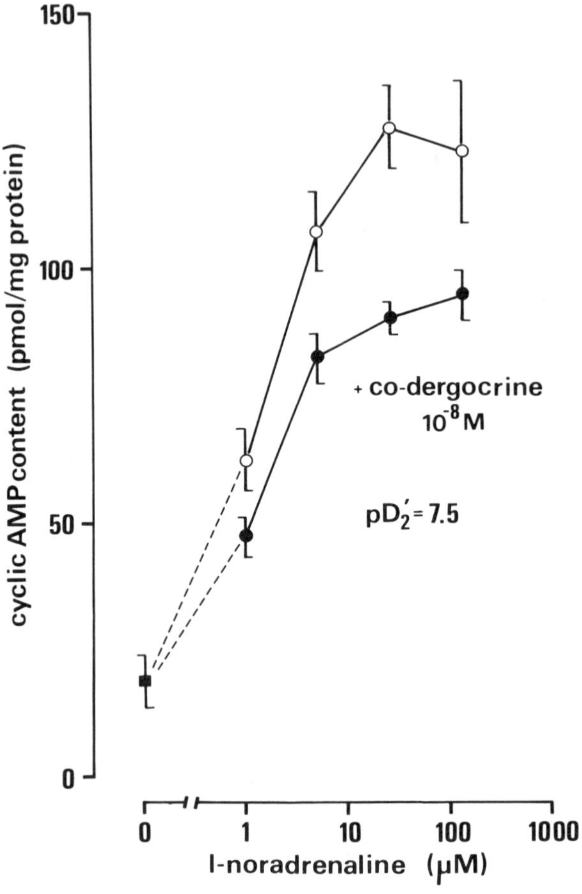

Figure 5
Antagonistic effects of co-dergocrine (Hydergine) on alpha-1-adrenoceptors. Effects of various concentrations of l-noradrenaline on cyclic AMP content (pmoles/mg protein) in rat cerebral occipital cortex slices in the absence (O) and presence of 10^{-8}M co-dergocrine (●). The slices were preincubated for 15 min. with co-dergocrine before l-noradrenaline was added. Incubation time with l-noradrenaline was 8 min. Cocaine (10^{-5}M) was present throughout the experiment. Values are means $\pm$ S.E.M. of triplicate experiments. p D`2 = p D`x + log (x-1) (Markstein et al., 1983).

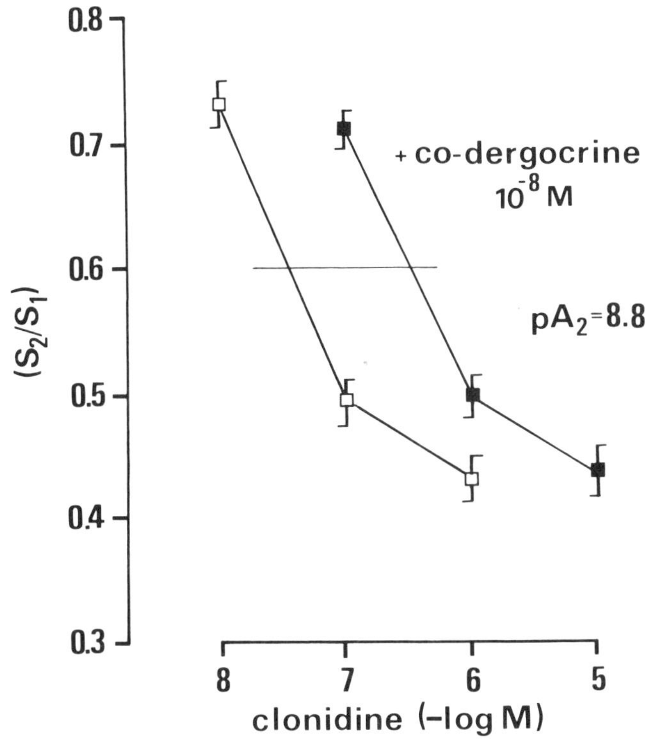

Figure 6
Antagonistic effects of co-dergocrine (Hydergine) on alpha-2-adrenoceptors. Effects of various concentrations of clonidine alone (□) and in combination with 10^{-8}M co-dergocrine (■) on electrically evoked tritium overflow from rat cerebral occipital cortex slices. After preincubation with 1-[^{3}H]noradrenaline, slices were superfused and stimulated twice each at 2Hz for 2 min. (S_1/S_2). Drugs were added 30 min. before S_2. Values are the ratios of tritium overflow evoked by S_2 and S_1 and are means ± S.E.M. of quadruplicate determinations. pA_2-value was calculated from the shift of the concentration-response curve of clonidine induced by co-dergocrine according to the equation $pA_2 = pB + \log (x-1)$ (Markstein et al., 1983).

Since an imbalance between the various neurotransmitter systems involved in SDAT is viewed to be crucial for the impaired functions rather than the mere changes in concentration of the one or other neurotransmitter, such a multiply active "buffer substance", capable of restoring balance, may be of particular therapeutic interest.

Regarding the influence of a substance, acting on monoaminergic systems, on hippocampal and striatal cholinergic neuronal function it is also interesting to know that chronic administration of co-dergocrine to 26 - 36 months old rats showing normally a decline in cortical and hippocampal CAT activity, resulted in an elevation of this enzyme`s activity (Dravid, 1983) in these structures.

In addition, it may be remarked that the administration of co-dergocrine to rats caused a significant improvement of maze-learning and other behavioral parameters linked to cognitive function in the rat (Jäggi and Loew, 1976, Judge and Quartmain, 1981, Loew et al., 1980).

In an overall conclusion, the pharmacological rationale for the treatment of SDAT, at least in mild-to-moderate stages, appears to be provided for the co-dergocrine on the basis of its multiple interaction with central monoaminergic systems.

REFERENCES

Adolfsson R, Gottfries CG, Roos BE, Winblad B, (1979). Changes in the brain catecholamines in patients with dementia of the Alzheimer type. Br J Psychiatry 135: 216.

Bartus RT, Dean III RL, Beer B, Lippa AS, (1982). The cholinergic hypothesis of geriatric memory dysfunction. Science 217: 408.

Bondareff W, Mountjoy CQ, Roth M, (1982). Loss of neurons of origin of the adrenergic projection to cerebral cortex (nucleus locus caeruleus) in senile dementia. Neurology 32: 164.

Bowen DM, Spillane JA, Curzon G, Meier-Ruge W, White P, Goodhardt MJ, Iwangoff P, Davison AN, (1979). Accelerated aging or selective neuronal loss as an important cause of dementia. Lancet i: 11.

Carlsson A, Adolfsson R, Aquilonius SM, Gottfries CG, Oreland L, Svennerholm L, Winblad B, (1980). Biogenic-amines in human brain in normal aging, senile dementia, and chronic alcoholism. In Goldstein M, Calne DB, Liebermann A, Thorner MO, (eds): "Ergot Compounds and

Brain Function", New York: Raven, p 295.
Carruthers-Jones DI, Deporteere H, Loew DM, (1978). Changes in the rat electrocorticogram following administration of two dihydrogenated ergot derivatives.Gerontology 24 (Suppl. 1): 23.
Copeland RL, Bhattacharya AK, Aulakh CS, Pradhan SN, (1981). Behavioral and neurochemical effects of Hydergine in rats. Arch Int Pharmacodyn 252: 113.
Corkin S, (1981). Acetylcholine, aging and Alzheimer`s disease. Implications for treatment. T I N S (December): 287.
Coyle JT, Price DL, De Long MR, (1983). Alzheimer`s disease: A disorder of cortical cholinergic innervation. Science 219: 1184.
Davis KL, Mohs RC, Tinklenberg JR, Pfefferbaum A, Hollister LE, Kopell BS, (1978). Physostigmine: Improvement of long-term memory processes in normal humans. Science 201: 272.
De Boni U, Crapper DR (1980). Senile Dementia and Alzheimer`s Disease: A current view. Life Sci 27: 1.
Deporteere H, Loew DM, Vigouret JM, (1975). Neuropharmacological studies on Hydergine. Triangle 14:73.
Drachman DA, (1978). Memory, dementia and the cholinergic system. In Katzman R, Terry RD, Bick KL (eds): "Alzheimer`s Disease: Senile Dementia and Related Disorders," New York: Raven, p 143.
Dravid AR, (1983). Deficits in cholinergic enzymes and muscarinic receptors in the hippocampus and striatum of senescent rats: Effect of chronic Hydergine treatment. Arch Int Pharmacodyn Ther : In press.
Ermini M, Markstein R, (1982). Hydergine therapy: Mechanism of action. Br J Clin Pract (Suppl. 16): 27.
Exton-Smith AN, Piper M, Phillips M, Simpson J, (1983). Clinical experiences with ergot alkaloids. In Agnoli A, Crepaldi G, Spano PF, Trabucchi M, (eds): "Aging Brain and Ergot Alkaloids", New York: Raven, p 323.
Fanchamps A, (1983). Dihydroergotoxine in senile cerebral insufficiency. In Agnoli A, Crepaldi G, Spano PF, Trabucchi M, (eds): "Aging Brain and Ergot Alkaloids", New York: Raven, p 311.
Flückiger E, Del Pozo E, (1980). Ergot derivatives and pituitary hormones. In Muller EE, (ed): "Neuroactive Drugs in Endocrinology: Physiologic, Diagnostic and Therapeutic Aspects", New York: Elsevier/North Holland, p 169.
Gottfries CG, (1980). Biochemistry of dementia and normal ageing. T I N S (March): 55.
Gottfries CG, (1982). The metabolism of some neurotrans-

mitters in ageing and dementia disorders. Gerontology 28 (Suppl 2): 11.
Hofmann M, Tonon C, Spano PF, Trabucchi M, (1979). Mechanisms of dihydroergotoxine`s effect on prolactin release J Pharm Pharmacol 31: 42.
Jäggi UH, Loew DM, (1976). Central dopaminergic stimulation and avoidance performance under hypoxia in rats. Experientia 32: 779.
Judge ME, Quartermain D, (1981). Reversal of anisomycin-induced amnesia by the ergot derivative Hydergine. Neurosci Lett 24: 313.
Kühns K, (1949). Untersuchungen über die Wirkung eines neuen Sympathicolyticums (Hydergin) und anderer vegetativer Pharmaka auf Elektrokardiogramm und Herzfrequenz des wachen Kaninchens. Helv Med Acta 16: 90.
Loew DM, Deporteere H, Bürki HR (1976). Effects of dihydrogenated ergot alkaloids on the sleep wakefulness cycle and on brain biogenic amines in the rat. Arzneim Forsch (Drug Res.) 26: 1080.
Loew DM, Spiegel R, (1976). Polygraphic studies in rats and humans. Their use in psychopharmacological research. Arzneim Forsch (Drug Res.) 26: 1232.
Loew DM, Vigouret JM, Jaton A, (1980). Neuropharmacology of bromocriptine and dihydroergotoxine (Hydergine). In Goldstein M, Calne DB, Liebermann A, Thorner M (eds) "Ergot Compounds and Brain Function", New York: Raven, p 63.
Loew DM, Weil C, (1982). Hydergine in senile mental impairment. Gerontology 28: 54.
Mann DMA, (1983). The locus caeruleus and its possble role in ageing and degenerative disease of the human CNS. Mech Ageing Devel, in press.
Mann DA, Yates PO, Hawkes J, (1982). The noradrenergic system in Alzheimer and multi-infarct dementias. J Neurol Neurosurg Psychiat 45: 113.
Marchbanks RM, (1982). Biochemistry of Alzheimer`s dementia J Neurochem 39: 9.
Markstein R, (1983). Dopamine receptor profile of co-dergocrine (Hydergine) and its components. Europ J Pharmacol 86: 145.
Markstein R, Wagner H, (1978). Effect of dihydroergotoxine cyclic AMP generating systems in rat cerebral cortex slices. Gerontology 24 (Suppl 1): 94.
Markstein R, Closse A, Frick W, (1983). Interaction of ergot alkaloids and their combination (co-dergocrine) with alpha-receptors in the CNS. Europ J Pharmacol: in press.
Olpe HR, Steinmann MW, (1981). The activating action of

vincamine, piracetam and Hydergine on the activity of the noradrenergic neurons of the locus coeruleus. Behav Neurol Biol 33: 249.

Olpe HR, Steinmann MW, (1982). The effect of vincamine, Hydergine and piracetam on the firing rate of locus coeruleus neurons. J Neural Transmission 55: 101.

Papp RH, Hawkins HB, Share NN, Wang SC, (1966). Emesis induced by the intracerebroventricular administration of Hydergine and mechlorethamine hydrochloride. J Pharm Exp Ther, 154: 333.

Perry EK, Tomlinson BE, Blessed G, Bergmann K, Gibson PH, Perry RH, (1978). Correlation of cholinergic abnormalities with senile plaques and mental test scores in senile dementia. Br Med J 2: 1457.

Poschel BPH, Ninteman FW, (1981). Exitatory effects of Hydergine on intracranial self-stimulation. Drug Devel Res 1: 163.

Rossor MN, (1981). Parkinson`s Disease and Alzheimer`s disease as disorders of the isodendritic core. Br Med J 283: 1588.

Rossor MN, (1982). Dementia. Lancet: ii: 1200.

Susic V, Masirevic R, (1981). Effects of repeated administration of dihydroergotoxine (Redergine) on the sleep-wakefulness cycle in the cat. Gerontology 27: 1.

Thal LJ, Rosen W, Sharpless NS, Crystal H, (1981). Choline chloride fails to improve cognition in Alzheimer`s disease. Neurobiology of Ageing 2: 205.

Wang SC, Glaviano VV, (1954). Locus of emetic action of morphine and Hydergine in dogs. J Pharm Exp Ther 111: 329.

Züger PE, Vigouret JM, Loew DM, (1978). Inhibition of reserpine induced PGO-waves in the cat by ergot derivatives. Experientia 34: 637.

IX. EPIDEMIOLOGY OF SENILE DEMENTIA

Presided by T. Abelin (Berne)

Senile Dementia: Outlook for the Future, pages 383–393

AN EPIDEMIOLOGIST'S VIEW OF THE SENILE DEMENTIAS--PIECES OF THE PUZZLE

Jacob A. Brody, M.D.

Associate Director for Epidemiology, Demography, and Biometry Program, National Institute on Aging, National Institutes of Health, Bethesda, MD 20205

Epidemiologists await with eager expectation the confirmation that loss of neurons in the medial septum, diagonal band of Broca and the nucleus basalis of Meynert and the accompanying reduced presynaptic cholinergic activity (Coyle, Price, and DeLong 1983) will ultimately provide a clear separation between the normal aged and those with the senile dementias. We hope that this new information will deliver us from our present frustrating state of knowledge in which neither specific patterns of disease nor specific risk factors for senile dementias have not been defined (Brody 1982).

Thus far only age appears to clearly correlate with development of the senile dementias. The age factor is ominous since international demographic trends indicate how very rapidly the most susceptible portion of our population has increased during this century and will continue to grow. In the United States alone (Census 1979, Census 1980) there was a greater than eightfold increase from approximately 3.1 million people aged 65 years and over in 1900 to 26 million in 1980. This represents a rise from 4.1 to 11.3 percent of the total population. The U.S. Bureau of the Census projects that the number of persons over age 65 will reach 33.5 to 36.6 million by the year 2000, then accounting for about 13 percent of the total population (Census 1980). It is anticipated that the number and proportion of Americans 65 and older will continue to increase over the next 43 years as the post World War II baby boom ages, reaching a peak of approximately 58.5 million (20 percent) by the year 2025. Currently one-third of the entire population in the developed countries will survive to at least 80 years of age when the risk of having a senile dementia reaches 20 percent.

For this discussion emphasis will be placed on those conditions associated with pathologic changes described in Alzheimer's disease which includes both senile and presenile forms. Our primary concerns are the senile forms generally embraced by the term senile dementia of the Alzheimer's type but some overlap with the presenile form cannot be avoided. Further, at autopsy at least 30 to 40 percent of patients with clinically diagnoseable senile dementia do not have the pathologic changes found in Alzheimer's disease (Terry 1978). Therefore, in surveys and most clinical studies the specificity of the diagnosis is uncertain, and restricting the study population to senile dementias of the Alzheimer's type is not feasible.

The issue as to whether Alzheimer's disease is one entity with a presenile form and a senile form cannot be resolved. There are those who argue that the early form and the late form involve the same disease both clinically and pathologically, but at different ages, and thus should be considered one entity. Rigorous data do not exist which would suggest that the pathogenesis and natural history of the early form are indeed identical with that of the senile form. Further, etiologic research is better served if we consider the entities as separate. If one is caused by factor X and the other is not, we could miss the critical association by case dilution; while if both are caused by factor X it will be manifest in both groups.

EPIDEMIOLOGY

The magnitude of the problem and clues to pathogenesis are described and sought by epidemiologists through comparisons of incidence, prevalence and mortality among groups of individuals categorized according to clinical and demographic characteristics and types of environmental exposures, etc. All procedures used to describe disease frequency have their own sets of methodologic problems. Mortality data is generally not useful in dementia research because of great underreporting and the lack of universality of findings. The validity of prevalence estimates depends on several factors relating to the identification of all cases in the population. Approaches which depend upon recognition of dementia during conventional medical contacts are of unacceptably limited utility because of the nature of the condition and because of the many cultural, social, and behavioral factors which cause some patients and their families to seek early professional attention and others to delay or avoid physicians and other care givers. For example, the individual who lives with his family in a sheltered environment is less likely to come to medical attention than another who does not have these advantages. A further difficulty is that the degree of impairment is often variable, with individuals slipping into and out of states of impaired cognitive functioning (Busse, Wang 1973). This may lead to underdiagnosis or to ambiguity of the diagnosis. Varying education and language backgrounds also influence the expression and/or recognition of cognitive disability (Gurland 1981).

Estimates of the incidence of dementia have been few and of uncertain comparability. Kokmen and Schoenberg have reported an annual incidence of 110 new cases per 100,000 among the residents of Rochester, Minnesota over 29 years of age (Kokmen and Schoenberg 1980). Their figures were based on clinically restrictive criteria applied to individuals whose condition had been recognized and documented by physicians in medical facilities in that area over a 5-year period. In a study carried out in Sweden, Akesson estimated the annual incidence of "senile psychosis" among persons age 60 and older as 380 per 100,000 (Akesson 1969). His estimate for the incidence of dementia due to "severe arteriosclerotic psychosis" was 520 per 100,000 in the same population.

There is no clear indication that trends exist or that rates have changed over time. Descriptions compatible with the clinical features of SDAT exist in literature and medicine from earliest writings. Obviously, with the increasing number of persons surviving to later age, the absolute number of cases is increasing rapidly. The possibility that changes in reported mortality and prevalence of dementia might actually reflect a changing incidence within a single community was considered by Gruenberg with reference to a study carried out in Southern Sweden between 1947 and 1957 (Gruenberg 1978). His conclusion was the improvements in medical treatment had increased the duration of illness and (thereby) the point prevalence, but that these did not indicate a true increase in disease incidence. It seems generally accepted that the frequency of dementia in the elderly is, in fact, fairly constant over time and over large geographic areas.

Estimates of the prevalence of dementia from population studies in Northern Europe have ranged from 3.9 to 21.6 percent (severe dementia, 1.3 to 6.2 percent; mild impairment 2.6 to 15.4 percent) among the elderly (Bollerup 1975; Broe, Akhtar, Andrews, Caird, Gilmore, and McLennan 1976; Essen-Moller, Larsson, Uddenberg, and White 1956; Kay, Bergmann, Foster, McKechnie, and Roth 1970; Kay, Beamish, and Roth 1964; Nielson 1963; Primrose 1962). A recent study conducted in Copiah County in rural Mississippi resulted in an estimate of 1 percent for severe dementia among county residents age 40 and older, climbing to a 7 percent prevalence among residents age 80 or older (Schoenberg 1981). These figures reflect stringent criteria and the inclusion of only severe cases. In Akesson's study, the age-specific prevalence of severe dementia at age 80 and above was 4.8 percent (Akesson 1969). Less restrictive criteria have resulted in higher age-specific prevalence figures such as 12.6 percent (Nielson 1963), and 22 percent (Kay, Beamish, and Roth 1964) among persons age 80 or older. In general, there appears to be a 10 to 20 fold increase in age-specific prevalence between the ages of 60 and 80, exceeding 20 percent by 80 to 85 years. It is also generally agreed that these figures are probably underestimates of the true prevalence.

Senile dementias probably have a life shortening effect. Available studies, however, have not shown this to be a consistent finding. More frequently age, male sex, and poor general physical condition at time of diagnosis of senile dementia are associated with early death. This does raise the possibility that senile dementia itself is not a fatal condition (Brody 1982).

Clinicians tend to agree that females are more susceptible than males to senile dementia. Surely clinicians see more female patients since females far outnumber males in the older and more susceptible age groups. Further, elderly females are more likely to be widowed and living alone than elderly males, and hence would require institutionalization in the absence of social supports. In the United States over age 65 there are about 5.5 million females living alone as opposed to 1.6 million males. It is unlikely from the information available that a true sex difference in age-specific incidence has been documented, although one may exist.

Among the Chamorro people of Guam and the other islands of the Mariana group there is a focus of dementia resembling presenile Alzheimer's disease associated with extrapryamidal features (Brody, Stanhope, and Kurland 1975). There is no other known focus or geographic localization by country, latitude, or urban-rural status, although suggestions of small clusters in Japan and New Guinea are under study (Yoshimasu, Yasui, Yase, et al. 1980; Gajdusek and Salazar 1982). No one would claim that this topic has been addressed systematically but wherever people are old and studied, senile dementia has been reported.

Because of thier potential importance demographic factors merit further attention. If one considers that in the U.S. white females have a threefold greater chance of surviving to be 70 years of age than black males of the same birth cohort then comparative incidence rates would be highly instructive. The apparent absence of differences in age-specific dementia rates suggests that the factors which determine risk for dementia are dissimilar from the major factors responsible for race and sex differences in morbidity and mortality. This line of reasoning focuses attention away from lifestyle, obesity, smoking, stress, diet, medical care, social and economic status, toward genetic and early common life experiencies, and most strikingly on late life characteristics and exposures.

Clusters of cases with common exposures or occupations have not been reported. One exception to this is found among prize fighters who develop a syndrome, dementia pugilistica, which shares much in common with Alzheimer's disease. Thus, trauma, at least that of the severity to which prize fighters are exposed, also provides a deviation from the absolute random pattern of observed dementias.

RELATED OBSERVATIONS

In recent years scientists studying senile dementia of the Alzheimer's type have provided a wide range of stimulating observations. While none has been definitive etiologically several offer attractive areas to pursue. Aluminum studies in cats, tissue culture, and neurons containing neurofibrillary tangles seem to offer a lead. Most data tend to confirm a higher concentration of aluminum in specific CNS tissues in patients with senile dementia of the Alzheimer's type (Crapper, Karlik, and DeBoni 1978). The significance is far from clear since the people with the greatest exposure to aluminum, such as aluminum workers and individuals on renal dialysis, do not necessarily develop neurofibrillary tangles or senile dementia of the Alzheimer's type (Dunea, Mahurkar, Makdani, et al. 1978). Perhaps, however, aluminum is an indicator of some metabolic process involving the parathyroid and metallic ions which is either causally or passively associated with the disease.

Many scientists look at genetic influences in thinking about presenile and senile forms of Alzheimer's disease (Mortimer 1980). However, clear genetic patterns have not been demonstrated except in the rare, but well documented form of familial, dominantly inherited, Alzheimer's disease in which many of the cases have onset in the presenile age range (Weelan and Race 1959). In the Guam form of dementia which occurs at an extraordinarily high rate in a population isolate, no Mendelian pattern of inheritance has emerged.

The clinical observation that senile dementias occur in family clusters may be valid. Longevity also appears to have a familial distribution. These longevous families would naturally have more family members in the highly susceptible age range, and hence give the impression, correct or false, of a genetic factor in the etiology of senile dementias.

Recent studies of the families of autopsied patients with Alzheimer's disease of presenile and senile forms have encountered an elevated frequency of Down's syndrome in close relatives. Data at present suggest that this association is much stronger when the Alzheimer's disease appeared in its presenile form (Heston and Mastri 1977).

The possibility that senile dementia of the Alzheimer's type is caused by a slow virus cannot be dismissed. Studies among Guamanians with dementia were coupled with the original kuru studies in the first primate experiments. Thus far, the Guam material has been entirely negative using the same techniques which did transmit kuru and other human slow virus diseases. In the late 1960's material from several unusual patients with familial Alzheimer's disease produced a spongiform degeneration in chimpanzees indistinguishable from the neuropathology encountered with inoculations of kuru brains. Numerous attempts to reproduce these transmissions from the original material and from many other patients with familial and nonfamilial dementias of the presenile and senile forms have been negative to date (Goudsmit, Marrow, Asher, et al. 1980). The early observations, thus, are essentially uncorroborated by the scientists who performed the original work and at present virus studies must be considered negative.

Other areas where active research may provide critical insights concerning the senile dementias include chromosomal studies (Ward, Cook, Robinson, et al. 1979), histocompatibility typing (Walford and Hodge 1980), and various immunologic parameters (Eisdorfer, Cohen, and Buckley 1978; Stam and Op den Velde 1978).

CONCLUSIONS

Epidemiologic studies of the senile dementias are faced with difficult structural and conceptual problems (Mortimer, Schuman, and French 1981). It is necessary to use strict epidemiologic methodology and to proceed according to the rules, with logic, and at times, with tedious dedication. Some impediments to direct acquisition of information have been mentioned. A primary need is for a series of viable clinical and psychometric instruments which achieve general acceptance through careful testing and follow-up. These must include instruments which can be used for field testing, others which can be used in hospitals and clinical settings, and others which are useful for following patients over time. There is need for an acceptable rating score such as that which is referred to as the Kurtzke Scale for multiple sclerosis which quantifies severity over a range of clinical signs and symptoms.

Many sound epidemiologic investigations are under way. Our group at the National Institute on Aging is working directly with a large number of investigators in a series of research efforts. Since our studies are all at an early stage, we do not have results. All involve noninstitutionalized populations. We are conducting a prevalence survey in New Haven, Connecticut with Yale University and the Center for Epidemiologic Studies of the Division of Biometry and Epidemiology, National Institute of Mental Health involving 2,500 people 65 and over, using the mini-mental status examination of Folstein, Folstein, and Mc Hugh. Two interviews are scheduled 18 months apart (Weissman et al. 1982).

In Boston, Massachusetts we are conducting a study with the East Boston Neighborhood Health Center, Peter Bent Brigham Hospital, an affiliate of Harvard Medical School, on the natural history of senile dementias detected through population screening. One hundred to one hundred fifty putative early cases will be matched with normals and carefully evaluated using medical, neurologic and neuropsychologic personnel, a CT scan, sequential cognitive and memory testing, and observation for a 5-year period.

A major effort with the Epidemiology and Biometry Program of the National Heart, Lung, and Blood Institute of the National Institutes of Health and Boston University Medical Center will utilize the Framingham Heart Study cohort which now consists of about 3,000 men and women age 65 to 90 (Dawber 1980). We are routinely screening the population using the mini-mental status exam. Mental status will be followed and integrated with the extensive data on all aspects of prior health, collected during the 17 biennial examinations which have been conducted in the Framingham cohort since 1953.

Perhaps during this challenging and lengthy evolutionary phase a pathologist and immunologist or a chemist will get lucky and speed our research efforts. This, of course, would be fine news indeed. I do, however, admit to the prejudice that the hippocampus and the nucleus basalis of Meynert are harder to get to than a well studied series of populations.

Akesson HO (1969). A population study of senile and arteriosclerotic psychoses. Human Hered 19:546.

Bollerup TR (1975). Prevalence of mental illness among 70-year-olds domiciled in nine Copenhagen suburbs: the Glostrup survey. Acta Psychiat Scand 51:327.

Brody JA (1982). An epidemiologist views senile dementia--facts and fragments. Am J of Epidemiol 115:2.

Brody JA, Stanhope JM, and Kurland LT (1975). Patterns of amyotrophic lateral sclerosis and parkinsonism-dementia on Guam. In Hornabrook RW (ed): "Topics on tropical neurology, contemporary neurology series," Philadelphia: FA Davis Co., p 45.

Broe GA, Akhtar AJ, Andrews GR, Caird FI, Gilmore AJJ, and McLennan, WJ (1976). Neurological disorders in the elderly at home. J Neurol Neurosurg Psychiat 39:362.

Busse EW and Wang HS (1973). Multiple factors contributing to dementia in old age. In DelaFuenta R, and Weisman MH (eds): "Psychiatry II," New York: American Elsevier Pub. Co., p 68.

Coyle JT, Price DL, and DeLong MR (1983). Alzheimer's Disease: A disorder of cortical cholinergic innervation. Science 219:1184.

Crapper DR, Karlik S, and DeBoni U (1978). Aluminum and other metals in senile (Alzheimer) dementia. In Katzman R, Terry RD, and Bick KL (eds): "Aging, Vol. 7, Alzheimer's disease: senile dementia and related disorders," New York: Raven Press, p 471.

Dawber T (1980). "The Framingham Study--The Epidemiology of Artherosclerotic Disease," Cambridge: Harvard University Press.

Dunea G, Mahurkar SD, Makdani B, et al. (1978). Role of aluminum in dialysis dementia. Ann Intern Med 88:502.

Eisdorfer C, Cohen D, and Buckley CE III (1978). Serum immunoglobulins and cognition in the impaired elderly. In Katzman R, Terry RD, and Bick KL (eds): "Aging, Vol. 7, Alzheimer's disease: senile dementia and related disorders," New York: Raven Press, p 401.

Essen-Moller E, Larsson H, Uddenberg C and White G (1956). Individual traits and morbidity in a Swedish rural population. Acta Psychiat Neurol Scand Suppl 100.

Gajdusek DC and Salazar A (1982). Amyotrophic lateral sclerosis and parkinsonism syndromes in high incidence among the Auyu and Jakai people of West New Guinea. Neurology 32:2.

Goudsmit J, Marrow CH, Asher DM, et al. (1980). Evidence for and against the transmittability of Alzheimer's disease. Neurology 30:945.

Gruenberg EM (1978). Epidemiology of senile dementia. In Schoenberg BS (ed): "Neurological Epidemiology: Principles and Clinical Applications," New York: Raven Press, p 437.

Gurland BJ (1981). The borderlands of dementia: The influence of sociocultural characteristics on rates of dementia occurring in the senium. In Miller NE and Cohen GD (eds): "Clinical aspects of Alzheimer's disease and senile dementia," New York: Raven Press, p 61.

Heston LL and Mastri AR (1977). The genetics of Alzheimer's disease. Associations with hematologic malignancy and Down's syndrome. Arch Gen Psychiatry 34:976.

Kay DWK, Bergmann K, Foster EM, McKechnie AA and Roth M (1970). Mental illness and hospital usage in the elderly: a random sample followed up. Comp Psychiat 11:26.

Kay DWK, Beamish P and Roth M (1964). Old age mental disorders in Newcastle upon Tyne. Part I. A study of prevalence. Br J Psychiat 110:146.

Kokmen E and Schoenberg BS (1980). Epidemiological patterns and clinical features of dementia in a defined U.S. population (Abstract). Ann Neurol 8:116.

Mortimer JA (1980). Epidemiologic aspects of Alzheimer's disease. In Maletta GJ and Pirozzolo FJ (eds): "Advances in Neurogerontology Vol. 1, The aging nervous system," New York: Praeger, p 307.

Mortimer JA, Schuman LM and French LR (1981). Epidemiology of dementing illness. In Mortimer JA and Schuman LM (eds): "The Epidemiology of Dementia," New York: Oxford University Press, p 3.

Nielson J (1963). Geronto-psychiatric period-prevalence investigation in a geographically delimited population. Acta Psychiat Scand 38:307.

Primrose EJR (1962). "Psychological illness. A community study." Springfield, Ill: CCThomas.

Schoenberg BS (1981). Personal communication.

Stam FC and Op den Velde W (1978). Haptoglobin types in Alzheimer's disease and senile dementia. In Katzman R, Terry RD, and Bick KL (eds): "Aging, Vol. 7, Alzheimer's disease: senile dementia and related disorders," New York: Raven Press, p 279.

Terry RD (1978). Aging, senile dementia, and Alzheimer's disease. In Katzman R, Terry RD, and Bick KL (eds): "Aging, Vol.7, Alzheimer's disease: senile dementia and related disorders," New York: Raven Press, p 11-14.

U.S. Bureau of the Census, Current Population Reports Series P-23, No. 85, U.S. Government Printing Office, Washington, D.C. 1979.

U.S. Bureau of the Census, 1980 Provisional Data.

Walford RL and Hodge SE (1980). HLA distribution in Alzheimer's disease. In Peresaki PI (ed): "Histocompatibility testing, 1980," Los Angeles: UCLA Tissue Typing Lab.

Ward BE, Cook RH, Robinson A, et al. (1979). Increased aneuploidy in Alzheimer disease. Am J Med Genet 3:137.

Weisman MM, Tischler G, Holzer CE, Orvaschel H, Leaf PJ, and Myers JK (1982). Psychiatric disorders (DSM III) in the elderly: 1980-1981. Presented at the American Psychiatric Association - 1982 Annual Meeting in Toronto.

Wheelan L and Race RR (1959). Familial Alzheimer's disease, note on the linkage data. Ann Hum Genet 23:300.

Yoshimasu F, Yasui M, Yase Y et al. (1980). Studies on amyotrophic lateral sclerosis by neutron activation analysis--2: comparative study of analytical results on Guam PD, Japanese ALS and Alzheimer disease cases. Folia Psychiatr Neurol Jpn 34:75.

Senile Dementia: Outlook for the Future, pages 395–403

CENTRAL NERVOUS SYSTEM FUNCTION IN A SAMPLE SURVEY OF OLD PEOPLE

Theodor Abelin, M.D., M.P.H.

Dept. of Social and Preventive Medicine,
University of Berne
Finkenhubelweg 11, CH-3012 Berne

Efforts at prevention are guided by two major objectives: one is to reduce mortality and increase life expectancy, and the other to reduce disability.

Although life expectancy of persons with senile dementia is reduced (Müller 1981; Roth 1978), the concern with this condition is guided mainly by the hope of reducing disability and enabling a larger proportion of the Aged to lead an independent life.

This presentation is to serve two purposes. One is to estimate the impact that senile dementia has by reducing the independence of old people and increasing their need for care. The other is to add to the still limited and to some extent contradictory information on the distribution of senile dementia in the population.

Method

The data were taken from a community sample survey of persons over the age of 65 years, conducted in 1977 and 1978 in the City of Basle and a circle of suburbs around the City of Berne. A stratified random sample was drawn from the files of the various city and town population registers, providing for equal numbers of persons in all five-year age

Acknowledgement. Support for this project has been provided by a grant from the Swiss National Foundation for Scientific Research, Project-No. 3.999-0.82

groups from 66 to 91 and over, in both sexes, and in both geographical areas. It was possible to examine and conduct interviews with 480 persons or 80.4 % of the original sample. Participation among those reached was 84,8 %. Interviews and tests were conducted by senior medical students and recent medical graduates after undergoing special training in interviewing and measurement techniques.

The precoded interview was concerned mainly with the capability of conducting activities of daily living, with medical conditions, with the housing and family situation, and with social activities. In a physical examination following the interview, neurological functioning was tested, and blood pressure, weight and height were determined.

As a measure of senile dementia, performance in a set of questions on orientation concerning time, space and person was used (Berg, Svensson 1980; Kahn et al 1960). Most probands answered all eight questions, but a few being asked only 6 or 7 were also included in the analysis. Persons failing to answer one or more questions correctly, were classified as poor performers. The results will be compared to the performance in a "digits backward" test of short-term memory. Results will always be presented after correction for the stratification procedure.

Results

Table 1 presents the prevalence of persons not able to perform correctly on the two tests. Prevalence is higher for women than for men, and increases with age. Very clearly, the age gradient is stronger for the orientation than for the short-term memory task.

In order to measure dependence on other persons' help, a scale of need for daily nursing help was constructed that will be described in detail elsewhere. Briefly, a person was classified as needing daily nursing help if he or she needed assistance from another person on one or more of the following tasks: getting up from bed; getting dressed; washing the upper part of the body, using the toilet, eating and drinking; and if he or she could not be left alone at night. Based on those who completed the questions on memory and orientation, 5 % of the population over 65 were classified as needing daily nursing care. As table 2

Table 1 Prevalence (%) of persons performing poorly on tasks of orientation and short-term memory, by age and sex

Task	Age (yrs.)[1]			
	66-75	76-85	86+	All ages 65+
a. Orientation[2]				
Men	3.4	4.2	23.1	4.4
Women	2.4	14.8	31.8	8.4
both sexes[3]	2.8	11.5	29.5	6.9
b. Short-term Memory[4]				
Men	8.8	3.4	14.4	7.5
Women	12.9	23.6	29.6	17.0
both sexes	11.2	16.1	25.4	13.3

1) Adjustment by 5-yr age groups and region
2) 1+ incorrect answers in sequence of (6-)8 questions
3) Adjustment by 5-yr age groups, sex, and region
4) Failure to recall 3+ one-digit numbers in reverse order

Table 2 Need for daily nursing care and performance on tasks of orientation and short-term memory

Task	Prevalence of need for daily nursing care	
	%	Prevalence Ratio
a. Orientation		
Good performance	2.3	1.0
Poor performance	40.6	17.7
b. Short-term memory		
Good performance	2.9	1.0
Poor performance	5.4	1.9

- see footnotes to table 1

shows, among those performing well in the orientation test, 2.3 % were classified as needing daily nursing help, whereas among those not performing well, the figure was 40.6 %, or almost 18 times higher. In contrast, performance in the memory test discriminated only marginally between those needing daily nursing care and those who did not, the ratio being 1.9.

In table 3, the prevalence ratios of being in need of daily nursing care are presented with respect to different types of functional impairment. By far the most important impairment in this context is that of orientation with a prevalence ratio of 17.7. Urinary incontinence is second with a prevalence ratio of 7.0, followed by visual impairment, difficulties of chewing and swallowing, troubles of balance, fecal incontinence, etc.

Table 3 Need for daily nursing care and types of functional impairment

Type of functional impairment	Need for daily nursing care (Prevalence Ratio)
Orientation	17.7
Urinary incontinence	7.0
Visual impairment	5.2
Chewing / swallowing	3.8
Balance	3.7
Fecal incontinence	2.7
Upper limbs	2.3
Lower limbs	2.3
Dyspnoe	2.2
Short-term memory	1.9

- see footnotes to table 1

Table 4 Type of residence and performance on tasks of orientation and short-term memory

Task	Type of residence: Private home	Residential home	Nursing home	All
a. Orientation				
Good performance %	94.2	3.7	2.1	100.0
Poor performance %	53.3	13.6	33.2	100.1
(Prevalence Ratio)	(0.6)	(3.7)	(15.8)	
b. Short-term memory				
Good performance %	94.9	3.2	1.9	100.0
Poor performance %	81.5	10.7	7.8	100.0
(Prevalence Ratio)	(0.9)	(3.3)	(4.1)	

- see footnotes to table 1

There is also a strong association between deterioration on the orientation task and residence in a home. Among all persons over age 65, 90.2 % were living in private households, 4.3 % in residential homes for the aged and 5.5 % in nursing homes or hospitals. As table 4 shows, among those who performed well on the orientation task, 3.7 % were living in residential homes and 2.1 % in nursing homes, as against 13.6 % and 33.2 % respectively of those with deteriorated orientation. The prevalence ratio associated with deteriorated orientation was 3.7 for living in a residential home for the aged and 15.8 for living in a nursing home, or, to say it differently, assuming that the association between deteriorated orientation and living in a residential or nursing home is of a causal nature, it can be calculated that 32.8 % or about a third of the beds occupied in homes are attributable to more or less severe forms of senile dementia. In table 5, the association between indicators of senile dementia and residence in homes is presented differently, in that it shows that among those living in nursing homes, 54 % suffer from impairment of orientation as measured in this study. Among those living in private households, this is the case in only 4 %.

Table 5 Performance on tasks of orientation and short-term memory in relation to type of residence

Type of residence	Impairment of Orientation %	Impairment of Short-term memory %
Private	4.0	11.5
Residential home	21.4	33.9
Nursing home	54.0	38.5

- see footnotes to table 1

The other question to be treated briefly here concerns the distribution of senile dementia in the population. As can be seen from table 6, there is a certain social class gradient in performance in both of these tests, with about 4 times as many poor performers in the economically lower groups than among the better-off. A similar gradient for orientation results if educational rather than economic criteria are looked at, whereas for the memory test, a very clear association with educational level can be observed, with a prevalence ratio of 16 for graduates of primary school as compared to those with a higher education.

Table 6 Performance on tasks of orientation and short-term memory in relation to standard of living and education

	Impairment of Orientation		Impairment of Short-term memory	
	%	Prevalence Ratio	%	Prevalence Ratio
a. Standard of living				
Upper + upper middle	2.3	1.0	5.7	1.0
lower middle	8.7	3.8	15.1	2.6
lower	9.9	4.3	20.6	3.6
b. Education				
Baccalaureat; technical	2.5	1.0	1.5	1.0
Secondary School	5.1	2.0	12.2	8.1
Primary School	13.5	5.4	24.0	16.0

- see footnotes to table 1

Finally, the question of an association between elevated blood pressure levels and the presence of signs of senile dementia was examined. As table 7 shows, no such association could be detected.

Table 7 Performance on tasks of orientation and short-term memory in relation to blood pressure

	Impairment of Orientation		Impairment of short-term memory	
	%	Prevalence Ratio	%	Prevalence Ratio
No Hypertension	8.2	1.0	15.7	1.0
Hypertension[1)]	6.2	0.8	12.0	0.8

1) 160+ mmHg syst. and/or 95+ diast. and/or in treatment

\- see also footnotes to table 1

Discussion

What considerations should be made in interpreting these results? Given the fact that the survey was not conducted primarily with senile dementia in mind, and that no attempt was made to establish diagnoses of senile dementia, there will remain some uncertainty as to the clinical meaning of the findings reported here. On the other hand, the advantage of using simple, replicable tests of intellectual functioning as measures of the presence or absence of senile dementia in epidemiological studies has been emphasized in earlier discussions (Katzman, Terry, Bick 1978) and becomes apparent here, where many interviewers were involved. Studies by other authors have shown that simple orientation scales had a high reliability and were able to differenciate between patients with senile dementia and other patients in geriatric hospitals (Berg, Svensson 1980). In the present study, a similar orientation scale was applied to a stratified random sample of the entire population over age 65, and when giving one or more wrong answers is used as a criteria, the prevalence of 6.9 % turns out to correspond well to that found in other studies of senile dementia among elderly populations (Mortimer, Schuman, French 1981; Roth 1978). The marked increase of prevalence with age shown in this study was typical wherever the question had been looked at. The higher prevalence in women than in men was also previously found.

One of the impressive findings of this study is the strong association between poor performance on the orientation task and the loss of independence, expressed either in terms of need for nursing help or in terms of residence in a nursing home. As a matter of fact, assuming a causal relationship, 30 % of the aged living in residential or nursing homes can be accounted for by senile dementia as measured in this survey. A question not yet examined in detail is, however, whether the assumption of a causal relationship is valid, or whether being in a home has reduced the ability to answer questions such as concerning place and time.

It had been shown by others before that performance on an orientation task depended on educational level (Pfeiffer 1975), whereas an association with social class was not always found (Miller 1977). In the present study, a certain social class gradient was shown. If a 'standard of living'-classification is used, the gradient is similar whether performance in orientation or performance in a short-term memory-test is considered. However, when educational level is used, a much higher gradient results in this study for the complex intellectual task of recalling digits in reverse order, than for orientation. As expected, an association between our indicators of senile dementia and hypertension could not be shown.

In summary then, this survey of elderly inhabitants from a Swiss urban and suburban environment confirms earlier findings on the epidemiology of senile dementia. A differentiation between the various disease entities could not be attempted, but the immense role of senile dementia as a cause of dependence and of need for institutionalization of old people has become impressingly apparent. Clearly, it would be most desirable to be able to prevent this condition, but in order to reach this goal, much more research will be needed.

References

Berg S, Svensson T (1980). An orientation scale for geriatric patients. Age and Ageing 9:215.
Kahn RL, Goldfarb AI, Pollack M, Peck A (1960). Brief objective measures for the determination of mental status in the aged. Amer J Psychiat 117:326.
Katzman R, Terry RD, Bick KL (1978). Alzheimer's Disease. Senile Dementia and Related Disorders (Aging vol 7). New York: Raven Press, p 342.
Miller E (1977). Abnormal Ageing. The Psychology of Senile and Presenile Dementia. London: John Wiley & Sons, p 10.
Mortimer JA, Schuman LM, French L (1981). Epidemiology of dementing illness. In Mortimer JA, Schuman LM (eds): The Epidemiology of Dementia. New York: Oxford University Press, p 3.
Müller C (1981). Psychische Erkrankungen und ihr Verlauf sowie ihre Beeinflussung durch das Alter. Bern: Verlag Hans Huber, p 25.
Pfeiffer EA (1975). A short portable mental status questionnaire for the assessment of organic brain deficit in elderly patients. J Amer Geriatr Soc 23:433.
Roth Sir M (1978). Epidemiological studies. In Katzman R, Terry RD, Bick KL (eds). Alzheimer's Disease: Senile Dementia and Related Disorders (Aging vol 7). New York: Raven Press, p 337.

Senile Dementia: Outlook for the Future, pages 405–409

A COHORT COMPARISON OF FUNCTIONAL ABILITY AND MENTAL DISORDERS IN TWO REPRESENTATIVE SAMPLES OF 70-YEAR-OLDS

Alvar Svanborg, Stig Berg, Lars Nilsson and Göran Persson
Departments of Geriatric & Long-Term Care Medicine and Psychiatry, University of Göteborg, Göteborg, Sweden

This report is based on results from the longitudinal and geriatric study of 70-year-olds in Göteborg, Sweden (Rinder et al 1975, Svanborg 1977, Svanborg et al 1982). This paper will include:

1. A description of the purpose, procedure and design of the longitudinal study of 70-year-olds.
2. Some comments concerning the rate and manifestations of age-related changes in intelligence and memory based both on retrospective and prospective longitudinal information. These data also illustrate some of the diagnostic difficulties and risk of overdiagnosis of organic brain disorders with dementia - especially of dementias of mild to moderate degree.
3. Cohort comparisons at the age of 70 and 75 of cognitive functions as well as of mental health at the age of 70. This paper will also include prevalence figures for mental disorders longitudinally from age 70 to 79.

The study is performed on samples that, as far as we can judge, are representative for the total population. The original sample, studied in 1971/72 comprised 30 % of the 70-year-old population. In 1976/77 the survivors of this cohort were followed up, and at the same time a new 70-year-old cohort was sampled in order to make a cohort comparison. A new follow-up of the first cohort has been undertaken at the age of 79 and a third follow-up has recently been started at the age of 81. The second cohort of 70-year-olds has been followed up at age 75.

Because of the findings of certain important cohort differences within such a short period as five years, a third 70-year-old cohort born in 1911 to 1912 is just now being investigated. The

Swedish Research Council has, furthermore, given us resources to measure not only possible cohort differences towards this third 70-year-old cohort but also to make an extensive intervention study of this third cohort. Although our investigations cover wide areas of morphology, physiology, clinical medicine and behavioural performance, the organic brain disorders are one example where the diagnostic resources are limited and were the possibilities to distinguish physiological ageing from symptoms of definable diseases often are rather questionable. To our experiences we need to include interventions into the life situation of the elderly in our diagnostic program in order to lower the obvious risk for overdiagnosis.

The survey includes a home-call for each subject in order to establish basic personal data such as housing conditions, income, social and physical communications, previous addresses, educational level, previous and any present occupation, and the need for and the use of health care facilities. All subjects undergo subsequently an examination at the out-patient department of the hospital, including a general medical and ophtalmological examination, blood and urine tests, ECG and chest X-ray. Psychological, psychiatric, dental, somatometric and audiometric examinations are performed on representative subsamples. In addition, subsamples also undergo a dietary interview, body composition examination, detailed studies of lung function, cardiac function, immunoresponse capacity, as well as extensive neurophysiological examinations including EEG, echoencephalography and measurement of cerebral blood flow.

The psychological studies were performed by or under the leadership of Stig Berg (Berg 1980). The following intelligence and memory tests were performed: Synonyms or SRB 1 measuring verbal ability, Figure grouping or SRB 2 measuring inductive and logical reasoning ability, Block design or SRB 3 measuring spatial ability and Ps-if measuring perceptual speed, Digit span measuring primary memory and Thurstone memory test measuring secondary memory.

As far as the diagnosis of mental disorders were concerned, the diagnostic routine was mainly in accordance with the ICD classification. The psychiatric investigations were performed by the psychiatrists, Göran Persson or Lars Nilsson. The average length of the examination was one hour. The examination consisted of questions in the following order; childhood, education, profession, marriage, sexuality, alcohol consumption, sleep, previous and current psychiatric care and psychiatric symptoms during the month preceding the interview. Symptoms and signs were rated in accordance with the CPRS in four steps: absent, mild, moderate and severe with half steps between them. A global rating of mental health was also included.

The prevalence figures presented are, furthermore, considered in relation to the observations at the home calls and at the neurophysiological examinations mentioned above.

Cognitive Functions

Further studies at age 75 and 79 confirmed our previous conclusions from studies at the age of 70 (Berg 1980) that intelligence and memory are not significantly changed at the age of 70, but that the perceptual speed apparently has started to decline already early in adult life.

The discrepancy in the rate of change by age between the perceptual speed and the other measurable parameters of intelligence and memory is, according to our experience, the main reason for overdiagnosis of dementia/senility in the elderly. This is especially the case when the perceptual speed is further lowered because of sensory deprivation, as e g unwanted isolation, bereavement, different forms of somatic injuries and diseases as well as mental depression.

The cohort differences previously observed at age 70 (Berg 1980) are recently found to be obvious also at age 75. Furthermore, these age cohort differences seem to be at the same order of magnitude at age 75 compared to age 70. Originally we had not planned to follow the second cohort of 70-year-olds longitudinally more than to the age of 75. The fact that measurable cohort differences in intelligence and memory still existed at age 75 has, however, actualized the need of further cohort comparisons also at ages above 75.

Mental Disorders

In the second 70-year-old cohort the prevalence of psychoses was 3.5 % (2.2 % in men and 4.4 % in women), of neuroses of moderate-severe degree 8.9 % (6.2 % in men and 11 % in women) of neuroses of mild degree 8.7 % (5.1 % in men and 11.5 % in women) and of diagnosed alcoholism 1.5 % (3.4 % in men and 0 % in women). The total prevalence excluding personality disorders was 22.5 % (16.9 % in men and 26.9 % in women).

The prevalence of dementia was 1 % (included among the psychoses) and of asthenic neuroses 4.2 % (included among the neuroses of moderate-severe degree). The diagnosis asthenic neurosis corresponds to what is usually described in dementias of mild to moderate degree but without etiological implications. 5.9 % of the subjects given a psychiatric diagnosis were without treatment. According to the investigator's (L. Nilsson) opinion 1.7 % untreated subjects would benefit from psychiatric treatment. A detailed report concerning the prevalence of mental disorders in this second 70-year-old cohort is under publication (Nilsson 1983). No significant differences could be found between prevalence rates from this study and the 70-year-old sample born five years earlier and investigated by G. Persson (Persson 1980).

The longitudinal population study of 70-year-olds in Göteborg, Sweden, has demonstrated other cohort differences than the above mentioned differences in cognitive function. There are direct evidences of cohort differences as far as longevity, body weight, length, oral status and state of health in general are concerned (Svanborg et al 1982). Furthermore, the negative influence on ageing, health and longevity of smoking, alcohol abuse and bereavement are examples of other indirect evidences for differences between different age cohorts in our population (Mellström et al 1981, 1982). In Sweden, like in many other countries, the older olds are the ones that will increase absolutely and relatively most in the population in the future. As one example, the number of those 85 and above will double and the number of 95+ will have increased three times during the period from 1970 to the year 2000, and these group of elderly will increase even more up to the year 2025.

Up till now, our longitudinal study has only reached age 81. It seems to be of great importance to improve our knowledge not only concerning the incidence and prevalence of organic brain disorders but also of the concomitant impairment, disability and handicap as well as the need of care and support of these grand olds. We can, however, foresee further increasing diagnostic difficulties in the even older age cohorts as far as possibilities to distinguish between physiological changes, environmentally provoked alterations and definable organic brain disorders are concerned.

Berg S (1980). Psychological functioning in 70- and 75-year-old people. A study in an industrialized city. Acta Psychiat Scand Suppl 288

Mellström D, Rundgren Å, Svanborg A (1981). Previous alcohol consumption and its consequences for ageing, morbidity and mortality in men aged 70-75. Age and Ageing 10:277.

Mellström D, Rundgren Å, Jagenburg R, Steen B, Svanborg A (1982). Tobacco smoking, ageing and health among the elderly: A longitudinal population study of 70-year-old men and an age cohort comparison. Age and Ageing 11:45.

Mellström D, Nilsson Å, Odén A, Rundgren Å, Svanborg A (1982). Mortality among the widowed in Sweden. Scand J Soc Med 10:33.
Nilsson LV (1983). Prevalence of mental disorders in a 70-year-old urban sample. A cohort comparison. J Clin Exp Gerontol, accepted for publication.
Persson G (1980). Prevalence of mental disorders in a 70-year-old urban population. Acta Psychiat Scand 62:119.
Rinder L, Roupe S, Steen B, Svanborg A (1975). 70-year-old people in Gothenburg. A population study in an industrialized Swedish city. I. General presentation of the study. Acta Med Scand 198:397.
Svanborg A (1977). Seventy-year-old people in Gothenburg. A population study in an industrialized Swedish city. II. General presentation of social and medical conditions. Acta Med Scand Suppl 611:5.
Svanborg A, Landahl S, Mellström D (1982). Basic issues of health care. In Thomae H, Maddox GL (eds): "New Perspectives on Old Age. A Message to Decision Makers". New York: Springer Publishing Company, p 31.

Senile Dementia: Outlook for the Future, pages 411–425

EPIDEMIOLOGICAL ELEMENTS IN PRESENILE ALZHEIMER'S DISEASE

Michel Gaillard

Service Universitaire de Psycho-Gériatrie

Prilly, 1008 Suisse

Since 1970, many studies have been made, most of them quite sophisticated, on Alzheimer's disease. They have touched on various domains, notably ultrastructural anatomo-pathology, genetics, the biochemistry of neurotransmitters, cerebral metabolism, immunology and virology (Schneck 1982).

In 1977, the Congress on Alzheimer's Disease, Senile Dementia and Related Disorders at Bethesda, Maryland, made a synthesis of these studies and noted that it was more and more widely recognized that patients suffering from senile dementia (onset after 65 years) and those with presenile Alzheimer's disease (onset before 65 years) presented the same pathological cerebral changes. Even though the clinical and pathological manifestations of these two conditions were identical, differing but still unknown etiological factors might have to be considered. So as not to prejudge the possibilities of a common etiology, it was proposed that the terms presenile Alzheimer's disease and alzheimerized senile dementia should be employed. Various etiological hypotheses were considered. Attention was first given to the genetic hypothesis, supported by numerous observations, dating from as early as 1934, and by recent correlations established between Alzheimer's disease, Down's syndrome and the haptoglobin gene of chromosome 16. The neurotransmitters were also implicated, probably in connection with a deficiency in the cerebral cholinergic system. The importance of heavy metals was suggested by the discovery of high levels of aluminium in the cerebral tissue of patients with Alzheimer's disease, but it was not known whether this was a primary or secondary phenomenon.

The hypothesis of a slow virus was suggested, after contaminating primates with tissues from patients suffering from Alzheimer's disease, but the specific lesions of the disease were not identified It was believed that an immunological factor might also be involved and the hypothesis of anti-brain antibodies was proposed(Katzmann, Terry, Bick 1978).

At the Congress, it was considered that the major obstacle to identification of etiological factors and risk factors continued to be the absence of adequate epidemiological information.This concern was expressed by a number of authors (Schoenberg 1978, 1981; Mortimer, Schuman, French 1981; Gruenberg 1978) who raised the problems of annual incidence, sex, environmental factors, order of birth, race, religion and various socioeconomic factors.

In 1979, Liston, in a study of all cases reported in the literature during the preceding 40 years, found that the parameters most commonly mentioned, in diminishing order of frequency, were : age, sex, age at the time of the first diagnosis, duration of the disease and age at death. Race, order of birth, religion and economic status were never mentioned (Liston 1979).

PURPOSE OF STUDY

This study seeks to contribute to an understanding of the questions raised above, by studying a population of patients suffering from presenile Alzheimer's disease and by finding out in what respect this population can be distinguished from a general population, in order to specify possible risk factors and other elements leading to better understanding of the etiology of the disease.

SELECTION OF POPULATION

For this study, we took all patients who had stayed in the University Psychogeriatric Service and the University Clinic of Psychiatry between 1970 and 1980 with the diagnosis of presenile Alzheimer's disease, code 290.1 in the WHO International Classification of Diseases. The diagnoses were made on the basis of clinical symptomatology and evolution marked by the following characteristics: onset during the presenile period, an aphasic-apractic-agnosic syndrome beginning early and evolving dramatically, behavior disorders, neurological disturbances characterized by hypertonia with rigidity of opposition, synkinesis, stereotypes and resurgence of prefrontal signs in the form of archaic reflexes (grasping reflex, oral reflex, palm-chin reflex) (Müller, Wertheimer 1981; Constantinidis 1978). 49 patients were obtained in this manner, of whom 13 are still living.

THE INVESTIGATION

This was a retrospective epidemiological analysis in which an attempt was made, among other things, to take into consideration criteria which were generally omitted in the literature. The data included :

1. Date of birth
2. Place of birth
3. Sex
4. Order of birth in sib group and number of siblings
5. Religion
6. Family medical history
7. Educational level
8. Occupation
9. Marriage
10. Number of children
11. Drinking habits
12. Date of first symptoms
13. Civil status at time of hospitalization
14. Domicile at time of hospitalization and previous domiciles
15. Date of death

1. Date of Birth

Our patients were born between 1900 and 1922 and thus covered an age-range within the definition of presenile Alzheimer's disease.

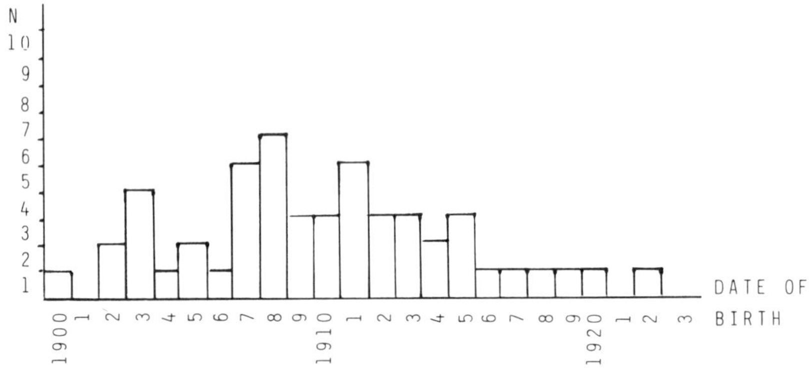

2. Place of Birth

The place of birth was found for 48 of the 49 patients. The proportions corresponded to those of the general population of persons more than 65 years old in 1980.

	Alzheimer's disease		General population + 65 years in 1980 *
	N	%	%
Lausanne	9	18,8	23,4
Vaud	18	37,5	33,0
Other cantons	11	22,9	28,6
Other countries	10	20,8	15,0

*General population in Lausanne

3. Sex

In our population, the female sex was preponderant (63%). This corresponds to the general population in the age group from 55 to 64 years. In 1970, the general population was that of the resident population of the canton of Vaud; in 1980 by the population of Lausanne.

Alzheimer's disease		General population* 55 to 65 years 1970		1980	
M	W	M	W	M	W
36,7%	63,3%	47%	53%	44%	56%

*General population: 1970 -Canton of Vaud
1980 -Lausanne

4. <u>Order of birth in sib group and number of siblings</u>

The number of brothers and sisters was known for 39 patients, but the order of birth for only 27. One group of 9 siblings was represented by 3 of its members. The average size of the group for the women patients was 4,8 and that for the men 3,8. In 2/3 of the population followed, the patient with Alzheimer's disease was either the first or second member of the group.

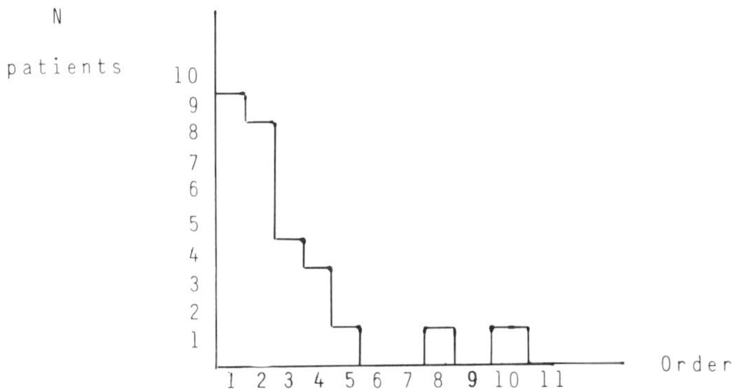

5. <u>Religion</u>

The religions of the patients were given as follows:

Protestant	61,2%
Catholic	28,6%
Others	2,0%
Not given	8,2%

To exclude a source of error resulting from South European Catholic emigration, these figures were compared to those of the Swiss population living in Lausanne (Protestants 59%, Catholics 32%).The distribution corresponded to that of the population studied.

6. Family medical history
The data for the families of patients were sparse we could usually obtain only the principal disease causing death. This was known for 29 of the fathers and 31 of the mothers. The frequency of dementia in the mothers of our patients was notable.

Principal disease causing death	Father	Mother
Cancer	7	2
Dementia	3	10
Stroke	3	3
Lung disease	3	1
Neurological disease	0	3
Cardiological disease	1	3
Endocrine disease	2	1
Viral infection	2	2
Others	8	6
	29	31

7. Educational level
The educational levels in our population corresponded closely to those in the general population. However, the proportion of patients with university education was higher than in the general population. The general population used for this purpose was that of residents in Vaud in the age group 55 to 64 years en 1970.

	Alzheimer's disease	General * population 55-64 years
Primary school	63,3	63,6
Lower secondary school	6,1	10,6
Upper secondary school	4,1	8,0
Professional school	14,3	5,5
Higher technical school	0	0,9
University	12,2	3,2
No education	0	0,3
Not given	0	7,9
	100%	100%

*General population: Canton of Vaud 1970

8. Occupation

In examing the records on occupations, it was striking to observe that 80% of the women had been employed. Among them, 35% had been manual workers or factory workers, 22,5% had special training as office workers, secretaries, sales personnel, etc. and 16% ranked as cadres, nurses, social workers, etc. These figures corresponded to those obtained in analyzing the female population hospitalized in the service between 1963 and 1974, combining all types of psychopathology. The figures obtained for the male population did not permit any special interpretation. It may be noted that there were no men who had worked in the aluminium industry. The medical branch was represented by 4 women nurses and 1 male dentist.

9. Marriage

In the total population, 43 patients had been married, 7 of them twice. The average marriage age of 19 of the 27 married women was 28,3 years and in 8 of the 16 married men, 33,1 years.

10. Number of children

The number of children was known in 39 cases. In

13 cases, there were no children. In the remaining cases, the distribution was as follows: 6 marriages with 1 child; 11 marriages with 2 children; 7 with 3 children and 2 with 4 children. On the average, the men had 1,3 children and the women 1,6. The fertility rate for all the women was 1,4. Among 30 of the 31 women for whom the number of children was known, or 40%, were childless.

11. <u>Drinking habits</u>
This is a difficult matter to evaluate and it is mentioned only when drinking may present a handicap. In this series, alcohol addiction was mentioned in 20,4% of the cases. It should also be noted that in 12,2% of the cases, the patient's partner was known to be an alcoholic.

12. <u>Date of first symptoms</u>
The time of the onset of the condition was obtained by anamnesis. It fell between 1958 and 1979 and was thus between the ages of 48 and 68 years. The mean age at onset was 58,8 years for the women and 62,4 years for the men.

Age at appearance of symptoms	M %	W %
54	0	16,7
55 - 59	16,7	30,0
60 - 64	44,4	40,0
65 - 68	38,9	13,3

Age at appearance of symptoms, by age groups and sex.

13. <u>Civil status at time of hospitalization</u>
Analysis of the civil status of the subjects showed that most of them were married, especially in the case of the men (88,9%). In comparison with the general population, married women were under-represented, whereas widows and divorcees

were over-represented.

	Unmarried M%	Unmarried W%	Married M%	Married W%	Widowed M%	Widowed W%	Divorced M%	Divorced W%
Alzheimer's disease	11,1	12,9	88,9	45,2	0	22,6	0	19,3
General population 1970	9	12	80	63,5	4	16,5	7	8
General population 1980	8,7	14,4	80,6	58,2	3,1	15,6	7,6	11,8

General population, 55-64 years: 1970 = Canton of Vaud
1980 = Lausanne

14. <u>Domicile at time of hospitalization and previous domiciles</u>

Domiciles at the time of hospitalization were as follows :

Lausanne	29
Vaud	16
Other cantons	1
Other countries	3

The domiciles of patients who had lived in Lausanne for some 10 years prior to hospitalization were considered from the point of view of relative population density and in terms of the different water distribution zones in which they were located (Truan 1978). The latter criterion was chosen on the basis of studies reporting increases in aluminium level in the brains of subjects suffering from Alzheimer's disease and descriptions of aluminium-related dementia in persons undergoing hemodialysis, on the hypothesis of an influence of the aluminium content of the water (Crapper,De Boni 1978; Dunea,Mahurkar 1978;Trapp,Miner,Zimmermann 1978). The 29 patients were uniformly distributed among the neighborhoods with high population density. The

14 water distribution zones covering part of the outskirts and the city itself accounted for 34 of our patients. It was found that 60% of our cases came from 2 of the distribution zones, but these were also the zones with the highest population densities (Rossier 1966).

15. Date of death
Of the entire patient population, 36 died between 1970 and 1982. The age at death ranged from 58 to 76 years. The mean age at death was 66,8 years for the women and 67,9 years for the men. The date of the first symptoms and the date of death enabled us to calculate the mean duration of the evolution of the disease as 7,5 years for the women and 5,5 years for the men.

Age at death	M %	W %
60	0	4,5
60 - 64	13,3	31,8
65 - 69	46,7	36,4
70 - 74	40,0	18,2
75 +	0	9,1

Age at death by age groups and sex

DISCUSSION OF RESULTS

The group chosen for this study was a population of hospitalized patients with Alzheimer's disease. Due to the generally dramatic evolution of this disease, hospital care is necessary for virtually all patients. In the absence of any other institution to assume responsibility for this pathology, the sample is representative of an area with a population of 250'000 inhabitants, 2/3 of whom live in the city. Because of the small number of autopsies, which were nevertheless positive for the pathology in question, there are relatively few anatomo-pathological correlations, but the very strict clinical criteria used in making the diagnoses compensate for this.

Items chosen for consideration, applicable to all cases, were sex, civil status, religion, place of birth, occupation, domicile, educational level, date of birth, date of first symptoms and date of death and, to a smaller proportion of cases, order of birth, number of siblings, number of children, family medical history and drinking habits.

The criterion of date of birth provided no particular information. The place of birth corresponded to the pattern of the general population.

For a long time, it has been believed that this condition affects women more than men (Roth 1978). Liston, in 1979, taking into account the male/female distribution in the United States, showed that the difference was not as great as had been supposed; this was indicative though not definitive, since, in his view, the male/female distribution in the United States did not necessarily correspond to that in northern Europe. In comparison with the general population in the age bracket in question, we found figures indicating a preponderance of women, taking into account that the proportion of women in the general population has been growing, decade by decade. This was confirmed by the fact that the male population, including all psychogeriatric pathology, is over represented in the hospitals in question in every age group, compared to the general population, except for the sample constitued by those with Alzheimer's disease.

With respect to the order of birth, the patients were fhe first or second children in 2/3 of the cases, but there is no comparison for this in the literature. The religious criterion showed no differences, compared to the general population. With respect to the family medical histories, which were known in only 60% of the cases, it is worthy of note that in the group studied there was one family with 9 children, 5 of whom suffered from presenile Alzheimer's disease, with 3 included in the study. It was also remarkable to find that 1/3 of the mothers of patients had degenerative or vascular dementia.

Educational levels corresponded almost exactly to the general population, but the over-representation of university graduates was noteworthy. Analysis of the occupations of the patients in the study showed no difference from those of psychogeriatric patients as a whole, except that a larger proportion of the women had been employed. The medical and paramedical professions were encountered in 5 cases, 10% of the total, but there was no basis for comparing this finding with the general population.

The criteria of marriage and number of children showed that the average number of children per marriage was low: 1.3 for the married men and 1,61 for the married women. The latter figure was below that for women in the general population between 1931 and 1945: 2,56 in 1931 and 2,35 in 1945. The fertility rate of the women was low at 1,4. Of all the women patients, 40% had no children. In 1945, the percentage of married women without children in the general population was 17,4% and in our sample, 29,6%.

Quantitatively, the problem drinking habits in our population were virtually identical with those in the general population.

With respect to the onset of the disease, the duration of its evolution and the age at death, our results corresponded to those in the literature. However, it appeared that the duration of the evolution for men was shorter than it was for women.

Distribution of patients according to civil status is close to that of the general population, if we take into consideration general trends toward a diminution in the number of married people and increases in the numbers of divorced and unmarried people. There was an under-representation of married women and an over-representation of divorced women.

Analysis of the place of significant domicile in the 10 years prior to onset of the disease shows that the Lausanne patients were uniformly distributed among neighborhoods with high population density. Study of the distribution of patients among water distribution zones in Lausanne showed that about

1/3 of those in Lausanne water district were in the same zone. The water in this zone has an aluminium content of 0,3 mg/liter and has a high mineral content and a hardness of 25 to 30°, with low contents in sodium, nitrates and phosphorus. The data are difficult to interpret, especially since a purification process using microflocculation with basic aluminium polychloride has been in use since 1977 and thus could not have played a role in relation to the population in the study. It may be possible in the future to make a better assessment of the influence of this heavy metal.

CONCLUSIONS

Within the terms of this study of a population of patients with Alzheimer's disease, with onset during the presenile period, following recommendations made to avoid prejudging the question of a common etiology for the presenile and senile forms, the following characteristics were observed in the patient population:

> A preponderance of women, a majority of whom had worked outside home; an early place in the order of birth in their siblings groups; a low fertility rate; a high frequency of dementia in the mother's ancestral line; a more rapid evolution of the disease in men. Observations of the onset of the disease, the mean duration of it evolution in both sexes and the age of death confirmed the data in the literature. It is necessary to compare these data with those obtained in an analogous study of the senile form of the disease to determine whether there are specific factors which distinguish them.

REFERENCES

Constantinidis J (1978). Is Alzheimer's Disease a Major Form of Senile Dementia? Clinical, Anatomical, and Genetic Data. In Katzmann R, Terry RD, Bick KL (eds): "Alzheimer's Disease: Senile Dementia and Related Disorders", New York:Raven Press p. 15.

Crapper DR, De Boni U (1978). Brain Aging and Alzheimer's Disease. Can. Psychiat. Assoc.J.23,229-233.
Dunea G, Mahurkar SD, Mamdani B, Smith EC (1978). Role of Aluminium in Dialysis Dementia. Ann. Intern. Med 88 :502-504.
Gruenberg E (1978). Epidemiology. In Katzmann R, Terry RD, Bick KL (eds): "Alzheimer's Disease: Senile Dementia and Related Disorders", New York: Raven Press, p. 323.
Katzmann R, Terry RD, Bick KL (1978). Recommendations of the Nosology, Epidemiology and Etiology and Pathophysiology Commissions of the Workshop Conference on Alzheimer's Disease - Senile Dementia and Related Disorders. In Katzmann R, Terry RD, Bick KL (eds): "Alzheimer's Disease: Senile Dementia and Related Disorders", New York : Raven Press, p.579.
Liston EH (1979). The Clinical Phenomenology of Presenile Dementia: a Critical Review of the Literature. J. Nerv. Ment. Dis. 167: 329-336.
Mortimer JA, Schuman LM, French LR (1981). Epidemiology of Dementia: Overview and Prospects. In Mortimer JA, Schuman LM (eds):"The Epidemiology of Dementia", New York: Oxford University Press, p. 173.
Muller C, Wertheimer J (1981). Abrégé de Psychogériatrie. Paris, Masson.
Office de statistique de l'Etat de Vaud (Lausanne 1978). Annuaire statistique du Canton de Vaud.
Office d'études socio-économiques et statistiques. (Lausanne 1982). Recensement fédéral du 2.12.1980: résultats lausannois et par secteur.
Rossier J,Berger W (1966). Cent ans d'histoire du Service des eaux Lausanne, Services Industriels.
Roth M(1978). Epidemiological Studies. In Katzmann R, Terry RD, Bick KL (eds): "Alzheimer's Disease: Senile Dementia and Related Disorders", New York: Raven Press, p. 337.
Schneck MK, Reisberg B, Ferris SH (1982). An Overview of Current Concepts of Alzheimer's Disease. Am. J. Psychiat 139: 165-173.

Schoenberg BS (1978). Neuroepidemiologic Considerations in Studies of Alzheimer's Disease-Senile Dementia. In Katzmann R, Terry RD, Bick KL (eds): "Alzheimer's Disease: Senile Dementia and Related Disorders", New York: Raven Press, p. 327.

Schoenberg BS (1981). Methodological Approaches to the Epidemiologic Study of Dementia. In Mortimer JA, Schuman LM (eds): "The Epidemiology of Dementia", New York: Oxford University Press, p. 117.

Trapp GA, Miner GD, Zimmermann RL (1978). Aluminium Levels in Brain in Alzheimer's Disease. Biol. Psychiat. 13: 709-718.

Truan JL, Apotheloz B, Gloor R (1980). Ville de Lausanne : Inventaire Urbain, Lausanne, Centre de documentation, Direction des travaux.

Senile Dementia: Outlook for the Future, pages 427–441

EPIDEMIOLOGY OF SENILE DEMENTIA

Daniel Coquoz

Hôpital psycho-gériatrique

Prilly, 1008 - Suisse

INTRODUCTION

The aging of the Swiss population has been persistent, especially since the 1920s. Mr. JJ Senglet, Director of the Federal Statistical Bureau, has commented on various causes of this development and has noted two indices for measurement of this trend:

- the proportion of "the number of aged persons in the total population (6% in 1880 and 1920, 14% in 1980)"
- the proportion of "the number of adults (53% in 1880, 56% in 1920 and 58% en 1980)", which brings into the picture "the burden imposed by the aged population on the active population".

Mortimer (1981), in his monograph on the epidemiology of senile dementia, emphasizes "the high incidence and economic impact of dementing illness" resulting from it and expresses his surprise that so little attention has been given to epidemiological approaches to it as compared with other diseases, even considering the difficulties of early diagnosis. The correlation between the aging of the population and the increased incidence of senile dementia is clear. Kay and Sir Martin Roth, in 1964 commented that there is no factor or characteristic which clearly augments the probability of developing senile dementia of the alzheimer type, other than advanced age.

Liston (1979), in his critical review of the literature on presenile dementia, notes that some epidemiological parameters are almost never mentioned, such as race, order of birth, religion and socio-economic status.

Our purpose was to study various factors specific to dementia and chosen according to criteria selected on the basis of earlier analyses, in order to identify risk factors and possible etiological indications. We considered such general data as sex, order of birth in the sib group, fertility; socio-economic and socio-cultural factors such as civil status, religion, place of birth, levels of education and social status; hereditary characteristics and factors serving to define the disease itself, such as age, time of evolution, the mode of appearance of the disease, the manner of its evolution, certain evolutional somatic factors and, finally, the diagnostic confirmations.

The study was concerned with the files on 151 cases treated at the Prilly Psychogeriatric Hospital, chosen according to the diagnostic criteria for the WHO codes 290.0, 290.2 and 290.3 and registered during part of 1980 and the whole of 1981. We did not include presenile dementia, psycho-organic syndromes of vascular origin or any other conditions which were not of degenerative origin. The type of epidemiological study was a retrospective one, with no other control group than the general population of persons of comparable ages analyzed in Federal censuses (1960-1980) and cantonal censuses (1970-1980). Consideration was also given to Lausanne urban data obtained from the Public Works Service and the Department of Architecture (EPFL) as the patient population came mainly from the City of Lausanne and its immediate surroundings (114 of 151 or 76%). Due to the sectoralizing of psychiatric activity in the Canton of Vaud, the Psychogeriatric Hospital serves the most highly urbanized area.

TABLE I. SEX

	Senile dementia	General population 75-84 years
F	80,1 %	68,6 %
M	19,9 %	31,4 %

$X^2 = 9,096$. $p < 0,01$. (Lausanne 1980)

TABLE 2. ORDER OF BIRTH

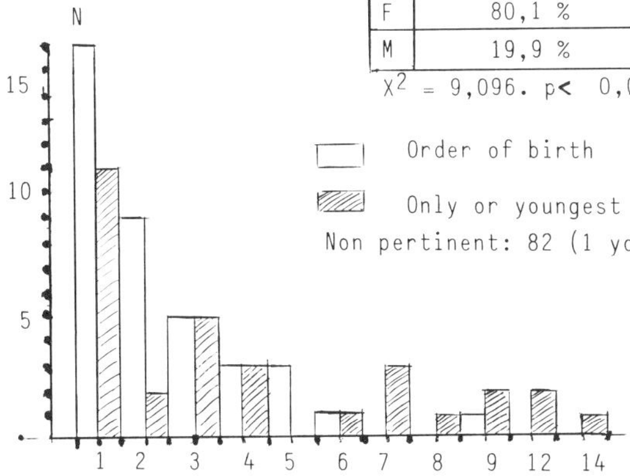

Order of birth

Only or youngest children

Non pertinent: 82 (1 youngest ch.) /151.

Analysis

1. Sex : 121 women and 30 men (Table 1)

2. Order of birth and number of children in the sib group :
   All patients : youngest children constituted the largest group (30,4%), followed by the eldest (23,2%), only children (16%), the second born (16%) and the remainder by order of birth (Table 2).
   The mean number of children in the families of origin of the women was 5,3, of the men 5.
   There were no known statistical data on family structure in Switzerland at the beginning of the 20th century.

3. Fertility : 38,8% of the women patients had had no children. Among women in the general population married between 1916 and 1920, 10,8% as of 1960, were without children. ($X^2 = 62,539$, $p < 0,001$).
   The married women patients had an average of 1,85 children. In comparison women in the general population married between 1916 and 1920, considered in 1960, had an average of 3,05 children (Table 3). The married men in the patient population had an average of 1,6 children. There were no corresponding data for men in the general

TABLE 3. Female fertility:

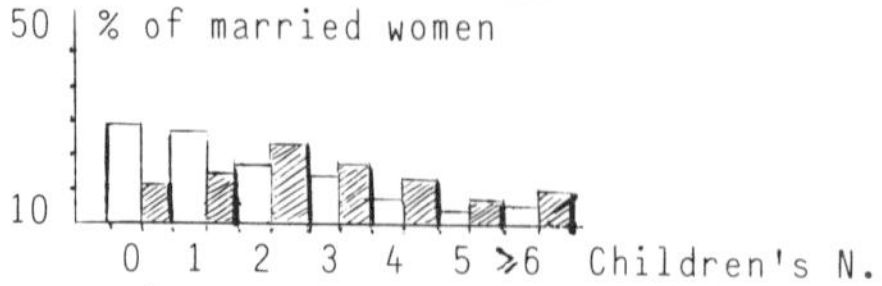

$X^2 = 50,43$, $p < 0,001$

TABLE 4. Place of birth:

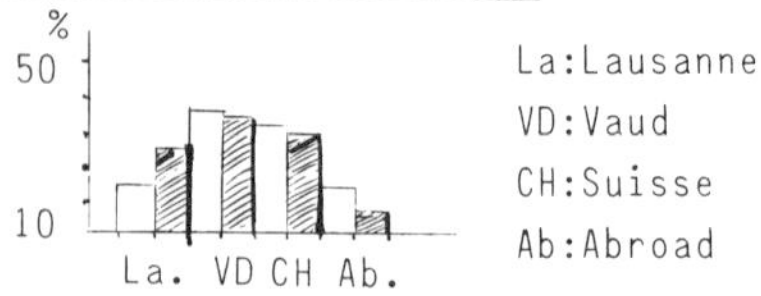

$X^2 = 15,460$, $p < 0,01$

TABLE 5. Educational level:

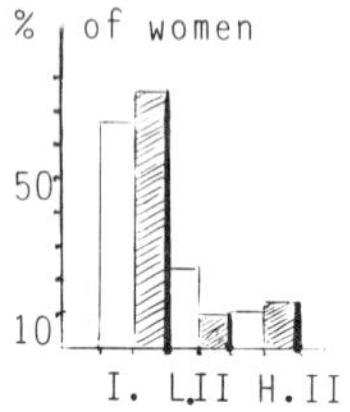

$X^2 = 21,878$, $p < 0,001$

TABLE 6. Educational level:

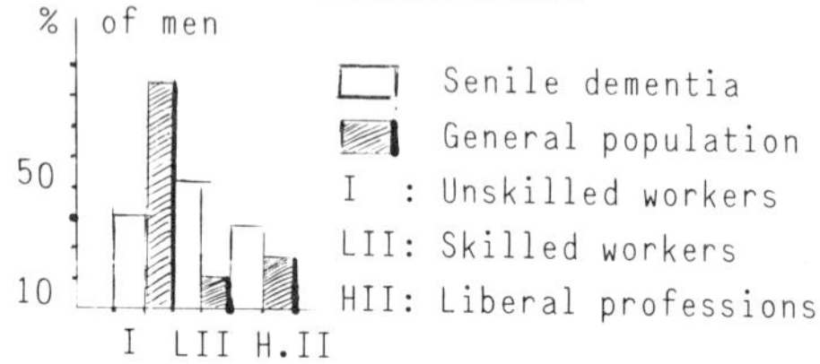

$X^2 = 42,626$, $p < 0,001$

population.

4. Civil status : 57,8% of the women patients were widows (58,7% in the general population of women between 80 and 84 years); 21,5% married (17,5%), 5,8% divorced (6,8%) and 14,9% unmarried (17%). ($X^2 = 1,550$, $0,50 < p < 0.90$).
   16,7% of the male patients were widowers (general population of men from 75 to 79 years, 18,5%) 80% were married (69,8%), 0 divorced (5,5%) and 3,3% unmarried (6,2%). ($X^2 = 2,517$, $0,30 < p < 0,50$).

5. Religion : Statistical data for 1980 for the general population did not show the distribution of religions by age groups and comparisons with the patient population would have little significance. We may note however that among the patients of both sexes there was a larger proportion of Protestants and a lower proportion of Catholics than in the general population.

6. Place of birth : Combining both men and women, we found that 14,5% of the patients were born in Lausanne, (25,1% in the general population over the age of 65), 36,6% born elsewhere in the Canton of Vaud, (35,7%), 33,8% elsewhere in Switzerland, (31%) and 15,1% in other countries,(8,2%), of whom 73% came from countries adjoining Swi-

tzerland, 13% from countries in the East and 14% from various other countries (Table 4). ($X^2 = 15.460$, $p < 0.01$).

7. Educational level and occupational status: Women who had only primary school education (I: housework, shop clerks without training, etc.) constitued 66,1% of the patient population (1970 statistics for the general population of women over 70, 76,7%), lower secondary school (L.II : housewives with some relevant training, secretaries, etc.) 23,2% (10,2%) and higher secondary school and university (H.II : teachers, nurses, etc.), 10,7% (13,1%) (Table 5). Regarding men, the table ($X^2 = 21,878$, $p < 0,001$). 6 gives the results.

8. Socioeconomic and urban characteristics : 117 patients, of both sexes, came from urban areas. Of these, 91, on the basis of their domicile prior to their first psychogeriatric hospitalization, were distributed in a pattern corresponding directly to the density of population per hectare by blocks of buildings (BEAU, Public Works Administration). This geographical distribution is difficult to interpret by age groups in view of the existence of a number of nursing homes. Corresponding to their socioeconomic conditions, our patients come predominantly from working class neighborhoods, generally composed of buildings with 4 or more stories and small apartments, rather than those with private houses or with apartments of 5 or more rooms, though the housing conditions were not particularly bad as a rule. There were for example more apartment houses with elevators than of old and delapidated buildings. (Système urbain lausannois, Département d'architecture EPFL).

9. Significant family antecedents :
   - Dementia : 14 out of 121 women, 11,6%, had family medical histories with senile psycho-organic conditions. The cases predominated among siblings (10 cases, 71,4%, including 6 involving one or more sisters, 3 with one or more brothers and sisters and 1 with a brother).

Among the mothers of patients there were 4 cases, one of the mothers having another daughter with the same condition. On the paternal side there were 2 instances, one in which the father and a brother were affected, the other being that of the paternal grandmother. There was 1 case in which a daughter suffered from presenile dementia. 2 men out of 30 had records of senile dementia in their families, affecting a brother in one case and both a brother and sister inthe other.

- Down's syndrome and leukosis : One of the men had a daughter with Down's syndrome. There were no cases of leukosis.
- Alcoholism : There were 9 out of 63 cases, 14,3% with alcoholic fathers. None of the mothers were known to be alcoholic. There were 2 cases among the siblings groups and 3 among the children of patients.

10. Somatic conditions of patients (absence of anterior and associated conditions, oncological and cardiac conditions) : These will be discussed mainly with respect to the differences between the men and women in the time of evolution, up to the time of death. It is noteworthy however that the frequency of epileptic episodes increases with the appearance of the disease (comitial crises before the disease, 2,5% for the women and 0% for the men; associated with the disease, 5,8% and 10% for the men). The frequency of pulmonary conditions also increased (bronchopneumonia prior to senile dementia, 3,3% for the women and 20% for the men). This was likely to be related to probable neurological difficulties in swallowing and the increase of cardiac pathology with age in both sexes (anterior cardiopathy, 13,2% for the women and 40% for the men; associated with the senile dementia, 47,9% for the women and 66,7% for the men).
With respect to previous psychic disorders, 14 women out of 121, or 11,6% had shown depressive symptoms and 3 men out of 30 had had psychiatric problems associated with alcoholism.

TABLE 7. Age groups at the onset of the condition, by sex:

Years:	Below 69.	70-74	75-79	80-84	85-89	over 90
F (%)	5	19	21,5	28,1	19	7,4
M (%)	6,7	20	40	20	10	3,3

TABLE 8.

Symptoms at the onset of the condition, by sex:

	F	M
Mnesic disorders	46,3 %	40 %
Depressive disorders	19 %	16,7 %
Disorientation	13,2 %	10 %
Behavioral disorders	7,4 %	26,7 %
Delirious symptoms	12,4 %	6,6 %
Maniac symptoms	1,7 %	0 %

11. Age groups at the onset of the condition, by sex (Table 7).

12. Symptoms at the onset of the condition, by sex (Table 8).

13. Type of evolution : The criteria of alzheimerization are : an obvious aphasic-apractic-agnosic syndrome or a slight aphasic-apractic-agnosic syndrome accompanied by prefrontal signs. Among the women, 55% were non-alzheimerized and 45% alzheimerized; among the men. 57% were non-alzheimerized and 43% alzheimerized.

14. Deaths :
    - Number of deaths by sex: 70 deaths out of 151 patients, or 47,7% including 46,3% of the women and 53,3% of the men. It was noted that 57,1% of the deceased women were alzheimerized and 56,3% of the men.
    - Age groups at death, by sex (Table 9).
    - Immediate causes of death : 40,3% died of bronchopneumonia, 79,3% were women and 20,7% were men. Of the total, 72,4% were alzheimerized. The distribution by sex, for each type

TABLE 9. Age groups at death, by sex:

Years:	70-74	75-79	80-84	85-89	90-94	over 95
F (%)	1,8	12,5	26,8	28,6	17,8	12,5
M (%)	18,8	12,5	37,5	18,8	6,2	6,2

of evolution, was similar. It was noted that 69,5% of the women and all of the men dying of bronchopneumonia had an associated cardiac pathology. 31,9% died of cardiac/respiratory arrest, with no other notable event. 82,6% were women and 17,4% men; 8,4% died of neoplasms, 83% of them women and 17% men; 6,9% of myocardial infarction, 20% of them women and 80% men; 5,6% of pulmonary embolisms, consisting only of women. The other deaths were due to a variety of causes.

15. Mean times of evolution in deceased patients:

- According to sex: the cases of the women evolved for an average of 5 years and those of the men for 4 years.
- According to type of evolution and sex: the cases of the alzheimerized women evolved for an average of 6 years (1 to 14), of alzheimerized men for 5 years (1 to 8), non-alzheimerized women for 4 years (1 to 20) and the non-alzheimerized men for 3 years (1 to 7).
- Mean time of evolution prior to alzheimerization, by sex: women, 4 years (1 to 13 years), men, 4 years (1 to 7 years).

16. Various evolutive factors :

- At the onset of their condition, the mean weight of the women was 52,7 kg, of the men 62 kg, In relation to sex and type of evolution, the mean losses of weight per year were : alzheimerized women, 2,6 kg, non-alzheimerized women 2kg, alzheimerized men 7,4 kg and non-alzheimerized men, 7,3 kg.

- Sensory organs : 61 out of 151 cases, 40%, had no sensory impairment. 50% of these were alzheimerized, of whom 70% died. Among the non-alzheimerized, more than 20% died. 90 cases out of 151, 60%, had sensory impairments. 37% of these had exclusively visual impairments, 1/3 of them having cataracts and 1/6 presbyopia. 31% had mixed lesions, both visual and auditory, and 32% had only impairments of he hearing, with hypoacousia in 1/4 of them and serious deafness in some cases. Whatever the sensory impairment, there were 59% non-alzheimerized, of whom 43% died, and 41% alzheimerized, of whom 49% died. The duration of alzheimerization was shortened by an average of 1 year, both in the women and the men.

17. Diagnostic confirmations :
- EEG : Of the 80 carried out, 85% showed diffuse bradyrhythmias and 1/4 indicated diffuse lesions with fronto-temporal predominance.
- Cerebral scans : Of the 24 made, there was only one which did not show cortico-subcortical atrophy.
- Brain autopsies : Of the 17 carried out, there were 12 which provided micro- and macroscopic diagnostic confirmation, 2 which offered only macroscopic confirmation and 3 with no morphologic substrate to support the diagnosis.

DISCUSSION OF RESULTS

Female predominance in senile dementia is statistically significant in comparison with the general population between the ages of 75 and 84 years (Table 1). Roth (1978) reported this for the degenerative condition, while noting that diffuse vascular lesions were predominant in men. The preponderance of the youngest, then the eldest and the only children need only be observed (Table 2). Statistically, the fertility of dementified women is significantly lower than that of the general population of women married in the same period as the group studied, and evaluated in the post-menopause period (Table 3). Kay, Beamish and Roth (1964) reported that dementified men had a larger number of children born and surviving, in comparison to functional patients and normal subjects, in a study at Newcastle Upon Tyne. There was no statistically significant difference with respect to civil status between the group of dements and the general population, taken by age groups, comparable to the ages of appearance of the disease in men and women. It was noted that in both sexes there was a somewhat larger number of married persons and fewer unmarried ones among the patients than in the general population. Larson and Sjögren (1963) reported that there was a higher proportion of demented patients who had never married, which was not the case in our population of patients. The birthplace of the dements, of both sexes, born in Lausanne and born abroad, was significantly different in comparison to the general population of persons over the age of 65. There were fewer born in Lausanne and more born abroad, especially in neighboring countries, among our patients. Those born in the Canton of Vaud and elsewhere in Switzerland constituted about the same proportion as persons in the general population (Table 4).

The levels of schooling and vocational training were significantly different in comparison to the general population over the age of 70. There were fewer dements, including both sexes, who had only primary schooling and no apprenticeship, but taking the women alone, we found a majority, with more than 60% being household workers without special training. The number of patients of both sexes who had lower secondary schooling was significantly higher in comparison to the general population, especially for the men. Male patients with a higher level of secondary education were also proportionately more numerous among the patients than in the general population of men over the age of 70, although this level was the least represented among the patients of both sexes (Tables 5 and 6).

Our hospital population was characterized by a low socio-economic status, although their housing conditions had not been especially poor. Gilliand, a swiss sociologist, in an analysis of recipients of social security retirement payments in 1976, noted that, "The proportion of very old persons is higher as their income is lower... 1% of the well to do retired are in hospitals or in other institutions, while the proportion is 15% for the poorest people". Kay, Beamish and Roth (1964) found no relation between social classes and the prevalence of the psycho-organic syndrome and also noted that persons of low socioeconomic status are predominantly in institutions.

Cases of senile dementia in the families present themselves mainly among the siblings of both men and women patients. Constantinidis (1978) commented that "familial senile cases are usually found within only one generation (sibs), favoring the hypothesis of recessive transmission. We also observed that both clinical forms (presenile and senile) may be found in the same family". This latter point was verified in one of our cases.

Heston (1981) referred to an apparent excess of Down's syndrome and leukosis in the families of persons suffering from Alzheimer's syndrome. We observed only one case of mongolism in the direct descendance of a demented man. The cases of paternal alcoholism are simply noted. With respect to psychic antecedents, Larson and Sjögren (1963) found no significant difference between the dementified and normal population in the same age groups.

The age of onset of the disease varies between the sexes. For women, the age groups are widely distributed between less than 69 years and more than 90 years, with a maximum of cases starting between the ages of 80 and 84 years. For men, the onset is distributed among **earlier age groups**, with a maximum of cases between 75 and 79 years. Female predominance is clear in the groups over the age of 80. On the contrary, in age groups below 79 years, there is a proportionately larger number of cases starting in men. Even though the relationship between the appearance of senile dementia and advanced age may be obvious, there is nevertheless a diminution in the number of cases after the age of 90 (Table 7).

The first symptoms noted, both for a majority of men and women, are memory difficulties. This has also been observed in the case of Alzheimer's disease by Liston (1979). Then, proportionately, women present predominantly depressive disorders while men primarily display behavioral problems of agressivity and agitation (Table 8). There is no notable difference between the sexes with respect to the type of evolution.

The number of deaths according to sex is proportionately greater among the men. This might be related to the fact that fewer men are free from anterior and associated somatic conditions (anterior, 6,7%, associated, 3,3%) as compared to the women (20,7% and 15,7%). Whatever the sex, there is a slightly higher proportion of deaths among alzheimerized subjects, which can correspond to an evolutive stage. The distribution of deaths by age groups, mainly between 85 and 89 years for the women and 80 and 84 years for the men, is not surprising in view of the ages at onset of the disease (Table 9).

The most common immediate cause of death is bronchopneumonia, primarily among the women and alzheimerized patients. Libow (1978) however reports that in a comparative study of dements and non-dements (Habot), "There was no significant difference between the two groups in the clinical occurence of pneumonia as the event preceding death".

The average periods of evolution and the difference observed between them, relating to sex on the one hand and to the type of evolution on the other, could be related to the somatic disorders present. As we have already seen, the men on the average were more affected by physical diseases than the women, both before and in the course of dementification. We can accordingly understand the shorter terms of evolution. In addition, the non-alzheimerized patients in our population advanced more rapidly toward death than those who were alzheimerized. This could be explained by the fact that, among the women oncological conditions affected only the non-alzheimerized patients (6,6% of the women suffered from breast cancer prior to the onset of dementia and 5% from various neoplasms associated with the dementia). In men, on the other hand, most of the cardiac pathology affected the non-alzheimerized subjects (40% for the anterior cardiac conditions, of which 75% were in non-alzheimerized patients and 66,7% for associated cardiac conditions, 60% of which were in non- alzheimerized patients).

The mean period of alzheimerization did not depend on sex.

The loss of weight per unit of time was greater when alzheimerization occurred. On the basis of the values observed, the hypothesis might be proposed that sensory deprivation does not necessarily accentuate an aphasic-apractic-agnosic syndrome but may shorten the evolution leading to its fatal outcome.

CONCLUSIONS

The study of 151 cases of senile dementia, analyzed from hospital files and compared with the general population of comparable ages, demonstrates the following :

Female predominance is significant. Considered in relation to the age of onset of the disease, it is apparent in the age groups of 80 years and up, but is relative in the groups below the age of 79. Female fertility is statistically lower. The place of birth is differentiated significantly from the general population over the age of 65 by a larger number of persons born in countries bordering on Switzerland and a smaller number born in Lausanne, regardless of sex. The levels of schooling and vocational training differ significantly, in both sexes, by a larger number of persons who have reached an intermediate level (lower secondary school and various types of apprenticeship). There is no significant difference in the civil status of dements. The low socioeconomic level of the patients is only explicable by the institutionalized character of the population analyzed. The most common initial symptoms are mnesic disorders. The type of evolution (alzheimerized senile dementia) and the time leading to its installation do not depend on sex. Sensory deprivation is not determinant of the type of evolution, but precipitates the evolution especially in cases of an aphasic-apractic-agnosic syndrome. Bronchopneumonia is the most common cause of death, especially for alzheimerized women.

The predominance of youngest and oldest children in senile dements deserves more detailed study. The hypothesis of recessive transmission of the disease should also be studied. Along with Katzmann, Terry and Bick (1978), we might emphasize the interest there could be, in the search for etiological factors, in analyzing the diminution of the "incidence" of senile dementia after the age of 90 years, especially since advanced age is the only clearly established risk factor.

REFERENCES

Constantinidis J (1978). Is Alzheimer's Disease a major form of senile dementia?Clinical, anatomical and genetic data. In Katzmann R,Terry RD, Bick KL (eds): "Alzheimer's Disease : Senile dementia and related disorders", New York: Raven Press, p. 15.

Gilliand P, Eichenberger P (1982). Vieillir aujourd'hui et demain. Rentiers suisses en 1976. Analyse des correspondances sur le revenu net. p. 433.

Heston LL (1981). Genetic studies of dementia: With emphasis on Parkinson's disease and Alzheimer's neuropathology. In Mortimer JA, Schuman LM (eds): "The epidemiology of dementia", New York:Oxford University Press, p. 101.

Inventaire urbain (1979-1980). BEAU/Direction des travaux de la ville de Lausanne. p 2 et 29.

Katzmann R, Terry RD, Bick KL (1978). Recommendations of the nosology, epidemiology and etiology and pathophysiology. Commissions of the workshop. Conference on Alzheimer's disease, senile dementia and related disorders.In Katzmann R, Terry RD, Bick KL (eds) : "Alzheimer's disease: senile dementia and related disorders", New York:Raven press p. 579.

Libow LS (1978). Epidemiology-Excess mortality and proximate causes of death. In Katzmann R, Terry RD, Bick KL (eds) : "Alzheimer's disease: Senile dementia and related disorders", New York : Raven Press, p. 315.

Liston ED (1979). The clinical phenomenology of presenile dementia. A critical review of the literature. In nervous and mental disease. Vol 167, p. 329.

Marazzi A. Biostatistique, médecine sociale et préventive. Université de Lausanne

Mortimer JA, Schuman LM (1981). "The epidemiology of dementia", New York : Oxford University press,

Müller C, Wertheimer J (1981). Abrégé de psychogériatrie. Paris, Masson. p. 137.

Office fédéral des statistiques. (Division des statistiques de la population). Recensement fédéral 1960. Vol. 27. p. 150.

Office des statistiques du canton de Vaud. Annuaire des statistiques 1978. p. 302.

Recensement fédéral 1980 (1982). Résultats lausannois. p. 9-59.

Richert G, Bassand M, Maillard P (1982). Rapport de recherche no 31. Système urbain Lausanne (cahier 4). IREC. Départ. Architecture EPFL. p. 27.

Roth M.(1978). Epidemiological Studies. In Katzmann R, Terry RD, Bick KL (eds): "Alzheimer's disease: senile dementia and related disorders", New York Raven Press, p. 337.

Semple A, Smith CM, Swash M (1982). The Alzheimer's disease.Syndrome in Alzheimer's disease, a report of progress. Corkin & al. (ed) New York:Raven Press. p. 93.

Senglet JJ (1982). Vieillissement de la population: situation et perspectives pour la Suisse. Dans vieillir aujourd'hui et demain (travaux réunis par Gilliand P). Ed. Réalités sociales. p. 27.

Sluss TK, Grünberg EM, Kramer M (1981). The use of longitudinal studies in the investigation of risk factors for senile dementia-Alzheimer type. In Mortimer JA, Schuman LM (eds):"The epidemiology of dementia", New York: Oxford University Press, p. 132.

X. SOCIO-POLITICAL PROBLEMS OF SENILE DEMENTIA

Presided by G.R. Andrews (Westmead) and J. Deboise (Paris)

Senile Dementia: Outlook for the Future, pages 445–454

PUBLIC POLICY IMPLICATIONS OF AN INCREASING ALZHEIMER'S POPULATION

Msgr. Charles J. Fahey
Director
Third Age Center - Fordham University
113 West 60 Street
New York, New York 10023

The human tragedy of Alzheimer's is overwhelming for the individual suffering from it, those who surround the patient, as well as for society as a whole.

To lose that which makes one human, that which enables us to enjoy the beauty of the sky or of another human being is as threatening an evil as death itself.

Such a reflection not only gives impetus to research but also to efforts to engage the whole person and his or her social network in an effort to ease loss and pain, if not to reverse the disease itself.

While the etiology of the disease may lie in physiological phenomena, the person and all who surround him are intimately involved in the disease process.

One never has a single patient with Senile Dementia Alzheimer's Type; one has a family and society as a whole as a client.

As research tries to unravel the mystery of the disease, reflection and research are needed to better understand all its human dimensions both as it effects the person with the disease and those who surround him.

Clearly and understandably panic and denial are two dimensions of response to manifestation of the disease. A lack of insight on the patient's part complicates the establishment or maintenance of a caring, supportive milieu.

A lack of understanding makes a difficult task impossible for family members.

Such an obvious and simple reality is suggestive of several issues for all those in the field.

Diagnosis / Labeling

The malignant, inexoriable and unknown aspects of Alzheimer's suggest that early and accurate diagnosis is critical. Since Senile Dementia may be secondary to other pathology, it is important that accurate diagnostic activity be undertaken so that appropriate therapeutic measures may be applied to the primary cause of confusion when such can be established. For the "true case" of Alzheimer's, such is important for "case management" and also that data may be added to our meager knowledge of the disease.

However, as in so many human endeavors, unanticipated, concomitant effects may occur with increased emphasis on diagnosis: in this instance, it may be characterized oppression by label.

In the United States there is a great deal of labeling of people as "senile" without sound diagnosis. Often such is an expression of ageism; a remnant of the notion that dementia is an inevitable sequella of growing old. In other instances, it is another example of the unwillingness of society to invest in old, old people. This is manifested by inadequate training of health related personnel and in lack of commitment on the part of government, institutional service patterns and individual professions to the elderly.

Failing to identify the primary cause of the dementia not only precludes appropriate therapeutic intervention and regimens but also may further an involutional process which will result in irreversible conditions.

Accurate diagnosis carries it own perils: it may mean consigning patients to a "hopeless" catagory and precluding any assistance to the person or families and may create such despair that a potential helper becomes discouraged exacerbating an already difficult situation.

The World Assembly on Aging (Vienna 1982) helped highlight the greying of the world's population. Today, a majority of the World's over 60 population is in developing countries. What might heretofore have been considered a developed country disease is likely to become much more prominent as a world wide phenomenon as mortality rates improve in Third World countries.

As was noted in a dramatic intervention by one of our participants, Simon Bergman, it is essential that developing and developed countries alike seek human and economic ways to support and care for the mentally frail.

At this same conference, (as well as in preparatory material) speaker after speaker expressed concern about the economic impact of caring for severely disabled persons. Some even pointed to the potential rivalry between the well and the frail aged for a society's resources.

Since World War II, particularly in Western Europe and the United States, we have witnessed a tendency to monitize, professionalize, medicalize and institutionalize every human hurt. Each such movement has had its rationale and developed its own momentum. Each has emphasized "better care" but each has had its price both in economics and human terms.

The development of psychotropic drugs as well as cost consideration has seen a movement toward deinstitutionalization, and better, non-institutionalization in the United States. However, the total number of "beds" for frail old people has continued to increase at a dramatic rate just as have professional home care services.

The Technical Committee on Long Term Care Report, prepared for the 1981 White House Conference on Aging, called for a balanced societal approach to the growing challenge of the mentally frail elderly. Borrowing liberally from earlier work done by the Federal Council on Aging, as well as the work of the committee, the delegates to the conference called for a broad, systemic approach including elements of research, training as well as locally based long term care systems with substantial governmental support.

Each segment of society tends to lay exclusive claims upon society's resources. Services and programs can be developed to respond to needs based on age, (e.g., the young and the old) or need for a particular service, (e.g., in-patient or out-patient) or by reason of etiology of the disability, (e.g., developmental disability or mental impairment).

The United States is tending toward an approach which emphasizes the ability of a person to cope with the tasks of every day life rather than upon any of these specifing conditions. However, such a policy approach is not without its critics.

Mental - Physical Health

The very existence of two large systems, one with a focus on mental health and another which emphasizes physical health, tends to perpetuate a schizophrenic approach to the human being. This dichotomy is reduced to the absurd in the instance of the frail elderly whose disease entities are likely to be many but who is left to deal with different professional disciplines, different facilities, different programs, different financing patterns, and differing philosophies of care: a challenge to a well and vigorous person.

The result of such a long standing approach is two large systems (with nearly 2 million in-patients on a given day) each describing persons with its own nomenclature, and treating them with its own approach yet these are people with some frailty.

At least a portion of the labeling problem arises from the inability or unwillingness of the mental health community to be insinuated within and integrated with the general provision of primary health care.

Medical - Social Model

An analogous but separate issue is that of the relationship between medicine and the socially oriented approach. Clearly in the area of diagnosis and treatment there is a primary in the leadership role of physicians and allied health professionals. However, in the instance of many older persons with dementia there is a point when the everyday care of such persons becomes the dominant consideration. It requires a set of skills and an environment quite different than that of a medicine and hospital.

The culture of health tends to engender substantial appetites for resources. The pursuit of excellence can be very expensive. Dramatic growth in health expenditures has led to a call for restraint.

Increasingly there are efforts to restrict the use of medical resources to those who need a medical regimen for active diagnostic or treatment activities. Once stablized, the patient would move into a different ambience, i.e., their own home or some social alternative in which medicine would be the an ancillary factor.

Such a trend is fueled by economic and humanistic considerations.

Medical facilities and activities oriented to episodes of illness can be inhospitable to those who require long term support or a living arrangement. When such persons are part of an undifferentiated patient load, they often find themselves at a disadvantage. Furthermore, "the patient" role may encourage dependency.

Formal and Informal Care

Since World War II the United States has emphasized access to a basic level of services for all who need care. While there has been debate about the means to acheive this goal, few would eschew it, at least publically. Government has made efforts to eliminate invedious discrimination by which race, diagnosis or economic level has our stripped public commitment to finance programs and services. However, during this period primary emphasis has been placed on those in need of acute care. Only in recent days, with an exponential growth in the old, old, as they are sometimes called, has general public attention been focused on the chronically ill, older person.

In the past five years, there has been a dramatic growth of interest in Alzheimer's in the scientific commununity and in society generally.

Economics and humanitatian considerations are stimulating discussion and debate.

The United States nursing home industry is the fast growing part of the health care field. Persons over 65 utilize up to 40% of a primary care physician's time as well as 40% of all acute care hospital days.

Several studies have shown that for every disabled person in a formal system of care, there are two others who are primarily in the care of family, friends and neighbors. While typically such care is given by family, particularly daughters, much is also provided by friends and neighbors. (GAO)

Virtually every governmental jurisdiction, local, regional or national, is trying to understand this phenomenon so that the delicate ecology involved will not be upset.

While academics have studied this phenomenon rather extensively (e.g., Cantor, Sussman, Brody and Silverstone), it has not been widely considered by either Federal or State governments.

While the Federal Council on Aging issued two documents (The Frail Elderly and The Need for Long Term Care) and sponsored a number of seminars on the subject, only recently has it become a matter of interest to all governmental units.

The World Plan of Action developed in Vienna and adopted December 3, 1982 by the United Nations's General Assembly reflects the concept that frail persons should be maintained at home.

Policies to make the idea operational follow several lines: enhancing the income of poor elderly persons so they can purchase services, providing protective environments which are smaller and less formal than institutions, providing "home care" service and providing support to those who care for the frail informally.

A detailed explanation of these approaches can be found in the report of the Task Force on Informal Supports of the New York State Governor's Health Advisory Council.

The first three might well be characterized as formal societal intervention involving positive public action. The latter, while formal, is an attempt to maintain, encourage and enhance the informal system.

Why some people choose to care for a frail person and others do not is of great interest. Culture, custom religion, values and ethical elements as well as physiciological factors all come into play.

If one has never had the care of a frail person, it is likely that he or she will identify money as a significant factor in the decision making process. Few, if any, would admit to crass motives of seeking to profit from another's misfortune. They identify it as a resource needed to change one's home, to include another or to provide for added expenes ranging from food to periodic nursing care.

If one has the care of a frail person, the primary needed help is identified as that of respite, knowledge, support and training. A number of studies indicate this enormous psychological investment can give rise to resentment and in nearly all instances, exhaustion if the need to help persists for a long period of time.

The actual decision to help lies neither in the presence or absence of assistance nor in the hope for it, but rather in the prior relationship with the dependent person. If people sang, laughed, and wept together in the past, they are likely to assist one another in time of difficulty. If there was no relationship in the past, it is unlikely there will be one in time of difficulty, no matter what incentive to help is given.

Of special interest is the growth of self-help groups particularly among families of Alzheimer's victims. Small localized groups have developed into a national movement.

This organization offers individual assistance, particularly through group sessions as well as acting as a societal advocate for greater investments in Alzheimer related programs.

A number of reseach and clinical centers have given assistance to the development of the organization both on the local and national scene.

There is the begining of a literature outlining techniques to help families and friends cope with the disease as well as to assist the patient.

A number of American Foundations have funded activities in the area of natural support systems. The Robert Wood Johnson Foundation, the largest group devoted to health, has initiated several national grant programs designed to facilitate the joining of formal and informal systems in the support of frail older persons particularly those with dementia.

Epilogue

Alzheimer's tends to be a disease associated with developed societies since longevity is associated with economic well being. This paper's overview of United States societal trends is given with a keen awareness of how little we know and how much we need the insights of all human kind. Perhaps some of the success and failures of American efforts to deal with the management of this disease will serve as a stimulus and source of learning for others. Surely the insights of those at this conference serve such a function for us in the United States.

Would it not be an irony were we successful in our efforts to prolong life only to have it be the occasion of pain and suffering for so many. Surely we need the best minds and hearts of human kind to deal with this tragic disease.

Alzheimer's Disease, Questions and Answers. U.S. Dept of Health and Human Services, NIH Publication #80-1646, Reprinted June 1980.

Bulletin on Aging. Vol. VII, No. 2, United Nations Dept. of International Economic and Social Affairs, Vienna, V.82-3395, December 1982.

Cantor, Marjorie, "Caring for the Frail Elderly: Impact on Family, Friends and Neighbors." Paper presented at the 30th Annual Scientific Meeting, Gerontological Society, San Diego, California, November, 1980.

Doing Better and Feeling Worse, Health in the United States, John H. Knowles, M.D., Editor, W.W. Norton & Co., Inc., New York, 1977.

Enhancing and Sustaining Informal Support Network for the Elderly and Disabled. Conference Proceedings and Recommendations, Published by the New York State Health Advisory Council, November, 1981.

Final Report - The 1981 White House Conference on Aging, Vol. I, A National Policy on Aging, Nov. 30 - Dec. 3, 1981.

Final Report - The 1981 White House Conference on Aging, Vol. II, Process Proceedings, Nov. 30 - Dec, 3, 1981.

Final Report - The 1981 White House Conference on Aging, Vol. III, Recommendations, Post Conference Survey of Delegates, Nov. 30 - Dec. 3, 1981.

The Gerontologist. Vol. 23, No. 2, Hiram J. Friedsom, Editor, Washington, D.C., April 1983.

Mental Health and the Elderly. Recommendations for Action, U.S. Dept. of Health, Education and Welfare, Federal Council on Aging, #80-20960, 1979.

The Need for Long Term Care, A Chartbook for the Federal Council for Aging, Dept. of Health and Human Services Publication (OHDS) 81-20704

Public Policy and the Frail Elderly. U.S. Dept. of Health, Education and Welfare Publication (OHDS) 79-20959, Dec., 1978.

Report of Technical Committee on Social and Health Aspects of Long Term Care, White House Conference on Aging, 1981, U.S. Government Printing Office 720-019/6889, 1981.

Report of the World Assembly on Aging. United Nations Publication E.82.I.16 Vienna, July 26 to August 6, 1982.

Schechter, Mal and Shelby, Philip. Aging 2000 - A Challenge for Society. MTP Press Limited International Medical Publication, Lancaster, England, 1982.

Silverstone, Barbara and Hyman, Helen Kandal, You and Your Aging Parent - The Modern Family's Guide to Emotional, Physical and Financial Problems. Pantheon Books, New York, 1976.

Sussman, Marvin, "Social and Economic Supports and Family Environments for the Elderly." Final Report to Administration on Aging, AOA Grant #90-A-316, January 1979.

U.S. Congress House. Select Committee on Aging, Every Ninth American (1982 Edition) 97 Congress. 2nd Session, July 1982.

The Well-Being of Older Poeple in Cleveland, Ohio. Report to The Congress by the Comptroller HRD 77-70, U.S. General Accounting Office, Washington, D.C.

Senile Dementia: Outlook for the Future, pages 455-465

EFFETS INTELLECTUELS ET MORAUX DU VIEILLISSEMENT D'UNE POPULATION

Alfred SAUVY

Institut National d'Etudes Démographiques

27, rue du Commandeur, 75675 PARIS-CEDEX FRANCE

Vous êtes sans doute surpris de voir donner la parole, dans ce congrès, à un homme tout à fait étranger à la démence sénile, à l'exception peut-être, diront certains, la sienne propre. Non médecin, mais démographe et sociologue, je vais décrire la maladie fondamentale d'un ensemble d'hommes, d'une population sénescente „ maladie peu connue encore et qui, du reste, confine, par certains points, sinon à la démence, du moins à la déraison.

Définition du vieillissement d'une population.

Le vieillissement d'une population, c'est, par définition, l'augmentation de la proportion des personnes âgées. On prend, le plus souvent, comme base, soit la proportion de sexagénaires, soit celle des plus de 65 ans.

Quelle que soit cette limite, le vieillissement de la population n'a pas résulté jusqu'ici, comme on le croit souvent, de l'allongement de la vie moyenne. Celui-ci est le résultat de la baisse de la mortalité, laquelle a été bien plus forte, pour les âges jeunes, que pour les âges élevés. A elle seule, la baisse de la mortalité infantile, depuis deux siècles, a allongé la vie moyenne de prés de 15 ans.

Toutefois, il peut se faire que, maintenant, dans certaines populations très avancées (Europe, pays anglo-saxons) la baisse de la mortalité des jeunes devienne négligeable, alors que des possibilités thérapeutiques permettent de prolonger la vie humaine, aux âges très élevés. Il y aura donc, dans cette hypothèse, une nouvelle forme de vieillissement, cette fois par les âges élevés.

Le vieillissement d'une population peut être également la conséquence d'une émigration. Un tel mouvement porte, en effet, surtout sur les éléments jeunes et exerce, par contrecoup, une influence défavorable sur la natalité.

En Europe, à la veille de la Révolution, la proportion des sexagénaires avoisinait 6%; elle est aujourd'hui trois fois plus élevée (18%) et est appelée à augmenter encore, même si la prolongation de la vie se maintient dans d'étroites limites. En laissant de côté l'influence possible de l'immigration d'éléments jeunes, les pays d'Europe occidentale pourraient avoir 25% de sexagénaires, dans le cours du siècle qui vient, donc 1 personne sur 4, au dessus de 60 ans, proportion jamais observée dans l'Histoire.

En même temps, la proportion des jeunes diminue. Tout se passe donc comme si les jeunes étaient, peu à peu, remplacés par des vieux; il est donc bien permis de parler de sénescence.

Dans les pays peu développés, à fécondité naturelle, la proportion des sexagénaires est d'environ 4%; elle augmente légèrement, dans ceux qui commencent à recourir à la limitation des naissances et augmentera notablement (sauf catastrophe) dans le siècle qui vient.

Conséquences matérielles et morales.

Le vieillissement d'une population a des conséquences matérielles et des conséquences morales. Ce sont ces dernières qui nous intéressent surtout ici. Disons cependant, dès maintenant, que la sénescence d'une population se traduit par une diminution de l'aptitude à traiter les conséquences matérielles, particulièrement pour l'avenir. Nous retrouverons d'ailleurs ce point plus loin.

Pour les conséquences morales, nous pouvons procéder, soit par logique, soit par voie expérimentale.

Examen logique à priori.

Le vieillissement d'une population peut agir de deux façons, sur la mentalité générale:

1. Même si chaque catégorie d'âge, jeunes, adultes, vieux, conserve sa mentalité antérieure, l'ensemble se modifie, du seul fait du changement des proportions. Si l'on admet, par exemple, que le vieux a plus d'expérience et moins d'audace que le jeune, qu'il est plus porté à la sécurité qu'à l'aventure, on peut annoncer un changement de l'ensemble et même calculer son ampleur, dans le cas où telle ou telle qualité se prêterait à la mesure.

2. Il peut se faire aussi que, du fait du vieillissement, les qualités se modifient à un âge donné. Ce second changement est plus difficile à prévoir que le premier, mais on conçoit qu'il a plus de portée encore que l'autre.

Prenons un exemple: devenus plus nombreux, les vieux pèsent davantage, par leurs charges sociales, par la propriété des biens, par leur prépondérance dans les postes élevés, par leur poids électoral etc. Sans intention collective de leur part, ils tendent donc à soumettre les jeunes. Comment vont se comporter ceux-ci?

Il est possible qu'ils se révoltent ouvertement, secouant le joug des vieux, au détriment de ceux-ci, ou bien qu'ils se résignent passivement, enveloppés dans un implacable réseau de relations. Rien ne permet de prévoir l'issue, de façon générale, par la seule déduction.

Lorsque au vieillissement de la population s'ajoute une diminution du nombre, les effets doivent être plus sensibles encore, par un effet de contraction.

En outre, lorsque le vieillissement s'accentue, les hospices, les maisons de retraite, deviennent un secteur important de la construction, voire de l'investissement; on peut craindre que ces charges finissent par s'affaisser, en quelque sorte sous l'effet de leur propre poids et que les adultes n'acceptent pas indéfiniment l'écrasement. Seulement, une de leurs façons de réagir peut consister à réduire leur propre descendance, comme nous le voyons déjà aujourd'hui. Dans ce cas, le vieillissement se nourrirait en quelque sorte lui-même (moins de jeunes, plus de vieux) de façon irrémédiable.

L'expérience.

Contrairement à ce que l'on croit, l'histoire est assez riche en examples de vieillissement d'une population. Je vais examiner les principaux:

1. La Grèce.
   A la période d'essor démographique et de jeunesse, marquée par une colonisation intense en Méditerranée, a succédé une période brillante (c'est le siècle de Périclès) et de stabilité. Le déclin a aussitôt suivi, du fait de la baisse de natalité. Celle-ci a été dénoncée dans des termes sans équivoque, par des auteurs aussi différents qu'Aristophane, Platon, Aristote, Hérodote, Ménandre, Polybe, Strabon etc.

Or, c'est la baisse de la natalité qui, à cette époque, était la seule cause du vieillissement. Pour la Grèce d'ailleurs, il ne peut pas être question d'une baisse de mortalité. Il en découle qu'un vieillissement de la population, sans doute important, a eu lieu

Polybe s'exprime ainsi:
"La Grèce entière souffre d'un arrêt de procréation et d'une disette d'hommes telle que les villes sont dépeuplées, parce que les hommes de l'époque aiment le luxe, l'argent et aussi la paresse et qu'ils consentent, tout au plus, à avoir un ou deux enfants, pour les laisser riches et les nourrir dans le luxe".

Il est difficile de préciser le calendrier des diverses étapes de la décadence. La natalité a du commencer à baisser pendant la pleine période de gloire, le siècle de Périclès, à Athènes d'abord, puis à Sparte. Comme bien des questions démographiques, celle-ci n'a pas été étudiée par les historiens avec une attention suffisante, mais les efforts se multiplient aujourd'hui, notamment en Grèce.

2. Rome.

Nous avons ici un témoignage précis: les lois d'Auguste en faveur de la natalité et les efforts d'autres empereurs par la suite. Pour qu'Auguste ait décidé d'adopter des mesures aussi novatrices et onéreuses que la loi Papia Poppea, à une époque où ses finances étaient fort obérées, il fallait que le phénomène eût déjà une certaine ampleur. La baisse de la natalité est donc très antérieure à la diffusion du christianisme, qui a pu accélérer le phénomène,mais bien plus tard seulement.

Il est couramment admis que les lois d'Auguste n'ont pas été efficaces. Du reste, un siècle plus tard, Nerva, puis Trajan, ont créé les Alimentana, pour les enfants, sorte d'allocations familiales. Si la natalité avait remonté, sous l'influence des lois d'Auguste, cette mesure, qui a été continuée par les successeurs de Trajan aurait été jugée trop coûteuse et inutile. Nous en concluons que le vieillissement a dû s'accentuer encore. Reste à déterminer l'extension du phénomène dans le reste de l'Empire et particulièrement dans la population rurale. Nous pouvons toutefois rappeler le vieil argument, qui n'a pas rencontré d'objection valable: lorsque les Barbares se sont présentés aux frontières, il a été possible de trouver des terres à leur offrir, mais non des soldats à leur opposer; cependant ces Barbares étaient peu nombreux. Mais les conséquences morales du vieillissement de la population romaine se sont fait largement sentir: absence de volonté et désorganisation. Comme en Grèce, le vieillissement a précédé la décadence et la chute.

Du reste ce qui importe ici, c'est le vieillissement à la tête, à Rome même. Il a largement précédé la décadence, qui a abouti à l'effondrement.

Venise.

Voici un nouvel exemple historique, aussi célèbre que mal connu. Les évènements ont été heureusement éclairés par les études de M. Daniele Beltrami (La composizione economica e professionnale della popolazione di Venezia nel sec. XVII e XVIII). Disposant de statistiques sur la répartition de la population par âge, il a montré que le vieillissement de la population a précédé et provoqué la décadence. La proportion des sexagénaires était déjà 10,7% au début du 17è siècle, ce qui montre que la baisse de natalité et le vieillissement ont commencé dès le XVIè siècle. Cette proportion de sexagénaires est passée à 12,4% en 1661-1670 et 15,7% en 1731-1740. Le vieillissement est la cause première et fondamentale du déclin et de la chute de la République.

La France au XIXè siècle.

Au début du siècle, l'économiste J.B. Say a donné aux Français le conseil suivant: "Faites des épargnes plutôt que des enfants".

Ce conseil a été suivi à la lettre: la natalité en France,déjà inférieure à celle des autres pays,a encore baissé, si bien qu'en 1890 la proportion de sexagénaires était 8,0% en Allemagne et 12,5% en France, supérieure de plus de moitié.

Du fait de la croissance modérée de sa population, la France était théoriquement promise à un progrès économique plus rapide que dans les autres pays. La formation d'un enfant coûtait, en effet, à l'époque, 5 années de travail; le report, sur l'épargne et l'investissement, d'une fraction seulement des ressources libérées par les non naissances devait permettre à la France, toujours selon les calculs, d'avoir, en 1914, un niveau de vie à peu près double de celui des autres pays (Angleterre exceptée). Le logement, la santé et l'instruction des Français devaient bénéficier d'une supériorité considérable sur les autres pays.

Aucun de ces avantages n'a été constaté; à la veille de la première guerre, le niveau de vie était à peu près le même que dans les autres pays; aucune supériorité culturelle, matérielle ou sanitaire,ne se manifestait.

Ce démenti aux lois et calculs économiques s'explique par un facteur qui n'entre bien dans aucun modèle, le facteur humain. Du fait du vieillissement de la population, le comportement des hommes, jeunes et vieux a changé. La France vieillie était tournée vers le passé, au moment même où les autres pays, poussés par leur jeunesse,misaient sur l'avenir.

Le refus du progrès s'est manifesté partout, par exemple:

- Refus de l'enseignement agricole par le Parlement, d'où retard considérable qui n'est pas encore totalement comblé.

- Refus de la marine à vapeur au profit des navires à voile.

- Stagnation de l'industrie, exportation de matières premières.

- Epargne placée en fonds d'Etat et non dans l'industrie.

- Etc...

A la vieille de 1914, le premier ministre Méline préconisait même le retour total à la terre, l'abandon de l'industrie.

Wallonie et Flandre.

Voici un exemple bien caractéristique, parce que différentiel: dans la Belgique du XIXè siècle, c'est la Wallonie qui a donné le départ de l'élan industriel, prenant, sur la Flandre, une large avance. Dans la seconde moitié du siècle, la natalité a baissé en Wallonie, tout en restant élevée en Flandre. Dès lors, le pronostic économique était doublement favorable à la première:

- Industrie déjà avancée.
- Charges de jeunesse réduites, donc épargne possible plus forte.

Une accélération du développement de la Wallonie était dans l'ordre des choses, sous l'effet des investissements et de l'expérience acquise.

L'évolution a été cependant à l'inverse: L'expansion en Wallonie a été moins rapide qu'en Flandre et c'est celle-ci qui s'est industrialisée, au XXè siècle, rejoignant et dépassant même sa concurrente.

Ce paradoxe apparent a une cause naturelle, le vieillissement des hommes et des idées, d'un côté, alors que de l'autre l'a emporté le désir de vivre qu'éprouve une population jeune.

Aujourd'hui, dans les deux régions, la population est âgée et la vitalité réduite.

Les exemples pourraient être multipliés: Espagne aux XVIè et XVIIè siècles, Irlande et Danemark au XIXè siècle, Gascogne et Bretagne pendant cette même période. Partout le résultat est identique. Aucune exception, mais les historiens sont encore très peu au fait de ces phénomènes profonds.

Les villages sans jeunes.

Nombreux sont en Europe et en France surtout, des villages qui ont perdu leurs éléments jeunes. Les essais d'y implanter des techniques nouvelles n'y ont pas de succès, tant sont difficiles à vaincre les inerties, tant est faible le désir d'entreprendre. Pour progresser, il faut alors introduire de nouveaux éléments jeunes dans la population.

Le vieillissement ignoré.

A l'inverse d'une personne qui voit ou ressent,tous les jours, les effets de sa montée en âge, une population ignore ce fait, révélé par les seuls recensements, peu connus et moins encore commentés.

D'autre part, les auteurs de toutes branches hésitent à mettre l'accent sur ce fait déplaisant, dont l'évolution provoque, inévitablement, un détournement d'attention des auditeurs ou lecteurs. Ainsi, en dépit de l'abondance de la documentation, dans le passé et dans le présent, en dépit de l'importance proprement vitale du sujet, la bibliographie est très rudimentaire, le phénomène n'étant guère évoqué que sous l'angle des retraites de vieillesse. En outre, l'étude de cette dernière question est elle-même déviée, dans ses résultats, par dissimulation semi volontaire et parfois inconsciente, des difficultés, conséquence même du vieillissement.

Un exemple puissant et même tragique, peut être invoqué ici: Voici un ouvrage important,paru aux Etats-Unis en 1972, sous le titre: "La population et l'avenir des Etats-Unis" (Population and the american future). Dans cette oeuvre scientifique réalisée par une pléiade d'universitaires et de personnalités de haute valeur, 7 pages seulement sur 350 sont consacrées à la répartition selon les âges; en outre, l'idée conclusive est qu'il faut redouter les jeunes (p. 93).

En Europe occidentale, vouée à un vieillissement exceptionnel, l'attention se porte sur d'autres domaines, alors même que l'avenir est en jeu. Aucune allusion n'est portée au fait qu'une population, où les vieux forment une forte proportion du corps électoral, ne sera guère ouverte au progrès, ni aux idées nouvelles et cela dans un monde en plein mouvement.

Une autoanalgésie.

L'explication de cette ignorance ou de cette indifférence, nous la trouvons dans une singulière propriété de ce phénomène:

Le vieillissement démographique a la propriété redoutable de créer sa propre analgésie, une sorte de non conscience collective. Cette attitude d'indifférence est-elle chez l'individu, volontaire? Nous laissons aux psychologues le soin d'en juger. Toujours est-il que les plus perspicaces, les plus pénétrants, passent à côté du phénomène. Ceux qui en ont une certaine idée l'attribuent à l'allongement de la vie, préjugé indéracinable, en dépit de démentis prodigués.

Le relachement de nos tissus sociaux, la sclérose de nos organes,la dégénérescence de diverses institutions, tout cela peut être rattaché, directement, au vieillissement démographique, délétère et anesthésiant.

L'oubli ou l'omission du vieillissement de la population, c'est-à-dire de l'évolution la plus fondamentale ne s'explique que par cette autoanesthésie, cet engourdissement, cette perte de sensibilité.

Le navire.

Le vieillissement est d'ailleurs loin de ne toucher que les générations âgées; il affecte peut-être plus encore les générations jeunes, car, plongées dès leur naissance dans la population vieillie, elles ont en quelque sorte, une avance sur les générations précédentes (lorsque celles-ci étaient jeunes). Ceci explique sans doute la faiblesse de l'esprit constructif parmi les jeunes d'une population âgée. Insuffisants en nombre, ils baignent, depuis 20 ans, dans une atmosphère de vieillesse.

Dans une pièce de Sutton Vane "Au grand large", qui a fait les beaux jours du théâtre Louis Jouvet, il y a un demi siècle et qui a, du reste, été reprise depuis, l'intensité dramatique est exceptionnelle:

Des passagers se trouvent sur un navire de plaisance et vivent normalement, la seule anomalie étant le mélange des classes sociales.

Et voilà qu'un beau jour, le barman, seul membre visible de l'équipage, annonce aux passagers qu'ils sont tous morts et qu'ils roulent, dans ce bateau, vers quelque jugement céleste.

Seuls parviennent à s'échapper du bateau deux jeunes amoureux, qui s'étaient suicidés au gaz et qui, par un suprême effort de conscience et de volonté, reviennent à la vie.

Notre situation est étrangement semblable: "embarqués" sur le navire de la vieillesse, nous risquons de ne plus pouvoir en sortir, car le vieillissement se nourrit en quelque sorte de lui-même.

Ainsi, le refus de reconnaître, sinon l'existence du vieillissement, du moins ses conséquences, est lui-même un test. La question est alors de savoir comment ce cercle vicieux peut être brisé, comment peut être guérie cette maladie, vraiment mentale.

Sénilité et déraison.

Le sujet que je traite peut vous sembler, je le répète, en dehors de votre domaine; si la sénilité de la société occidentale est bien évidente, le terme démence pourrait être contesté. A tout le moins s'agit-il de déraison, de pertes de facultés mentales et d'un affaiblissement de l'instinct de conservation. De brefs regards dans l'ensemble du monde, avec projections sur le siècle qui vient, nous donnent à conclure à une défaillance mentale profonde de notre part qui appelle d'ailleurs une thérapeutique appropriée.

A l'inverse d'une personne, ai-je dit, une population ne se voit pas vieillir, mais, à l'inverse aussi, elle peut réaliser le rêve interdit aux individus, le rajeunissement. Encore faut-il que cette thérapeutique soit acceptée et qu'au préalable soit fait l'effort de conscience nécessaire. Il y a là beaucoup à faire.

Senile Dementia: Outlook for the Future, pages 467–477

THE SOCIAL AND SOCIETAL IMPACT OF SENILE DEMENTIA

Prof. Simon Bergman

University of Tel-Aviv, and
Brookdale Institute of Gerontology,
Jerusalem, Israel.

This conference has brought together basic researchers, clinical specialists, epidemiologists, social and behavioral scientists and professionals in the area of psycho-geriatrics to take a look at senile dementia in two dimensions of time - the present state of arts, and the projection for the future - the end of this century; and at three levels of impact and effect - that on the person afflicted: that on the system of which he is an integral part, namely the family; and that on the community and society as a whole.

The importance of the findings and of the progress in two areas - epidemiology and research in etiology of senile dementia - for the applied social scientist and social planner is self-evident. The human cost at micro level of the individual and of the family, and at macro level of society can hardly be quantitated or translated into economic terms; and the social and economic cost of supportive services and of the ever growing demands for further societal investments are staggering (Godber, 1982). Available estimates from the U.S.A., the U.K. and from other countries may vary in scope, but they express themselves in considerable percentages of the total cost of health and welfare services. Everything points to the certainty that growing amounts will be needed until the end of the century to maintain the existing needs; to assure the maintenance of the expectable and unavoidable developments resulting from the changing population structure (the increase of the grand-old group of 80+ in the elderly population); and to allocate the resources needed for expansion of research and of experimental methods of intervention leading to prevention or, at least, to beginning and promising treatments of the disease.

Epidemiology and research - have been widely reported and discussed at this conference. Both raise some very basic issues; some confirm the limits of our knowledge; some contain indications of promise and hope that we are not facing a hopeless task.

Brockelhurst (Hirshfeld, 1978), sees in the management of senile dementia old people the single most serious problem facing present health services. The Royal College of Physicians of the U.K. (1981) sees in the high prevalence of senile dementia and in the need for the majority of the cases to be treated in the community "one of the most pervasive social health problems of our generation". Plum (1979) defines dementia "an approaching epidemic" and warns that if we do not find measures to either prevent or treat senile dementia, the disease will impose burdens on society in the coming fifty years that will be enormous due to the dramatic increase in the number of older people over 80. He therefore demands that enormous increase in research into senile dementia be given priority in effort to prevent economic and personal catastrophes in the coming decades. In a recently published note, D. Cowell (1983) of the National Institute on Aging in the USA reviews cost estimates of care to older persons afflicted with senile dementia of Alzheimer's type and other dementias occurring in later life, based on the 1977 National Nursing Homes Survey which showed that a minimum of 32% of the population of the nursing homes, or 360,000 patients were considered to have some type of senile dementia. (The number of older people having senile dementia and living in the community is estimated to be almost twice as high). Current expenditure for senile dementia in Nursing Homes alone would amount to slightly over 5 billion Dollars. Senile dementia of Alzheimer's type is thought to account for about half of that amount.* The quoted figures do not include other direct costs for acute medical hospitalization or indirect costs reflecting lost earning power among victims of senile dementia. It is practically impossible to calculate the

---

* In Israel, the author's country, 50% of aged hospitalized in psychiatric settings are defined to be there due to O.B.S.

value of care provided in the home by family, nurses, companions, medical personnel, medications etc. I have no data from my own country.

If we consider epidemiological estimates for the next two decades as a result of the dramatic increase of the 75 and 80 plus with the 20% prevalence in the group 85 and over as well as the lengthened survivalship of senile dementia patients, the picture emerging from these frequently published estimates indeed conjures up images of dread which regretfully remains a reality society is bound to cope with.

This may reflect Gruenberg's (1977) concept of the "failure of success", meaning that health technology adds years to sick rather than healthy lives. Fries (1980) represents a more optimistic view that suggests a "compressed morbidity" over a relatively smaller proportion of the typical life span with a resulting decreased need for prolonged care. What the impact of this more optimistic trend will be on senile dementia in the upper age brackets is subject to guess in either direction.

For the social scientist and planner, it is important to know whether we speak only of a longer period of survivalship of those already afflicted with senile dementia since their earlier old age and into their 80's and beyond - on a continuum of progressive severity of the diseases; or that we speak also of a growing incidence of new cases as survivalship into grand old-age includes larger and larger groups of elderly not previously diagnosed as afflicted by senile dementia. Is there an upping curve? Or will this curve flatten and prevalence will level off and become "arrested" - so to say.*

---

* Figures from a recent study on the prevalence of senile dementia among those 65 and over, in a community of 40000 inhabitants in Israel, show a higher prevalence of chronic brain insufficiency among females, with a % almost twice as high among women at the level of severe insufficiency. The % of severely impaired in the group 85 and over was twice as high as that in the 65-69 group (22% as against 10%), and was close to the prevalence reported in foreign studies. The findings of the study will be tested in a few more communities and are at the moment serving as the base line for the planning and policy formulation stage of an important law to provide nursing care services to elderly in the community (Silberstein, 1981).

The relatively low prevalence of senile dementia in the community as established in surveys, when compared with the one in institutional settings, raises some important questions. Is the high prevalence in institutions a result of admission policy (preference for such cases)? Or is it inherent in institutional life? Or of more numerous studies of the "captive population" of nursing homes as compared to the paucity of community studies? Lawton (1980) stresses the importance of residential distribution of the population with senile dementia because availability of protectivity of environment and of care will vary greatly depending on the living conditions. In evaluating present or future needs and solutions we must seriously consider the environmental dichotomy of institutional versus community-home care.

This brings us to the consideration of the second major question posed in this paper: the impact of senile dementia on the individual, on the family system, and on the macro system of societal solutions and intervention.

Gerontological literature repeatedly points out the fact that old people tend to be rather easily diagnosed as having senile dementia. Clinical decisions tend to be biased against the older person. Butler (Hirshfeld, 1978) cautions against casual diagnosis of organic brain syndrome simply because a person happens to be over a certain age and because symptoms are stereotypically seen as concommitant to the aging process per se. Glassman (1980) warns against "wastebasket" diagnosis that serves to deny adequate medical care to confused elderly on the assumption that their situation is "hopeless anyway". Once labelled, the old person may be seen in terms of custodial care and so a premature process may be set in motion of passage from person to long term hopeless patient; of institutionalization, guardianship by family, and more than occasional abuse and victimization of the older person. Literature and social work practice abund in misdiagnosed cases who did not receive needed services although such services existed in the community. The dividing line between what is termed "benign forgetfulness of old age" and even a mild level of senile dementia is often overlooked in the process of assessment, diagnosis and the resulting labeling of the older person.

The creation of good diagnostic tools and the raising of the level of the professionals involved in the process of decision as to who is or is not labelled as a senile dementia case, is an obvious conclusion and necessity. Assessment is difficult because mental impairment in old age is frequently complicated by coexisting physical disease, multiple disorders, family and socio economic difficulties, life style, and the tendency to think of all problems as inevitable consequences of aging (Ernst, 1978). Psycho-social evaluation is particularly a "forte" of social work theory and practice and these professionals must make the most of it in their assessment of the individual situation (Glassman, 1980). Their role in the team process of diagnostic decision must become more crucial and decisive especially in the evaluation of such components as nutritional habits, type and use of medicines, social and personal network, quantity and quality of care and services received, observed behavioral changes, rapid or gradual , etc. Storand (1983), may be right in her observation that a social worker called in to investigate senile behavior may do well to start with the medicine chest and survey of the frigidaire.

The senile dementia patient ceases to be a rational source for feedback for the care providing environment. What we know about the inner impact and changes is what we observe from outside and measure by our values and yardsticks of normalcy and deviation. Literature contains no documentation of those who "returned from there". The partial, and particularly severe disengagement from reality of life, behavior, social norms, and reactions create a world of their own perception of which is difficult for us to absorb. In a most perceptive article on "The senile dementia in our midst" Hellenbrandt (1978) describes the world of senile dementia patients in an institution. "The locked door of the department may be a distress to the visitor, the family or even the staff, but it is a meaningless concept to virtually all patients deteriorated enough to require segregation". The description of the process of senile deterioration by Lyons (1982) is a moving and convincing document, personified in the form of a first-person story of gradual enstrangement from realtiy. Another document "The dying mind in a living body" (Bergman, 1979) is an equally moving and realistic presentation by a professional of a siblings gradual sinking into the world of reality oblivion. There are a few more attempts in Belle-letters and documentary literature to present the "inside" of the process and of the world of senile dementia aged. They may be helpful for understanding and visualization of what goes on - but they do not compensate us for the absence of personal reflections, feeling and perception of the individual victim of the "silent epidemic" of senile dementia. Those involved in interventive activities at micro-level of the afflicted individual are keenly aware of the serious limitations in the process of the therapeutic interaction or when intervention is attempted. The second level of impact of senile dementia is the one on the family system of which the older person is a part.

The universality of families caring for kin is undisputed. Simone de Beauvoir (1972) believes that the only protection aged have is the affection of their children. This is put to test many times, but possibly never more acutely than in conditions of senile dementia when far reaching changes in personality and behavior occur in the older parent. Living with and caring for relatives with senile dementia in a joint household has become one of the major tests of affection, need, family solidarity, or feeling of normative responsibility which many families are not ready to give up, whatever the price may be. Researches deal with the "undue strain" produced on carers of elderly with OBS, of physical, emotional, psychological, social and economic nature (Isaacs, 1973; Eisdorfer, Cohen, 1981). Where society and government are doing less, families are bound to do more. Existing services and policies seem to favour those without families, without compensation, support, or supplementation being offered on equal footing to supportive family systems. The British Royal College of Physicians (1981) estimates most OBS cases will have to be taken care of by families also in the future, until the late stage of the disease requiring more and more effort and tolerance by families. The degree of the dependence of the OBS elderly will be determined by the degree of acceptance by families. One man's right to be cared for at home becomes the other person's duty to care for him. Social dementia changes not only the victim but also the caregiver and involves obligations and risks potentially harmful to the older person or to the carers. The important question discussed in literature is not whether the family system plays a valuable role in senile dementia care, but how vulnerable this system has become and how much hope one can place on its continuity and effectiveness in face of rapid social changes. In her study on "Families living with senile brain disease", Hirshfeld (1978) found that in her sample the impairment of the cared for or of the care givers did not determine the family's ability to continue care at home. However, tension resulting from disease and care-giving situations did determine that ability.

Even if the principle of diminishing societal resources is defensible and has to be considered, families must not be pushed too far. One must not forget that those who live with others may be causing the greatest stress, and their right to societal support must not be less only because they do constitute a part of a family system. Any policy favouring home care for OBS patients must include care of care-providers as an integral component of its principles.

There have so far been too few researches on the impact of care of senile aged on the families. On the other hand, there have been too many punitive policies in regard to care-providing families. The expectation of filial responsibility raises a number of moral and social issues. Even if accepted, society must facilitate its implementation, not only in the name of equity, but from the point of view of calculated benefits resulting from the partnership between the familial and societal levels. Senile dementia is a personal affliction, a family problem, and most frequently, a tragedy, and a social issue which justifies policy clarification and provisions that would enable families to continue with carrying the burden which is so heavy to carry.

Many of the care givers are themselves not young; (in Isaacs study, 54% were over 50, and 18% over 70); incontinence, disorientation and risks of self-inflicted harm are hard to take. Some care-givers show somatic symptoms, sleep disturbances are other consequences of upset life-style resulting from tension-producing ongoing care-giving obligations.

There is no doubt that in our planning till the end of the century, home care by families of senile dementia older people will be of crucial importance, and societal intervention to maintain family system capacity and interest to provide care must be a vital component of social policy. Investment in preparing families for that role; provision of economic, social and psychological support; re-orientation of direction of health and social services; alleviation of the burden, and a policy of instrumental partnership between family, community, and society - are steps to be taken. A review of social legislation and of special services in different countries will provide ample evidence of what has been already done, or what is being debated as the line of policy to be introduced.*

In the long view, we must devote more resources to advancing our knowledge and understanding of how the family system works in care provision: where is the satiation and breaking point in the readiness to continue with care provision; means of preventive intervention; effects of care needing and care giving on the family system, etc. The results of such studies might be helpful in our coping with such principal but also practical questions, as where, when, how, and to what extent is, or should society intervene in its reaction to and its participation in the process of coping with consequences of increased prevalence of senile dementia in the years to come.

As for the societal level - we are facing a problem of growing dimensions affecting millions of people at various levels of severity of the disease and diminishing prospects of cure or effective care. Neither families, where they exist, nor voluntary organizations or voluntary efforts alone will be able to cope with the multi-dimensionality of needs and resources required. The role of the state in the next two decades will become progressively more central and decisive if we are to meet the needs of a most fragile, vulnerable, and hopeless group for whom present state of knowledge does not yet provide hope of prevention or of effective treatment in the nearest future.

There are several major areas in which the state will have to make major societal decisions and investments.

1. Provide economic support to existing support systems at individual, family, or organized voluntary service levels at home and in institutional settings (Bane, 1983; Sheldon, 1982).

---

* In Israel, the Nursing Services Law now being implemented will provide support to families caring for elderly chronics (including senile dementia) in the form of services, respite arrangements, and other incentives leading to greater "longevity" of family care and support.

2. Assure, supervise and protect the implementation of realistic but dignified standards of essential services in such settings.

3. Legislate, support, and protect societal arrangements for care and welfare of those afflicted with and suffering from the devastating effects of senile dementia.

4. Provide for ongoing monitoring of implementation of policies, legislation and services to assure their flexibility, reviewability and changes as needs change and as science and clinical experience supply the knowledge and the means for better coping with the disease.

5. Advance and develop working partnerships with all possible factors interested in and directly concerned with the well-being of the victims of senile dementia-families, voluntary bodies, human care professions, and scientific investigators concerned with etiology and treatment of the disease.

6. Give high priority to and allocate resources for research into the causes of senile dementia and for innovative and scientifically controlled treatment experiments in medical and psycho-social clinical areas (Wershow, 1977).

7. Elaborate and implement a policy of planning and coordination of efforts in research, treatment experimentation, service development and of societal investments in manpower education and training as well as cooperation with various factors in society for the purpose of formulating an agreed order to priorities, distribution of resources, avoidance of duplication and wastage of scarce resources, and for greater advancement in our coping with the devastating effects of the disease.

There is a growing awareness of the gravity of the problem in terms of human wastage and suffering, familial strain and tragedy, and individual and societal damage and cost. We are only beginning to appreciate the enormity of the task facing the scientist, the care provider, the clinicians in the helping professions, the social planner, society as a whole, and last but not least - the decision-maker and the legislator, in creating conditions in our societies in the years to come in which the effort to alleviate the suffering and the constant scientific search for its elimination and prevention will never cease.

As a result of increased scientific interest and public awareness, "the future looks brighter for the families of people with dementing disorders who were once told to proceed as best as they could with no hope and little support", (N.I.A.,1981). This is now possible because "... there are clues to senile dementias etiology, and there may be hope for its treatment", (Small, Jarvick, 1982).

Bibliography

Bane, M.J. Is welfare state replacing family. The Public Interest, 1983, Winter, pp. 91-101.

Beauvoir, S. de: Old Age, Deutsch Publications, London, 1972.

Bergman, R. The dying mind in the living human in de Vries, A. and Carmi, A.(eds): The dying human, Turtle-dove Publish., Ramat-Gan (Israel), 1979.

Cowell, D. Senile Dementia of the Alzheimer's Type: A costly problem, Journal of the American Geriatric Society, 1983, 1.61.

Eisdorfer, C. and Cohen D. Management of the patient and family coping with dementing illness, J. of Family Practice, 1981, 5:831-837.

Ernst, Ph. et al: Isolation and the symptoms of chronic brain syndrome, Gerontologist, 1973, 5, 468:497.

Fries, J. F. Aging, natural death and the compression of morbidity, New England Journal of Medicine, 1980, 130-135.

Glassman, A. Misdiagnosis of senile dementia: denial of care to the elderly, Journal of Social Work, 1980, 4:288-292.

Sir George Godber, Striking the balance: Therapy, prevent-ion, and social support. World Health Forum, 1982, No.3.

Gruenberg, E. M. The failure of success. Milkbank Memorial Fund Quarterly, 1977, 3-24.

Hellebrandt, F. The senile dement in our midst: A look at the other side of the coin. Gerontologist, 1978, 1:67-70.

Hirshfeld, M. Families living with senile brain diseases, Ph. D. Thesis, Univ. of California, 1978.

Isaacs, B. et al: Survival of the unfittest, 1973.

B.M.J. Dementia Senilis, British Medical Journal, 1981, 12.12

Lawton, P. Psychosocial and environmental approaches to the care of senile dementia patients, in: Cole, J.

and Barrett, J. (eds). Psychopathology in the Aged, Raven Press, New York, 1980, pp. 265-280.

Lyons, W. Coping with cognitive impairment: Some family dynamics and helping roles. Journal, Gerontological Social Work, 1982, 3/4:3-20.

N.I.A. "Progress Report on Senile Dementia of the Alzheimer Type", Washington D.C., 1981.

Plum, F. Dementia: an approaching epidemic, Nature, 1979, (279) 372-373.

Sheldon, F. Supporting the supporters: Working with the relatives of patients with dementia. Age and Aging, 1982, 184-188.

Silberstein, J. et al: Medical and social needs of disabled aged: Services needed and their cost (Bnei-Brak survey), National Institute of Insurance, Jerusalem, 1981, pp.105-120.

Small, G.W. & Jarvik, L. The dementia syndrome, Lancet, 1982, 1443-1446 (25. 12.1982).

Storandt, M. Understanding senile dementia: A challenge for the future. Int. Journal of Aging and Human Development, 1983, 1:1-6.

Wershow, H. Reality orientation for gerontologists. Gerontologist, 1977.

Senile Dementia: Outlook for the Future, pages 479–490

AGING AND DEMENTIA IN THE DEVELOPING WORLD - A CHALLENGE FOR THE FUTURE

Gary R. Andrews and Ann Harris Davidson,

Department of Community and Geriatric Medicine,
University of Sydney, Westmead Centre,
WESTMEAD, N.S.W. 2145, AUSTRALIA

INTRODUCTION

The availability of reasonably accurate information on population trends and age related risks of physical and mental impairments now provides a wealth of information to guide planners and decision makers. This is especially so in the identification of future community needs and the allocation of scarce resources to meet them (Maddox 1982). History, in our view, will judge the social and health planners of the present era severely if account is not taken of the overwhelming evidence that organic brain disease represents one of the most significant problems to be faced as a consequence of the continuing proportional and absolute increases of the aged in the world's populations. The phenomenon has been graphically described as the "quiet epidemic" (Leading Article, British Medical Journal, 1978).

There is evidence in the developed parts of the world that there is some realization of this potentially major challenge to social and health services. Indeed, this seminar itself illustrates the point. However, we have not been able to identify, at least in Asia, any corresponding level of realization in relation to the developing world. Yet the demographers have repeatedly stressed that the greatest impact of population aging will be upon the least developed parts of the globe (Myers 1982; Schade 1982; United Nations 1982).

This paper attempts simply to draw immediate attention to this issue. In the light of demographic and epidemiologic evidence the case is put for investment in research into the definition and prevalence of organic brain disease of the elderly in the developing nations of the world. The findings should then be considered in terms of the varying social, economic and cultural constraints. Given the rates of social and economic change which will occur at the same time, imaginative strategies will need to be devised if there is to be an effective response to the problems generated by the growing numbers suffering from organic brain disease.

THE DEMOGRAPHIC REALITIES

The aging of the world's population is now a well documented phenomenon (United Nations 1982). Attention has been drawn to the spectacular development in the growth of the older population which can be expected in developing countries (Schade 1982). Declining birth rates, reduced mortality and rising life expectancy are the determinants of these age structure changes, the rates of which are directly proportional to the rates at which birth rates are falling and life expectancy is increasing.

Throughout Asia, the cultural, religious, historic and economic diversity which exists results in varying consequences; the rates of increase in the aged population vary also, but the overall impact is inescapable with most Asian countries predicted to experience increases in those over 60 years in excess of 80% between 1980 and 2000 (Final Report, International Symposium, Hamburg 1981). Indonesia tops the list with a predicted increase of 134% (Table 1).

It is worth noting that the projected percentage increases in those 60 years and over are expected to be twice as great in the years 2000 to 2025 as the increase in the years 1975 to 2000 (Figure 1). A further important consequence of rising life expectancy will be that the older population itself will be aging as the rate of population increase will be greater in the older age groups (Table 2).

The figures in Table 2 include all the less developed regions of the world (as defined by Siegel, 1982) however, many Asian countries show even higher percentage increases in the 80 and over age group. The expression of these figures in percentages, while useful, does tend to reduce the impact of the problem. To reveal more graphically the

TABLE 1
EXAMPLES OF PROJECTED PERCENTAGE INCREASES IN POPULATIONS IN SELECTED ASIAN COUNTRIES

	Projected %↑ of the total population (both sexes, all ages) 1980 - 2000	Percentage of the population ≥60 years 1980	2000	Projected %↑ of those ≥60 years in the population 1980 - 2000
CHINA (People's Rep)	24.3	8.6	10.6	54.7
JAPAN	10.8	12.6	19.8	73.8
KOREA (Rep)	33.7	6.2	9.3	100.0
PHILIPPINES	63.6	4.8	5.6	89.2
MALAYSIA	48.0	5.4	6.6	80.1
INDONESIA	45.9	4.3	6.8	134.4

SOURCE: "Demographic Aspects of the Aging Population in the Asian and Pacific Region", (United Nations Centre for Social Development and Humanitarian Affairs, 1981).

TABLE 2
PERCENTAGE INCREASE IN THE OLDER AGE GROUPS, 1980 - 2000, FOR THE LESS DEVELOPED REGIONS* OF THE WORLD

	1980	2000	%↑
Total population numbers (In millions)	3300.8	4846.7	46.8%
Numbers ≥60 years	205.3	360.0	75.4%
Numbers ≥80 years	14.4	29.4	104.2%

* The less developed regions of the world included all of Africa, all of Latin America, Asia excluding Japan and the USSR, and Oceania excluding Australia and New Zealand

SOURCE: "Demographic Aspects of the Health of the Elderly to the year 2000 and Beyond", Siegel, WHO/AGE/82.3, 1982 (Adapted)

Figure 1

PROPORTION OF THE TOTAL POPULATION THAT IS 60 YEARS AND OVER, BY SELECTED SUBREGIONS, FOR 1950, 1975, 2000, 2025.

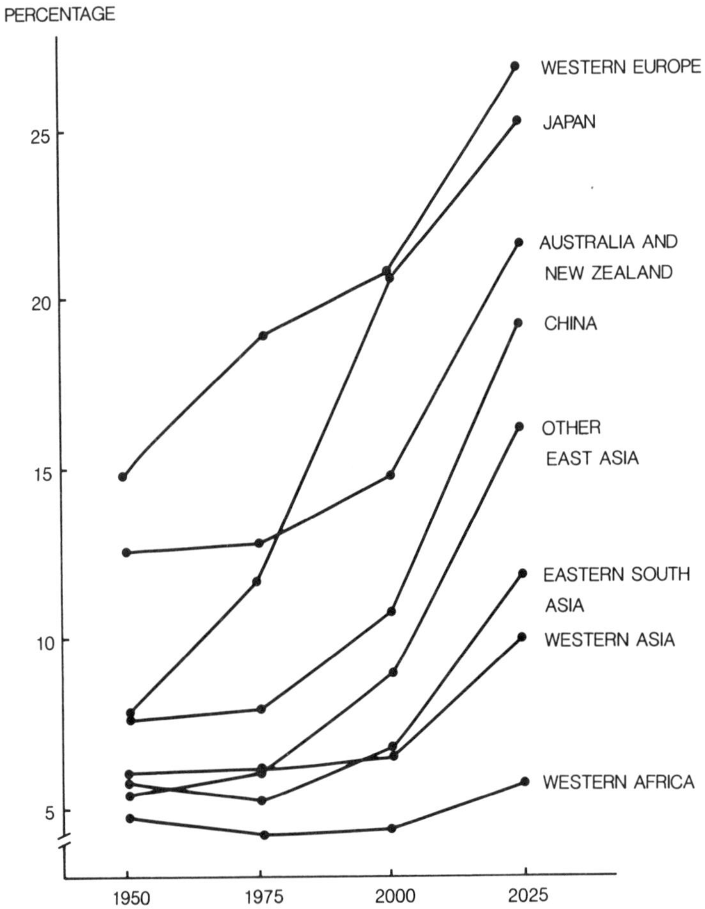

SOURCE: United Nations World Assembly on Ageing, 1982. "Introductory Document: Demographic Considerations." A/Conf.113/4.

issues to be faced and the resources and programs which will be required by a society to cope with the conditions and needs of the aged, absolute numbers should be used (Beattie 1978). This is especially true of Asia with its total population of over 2½ thousand million (United Nations Centre for Social Development and Humanitarian Affairs, 1981).

DEMENTIA IN AN AGING WORLD

Determining the precise prevalence of dementia is difficult. Different diagnostic criteria are sometimes used and confounding factors such as drug use may complicate the issue further as has been documented in reviews on the topic (Svanborg et al 1982; Gilmore 1981). The comparability of prevalence studies is further diminished as the age groups studied and the categorization of the severity of dementia often vary. For European countries, Svanborg et al (1982) estimated that the prevalence of moderate to severe dementia lies between 3 and 5% for the population aged 65 years and over. These figures include those suffering from the two most common forms of chronic brain syndrome; that is, multi-infarct dementia and senile dementia of the Alzheimer's type.

There is a dearth of such prevalence studies on Asian populations. Thailand is reported (Abaya 1982) as having pinpointed the ten most common afflictions of its elderly and of these, the first two were listed as senile change and involuntional change. If one applies the estimate of a 4% prevalence of dementia, based on the European figures while acknowledging their potential inappropriateness, and using the demographic projections for the Asian region, the numbers of those likely to be suffering from moderate to severe dementia in the year 2000 are startling (Table 3).

Further, as the classic studies of Kay et al (1970) indicated a dramatic rise in prevalence among the older age groups (eg. >20% for those ⩾80 years), the application of modest estimated prevalence rates to the total projected aged population will be an underestimate given the differentially greater increase in the very old in the population and the correspondingly disproportionate prevalence of dementia in that group (Figure 2).

FIGURE 2 PREDICTED NUMBERS OF DEMENTIA PATIENTS, BY AGE GROUP, 1980 - 2000 (in millions)

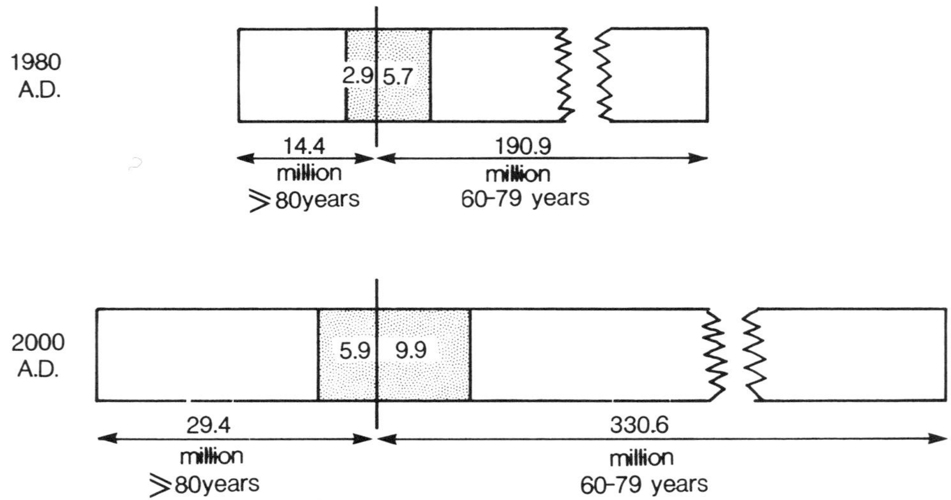

SOURCE: Designed using statistics from "Demographic Aspects of the Health of the Elderly to the year 2000 and beyond", J. S. Siegel, WHO/AGE/82.3, 1982

TABLE 3
ABSOLUTE NUMBERS OF THOSE 60 YEARS AND OVER,
AND THOSE WHO MAY BE EXPECTED TO HAVE DEMENTIA,
FOR SELECTED ASIAN COUNTRIES

	Projected numbers of those ≥60 years		Projected numbers of moderate to severe organic brain syndrome sufferers in 2000 AD (4% of those ≥60 years)
	1980	2000	
CHINA (People's Rep)	82,288,928	126,094,632	5,043,785
JAPAN	14,661,864	25,522,398	1,020,896
KOREA (Rep)	2,354,698	4,723,470	188,939
PHILIPPINES	2,447,808	4,672,304	186,892
MALAYSIA	736,560	1,331,946	53,278
INDONESIA	6,531,442	15,070,568	602,823
ASIA OVERALL	164,753,670	279,205,137	11,168,205

SOURCE: Figures computed from the numbers and percentages in Tables 2 and 3 of the UNCSDHA Report on the Technical Meeting on Aging for the Asian and Pacific Region, 1981.

AWARENESS IN THE DEVELOPING COUNTRIES OF ASIA

While the demographic and epidemiologic messages for Asia are clearly evident, it has been acknowledged that few Asian countries have considered what might be done for this total of over 11 million people who are likely to be manifesting moderate to severe organic brain disease by the year 2000. Some of the reasons for the failure in Asia to see aging and its consequences as a serious problem deserving immediate attention were mentioned in various papers in the proceedings of the Asian Regional Conference on Active Aging held in Manila, 1982:

1. Aging is but one of the critical problems facing developing countries. In countries where poverty affects the majority of the people, "the problem of old age ... is inseparable from the overall economic condition of the country." (Sharma 1982)

2. Developing countries tend to be immersed in population problems, thus, "The Asians' familiarity in dealing with huge numbers may be one reason for the refusal to take this issue seriously." (Abaya 1982)

3. Demographically, most developing countries still have very young populations. "In a country like India where about 60% of the total population is below 25 years and only a little over 3% of the population is over 65 years, the problems of children and youth dominate the scene." (Bose 1982) Even by the year 2000 AD, the majority of the countries will remain "young countries" by definition as less than 7% of their populations will be over 60 years of age.

This general lack of concern about the impact of an aging population is compounded by the fact that the greater majority of the aged, in all circumstances, are likely to live out their lives without the burden of dementia. It is thus not surprising that a condition which will not affect over 95% of the aged population has been given scant attention.

Again, it needs to be stressed that though the percentages with moderate or severe degrees of organic brain disease are small, the absolute numbers will be staggeringly large. Nor indeed is the lack of consideration for psychogeriatric problems unique to the developing countries. The New Zealand Report to the World Assembly on Ageing ("Ageing New Zealanders", 1982) noted, "While services to the physically sick and disabled elderly in this country are quite well advanced, psychogeriatric services are poorly developed." The pattern in other developed countries is reportedly similar (Office for Health Economics 1979).

THE CONSEQUENCES FOR DEVELOPING COUNTRIES

The consequences of age structure changes in any developing country, and the resulting increasing rates of dementia, cannot be logically assessed without a number of questions being considered:

1. How applicable are rates of dementia in developed countries to developing countries? That is, what is the prevalence of organic brain syndrome in different developing countries?

2. What is the present social impact of dementia in the context of a developing country? What support systems currently exist for dementia patients?

3. How will the major social changes, particularly the changes in traditional habits, which are being observed in developing countries (as reviewed in Schade 1982), influence the situation of older persons and especially the mentally incapable elderly?

4. What support should and could be provided if the demand for institutional care is not to increase dramatically as a consequence of the needs of this group?

Ready answers to these questions do not currently exist in most developing countries. In general, the burden of health provision for the aging has fallen, and falls heavily still, on the family. Factors which contribute to this situation are that, historically, older persons living in traditional societies were better integrated into the family; that institutionalisation of the elderly has been rare (Abaya 1982); and that there remains a lack of other alternatives. With the responsibility for the elderly, and the mentally incapable elderly, resting primarily with the family in developing countries, the impact of urbanization, fertility control, technological change and increased social mobility on family patterns cannot be ignored.

The reduction in birth rates has led to fewer children to support the now multigenerational families. In urbanized areas of South East Asia nuclear families are reported as being increasingly the rule rather than the exception (Abaya 1982), with corresponding increases in the numbers of aging living alone or as a couple. Furthermore, a study conducted by the Korean Institute of Gerontology, reported by Ahn (1982), concluded that the majority of the aging think that the time is over when parents rely on their children and 39.5 per cent considered that the State should support them. Irrespective of these social changes, the Report of the WHO Preparatory Conference for the UN World Assembly on Aging (World Health Organisation 1980) stated that, despite the efforts to incorporate community approaches, there will remain an "irreducible minimum" of mentally impaired people of advanced age, with no family, who will require institutional care. Given the increases in the prevalence of dementia, as documented, and the changing patterns of the family, this irreducible minimum is likely to become sizeable.

CONCLUSION

The main theme of this paper is an essentially simple one. We know the likely patterns of demographic change in the developing world; using these patterns, predictions can be made about the numbers of people who are likely to have dementia in the future. However, the fundamental question of whether in fact the prevalence rates for the major forms of organic brain syndrome are comparable between countries of the developed and the developing worlds and throughout the developing world, remains to be answered. Our understanding of senile dementia of the Alzheimer's type in particular may be significantly enhanced by such knowledge. Though even without precisely known prevalence rates, it is clear that one of the greatest challenges to health and social planners in the developing world over the coming decades will be the impact of the "quiet epidemic" of dementia.

We know far too little of the social and cultural aspects of dementia, particularly in terms of its consequences. Here it seems to us, is one of the most potentially fertile areas of research and we urge it be taken up especially as the information yielded may be of fundamental importance to social and health planners, policy and decision makers and will certainly have significant implications for the allocation of scarce resources in Asia and the rest of the developing world.

Abaya AG (1982). Some aspects of aging in Southeast Asia. In "The Elderly of Asia", conference proceedings of the Asian Regional Conference on Active Aging. Manila: Social Research Centre, University of Santo Tomas.

Ageing New Zealanders (1982). The New Zealand Report to the United Nations World Assembly on Aging, Vienna.

Ahn KR (1982). The situation of the aging in Korea. In "The Elderly of Asia" conference proceedings of the Asian Regional Conference on Active Aging. Manila: Social Research Centre, University of Santo Tomas.

Beattie WM (1978). Aging: The Developed and Developing World. Meeting on Aging, sponsored by the Institut de la Vie under the auspices of the United Nations Fund for Population Activities. Syracuse University, New York.

Bose A (1982). Aspects of aging in India. In "The Elderly of Asia", conference proceedings of the Asian Regional Conference on Active Aging. Manila: Social Research Centre, University of Santo Tomas.

Final Report, International Symposium (1981). Population Development and Social Security: Aging in Developing Countries. Organised by Carl Duisberg - Gesellschaft, Hamburg.

Gilmore AJJ (1981). Psychiatric illness of the elderly in the community. In Gilmore AJJ, Svanborg A, Marois M, Beattie WM, Poitrowski J (eds): "Aging: A challenge to Science and Society", Volume 2. Oxford: Oxford University Press.

Kay DWK, Bergman K, Foster EM, McKechnie AA, Roth M (1970). Mental illness and hospital usage in the elderly: A random sample followed up. Acta Sociomedica Scandinavia (suppl. 3)

Leading Article, British Medical Journal (1978). Dementia - the quiet epidemic. 6104 1:1-2

Maddox GL (1982). Aging people and aging populations: A framework for decision making. In Thomae H, Maddox GL (eds) "New Perspectives on Old Age. A Message to Decision Makers." New York: Springer Publishing Company.

Myers GC (1982). The aging of populations. In Binstock RH, Chow WS, Schulz JH (eds): "International Perspectives on Aging: Population and Policy Challenges." New York: United Nations Fund for Population Activities.

Office of Health Economics (1979). Dementia in Old Age. London.

Schade B (1982). Aging and Old Age in Developing Countries. In Thomae H, Maddox GL (eds): "New Perspectives on Old Age. A Message to Decision Makers." New York: Springer Publishing Company.

Sharma PR (1982). Old age in Nepal: Some preliminary observations. In "The Elderly of Asia", conference proceedings of the Asian Regional Conference on Active Aging. Manila: Social Research Centre, University of Santo Tomas.

Siegel JS (1982). "Demographic Aspects of the Health of the Elderly to the year 2000 and Beyond. World Health Organisation, WHO/AGE/82.3

Svanborg A, Landahl S, Mellstrom D (1982). Epidemiological Studies on Social and Medical Conditions of the Elderly. EURO Reports and Studies, 62. Copenhagen: World Health Organisation, Regional Office for Europe.

United Nations (1982). Introductory Document: Demographic Considerations. A/conf. 113/4. Prepared for the UN World Assembly on Aging, Vienna.

United Nations Centre for Social Development and Humanitarian Affairs (UNCSDHA 1981). Demographic Aspects of the Aging Population on the Asian and Pacific Region. Report of the Technical Meeting on Aging, Bangkok, ESP/P/WP.65

World Health Organisation (1980). Report of the WHO Preparatory Conference, for the United Nations World Assembly on Aging. Mexico City.

XI. GENERAL CONCLUSIONS

Senile Dementia: Outlook for the Future, pages 493–515

SENILE DEMENTIA AND RELATED DISORDERS

SIR MARTIN ROTH

Professor of Psychiatry
University of Cambridge School of Clinical Medicine
Addenbrooke's Hospital, Cambridge England.

An Overview of the Conference

Senile dementia which has been at the focus of interest at this conference is generally regarded as the largest and most pressing single problem facing present day health and social services in different parts of the world. The most authoritative population projections attempted have all made it plain that, failing major advances in treatment and prevention of the disorder, the burdens on society are bound to grow in coming decades. One of the most telling statistics to have been cited in recent years has been the estimate that about one third of the current population of developed countries will survive to at least eighty years of age beyond which the prevalence of all forms of dementia but mainly Alzheimer's disease, is approximately 20%.

Reliable figures regarding the prevalence of dementia in late life are essential for planning future services among other reasons. It is a striking fact epidemiological studies employing similar methods of case finding and diagnostic criteria have all reported prevalence figures that fall between 5 and 7.1% (mean 6.3%) for those aged 65 years and over (Kay and Bergmann 1980). Professor Abelin's figure of 6% falls within this range but Dr Svanborg's finding of a 1% prevalence of dementia among those aged 70 years of age is substantially lower than that recorded by most other investigators. Differences in the diagnostic criteria employed are likely to underlie such discrepancies.

Swedish figures for prevalence and incidence of dementia

in late life have recently aroused interest from another quarter. Hagnell et al (1981) have recently compared the age specific incidence and prevalence rates for senile dementia during the ten year period 1947-1957 and the fifteen year period 1957-1972. Their observations were derived from a twenty five year prospective study of the entire population of the city of Lundby. They reported a significant decline in incidence and in cumulative lifetime risk in the second period for both sexes. Women up to the age of 80 years in whom the incidence of multi-infarct dementia showed a slight increase, were the only group of dements to exhibit a reversal to general trend. But this group of cases was relatively small. Hagnell and his colleagues suggest that the overall decrease in respect of senile dementia has been due to improved nutrition and social circumstances and decline in alcohol abuse. However for the present generalisations would be unjustified from these findings. They clearly need to be repeated in other countries particularly in communities in which figures for incidence and prevalence of mental disorders in late life have been placed on record two or more decades ago.

The figure of approximately 6% that has emerged from most epidemiological investigations for prevalence of all forms of dementia among those aged 65 years and over has been validated by independent observations. In a prospective investigation of a random community sample 6.2% of those diagnosed as suffering from dementia of moderate or severe degree were found to have occupied institutional accommodation of every kind for significantly longer periods than a control group of subjects without mental disorder drawn from the general population of comparable age (Kay et al 1970). The weeks of residence during the period of study was higher in the dements by a factor of ten.

Validation has also come from studies of life expectation. Dr Jacob Brody has posed a question mark against the purported life shortening effect of senile dementia of Alzheimer's type. Valid observations bearing on this question can only be made in representative community samples. In a prospective investigation of such a sample in the North of England, those initially diagnosed as suffering from dementia were found to exhibit a highly significant decrease in life expectation as compared with individuals of comparable age but without psychiatric disorder or those diagnosed as suffering from non-dementing forms of illness. (Kay & Bergmann 1966)

CLINICAL DIAGNOSIS AND RELATED ASPECTS

The development of standardised methods of interviewing and diagnosis as for example the Geriatric Mental Schedule of Copeland et al (1976) which has been extensively tested and proves to have an acceptable degree of reliability have provided valuable tools for clinical and epidemiological research. But no methods which have proved sufficiently sensitive to detect the early stages of Alzheimer or other forms of dementia is currently agailable. And it is open to question whether the open clinical interview in the structured form usually employed nowadays should be jettisoned in all situations in favour of a standardised instrument that had been introduced for research purposes. The flexibility of a full psychiatric examination endows it with considerable advantages in clinical practice. No matter how well designed a standardised instrument may be it is tied to a sequence of pre-set procedures or algorithms. This creates the risk of error particularly in patients with dementia who may be difficult to examine. The opportunities enjoyed by the clinician for examining the behaviour and practical competence of patients in a whole range of situations over a period of time provides him with a rich body of data for the purpose of making decisions regarding diagnosis and treatment. He can also elicit information from independent observers regarding previous development and adaptation, mode of onset and evolution of the disorder, the competence displayed in dressing, washing, feeding, household tasks, handling of money, self-care and social conduct in general. However, as Dr Brady has pointed out, there is a need also for instruments which can be employed in field testing and reliable and valid rating scales which can quantify the severity of the clinical signs and symptoms and of cognitive impairment.

Professor Wertheimer has emphasised the need for an integration of evidence derived from such methods of investigation as the E E G, C T Scan and psychometric tests within a global clinical assessment. A large body of evidence has accumulated to validate an approach that does not readily allow the results of an over-all clinical appraisal to be over-ridden by any one laboratory investigation. The C T scan proved to have its false positives as did the conventional x-ray examination of the skull and none of the other ostensibly objective investigations including psychometric testing are devoid of pitfalls. The PET scan will provide a powerful adjunct in clinical investigation but not a substitute for it.

Dr Richards and his colleagues have made the point that the stringent delineation of the clinical profile of the patient for the purpose of a cross-sectional diagnosis does not suffice for a programme of action aimed at improving social adaptation. Psychiatrists are liable to focus on deficits and to leave assets out of consideration. A formulation is therefore needed which takes account of assets as well as fall outs in function and places the presenting clinical picture within the context of the patient's personality, social and familial setting, his physical health and vigour, his mobility, stance and vigour. Above all, what remains of the patient's inherent emotional characteristics is of vital importance. Even severe dements will often remain acceptable to the family and viable in a community setting provided enough survives of emotional features which enabled them to forge bonds with others and rendered them loveable. This is part of the explanation, for the survival of some individuals in the community where others with dementia of similar degree gravitate to institutional accommodation for the rest of their lives.

Reference has been made to the overlap in clinical symptomatology between Parkinsonism and senile dementia of Alzheimer's type (Dr Stahelin and colleagues). More evidence is required before firm conclusions are drawn. It is rare to find lesions in the nigro-striatal system in senile dementia and the difficulties of gait and involuntary movement observed in advanced Alzheimer's disease are not those typical of Parkinsonism in the majority of cases. Dementia is observed as a complication of Parkinsonism in its advanced stages. But stringent evidence to indicate that it is found in excess of normal expectation is lacking. Parkinsonism may be observed along with other neurological signs in patients with dementia due to multiple infarcts. Plaques, tangles and other changes may be found as was the case in three of the seven patients in whom Parkinson's disease was observed in association with dementia. But it is not clear whetherthe intensity of plaque and tangle formation in the brain is quantitatively comparable to that observed in Alzheimer's disease proper.

A series of related questions are posed in connection with the possible pharmacological causes for the dementia observed in patients with Parkinsonism. It has been suggested that the anti-cholinergic effects of anti-Parkinsonism. It has been suggested that the anti-cholinergic effects of anti-Parkinsonism drugs such as methyl-dopa were responsible. But the evidence to support this hypothesis is insubstantial. It has to be remembered that life expectation of patients with Parkinsonism has been increased by modern therapy. In consequence, they will often survive to an age at which they are at increasing risk of dementia. However, although there is neither pathological nor neurochemical evidence in favour of the hypothesis it poses an interesting challenge to be pursued with further enquiries. The underlying question could, in fact, be inverted to advance an alternative hypothesis. If patients with Parkinsonism treated with levo-dopa over many years do not develop dementia does this not call in question the validity of the cholinergic hypothesis in regard to the primary dementias of old age?

Finally, in this context the differential diagnosis between Alzheimer's disease and multi-infarct dementia can indeed be difficult in individual cases. But in the majority of patients a careful history and examination together with ancillary tests rarely leaves room for serious doubt. Pathological findings at post mortem agree very closely with clinical diagnosis made during life where this has been based upon observations of adequate scope and duration.

The purported extra-pyramidal complications associated with tricyclic compounds have also been attributed to their anti-cholinergic effect. These are, however, such a rare development within the vast population of those treated with anti-depressive drugs, that a latent tendency to Parkinsonism exacerbated by the anti-cholinergic effects of tricyclic compounds has to be considered as a possible explanation.

MORTALITY IN THE DEMENTIAS AND PROBLEMS OF AGEING

There are certain aspects of abridged life expectation in dementia that are of general biological interest and germane for the opening lecture Professor Danon devoted to theories of ageing. The causes of death in Alzheimer's disease are often unclear and liable to be expressed in vague terms. "Senility", "myocardial degeneration", "arteriosclerosis" which are liable to figure on the death certificates, seem more like confessions of ignorance than actual diagnoses of the conditions that led to the patient's demise. Even in multi-infarct dementia the terminal event is much more often an intercurrent infection or other illness than a stroke. In contrast, among other psychiatric disorders such as depressive illness, neurosis and schizophrenias of late life in which mortality is substantially lower, more clear and specific diagnoses are cited such as cardiac failure myocardial infarction, gastro-intestinal disease and various forms of carcinoma (Kay et al 1955, Roth & Kay 1956, Kay 1962) Of course patients with dementia suffer from well established cerebral degenerative disease and this might be responsible for their shortened life expectation. But we know as much or as little of the means by which cerebral degeneration hastens the end of life as we know about the manner in which 'Ageing' does so.

Professor Danon came to the conclusion that valid theories of Ageing will have to await better understanding of the manner in which molecules interact with other molecules. Only when we understand the manner in which dissonance evolves within the global harmony of systems of cells in the sense of Koch, can we hope to gain some glimmerings of insight into the nature of the ageing process. His prediction may be fulfilled. But is it not possible that as in other fields of biological endeavour, progress will occur in the reverse direction that is from more precise knowledge of pathology to clearer definition of the processes underlying physiological functioning.

In addition to diminished life expectation, the senile dementias are characterised by accentuation of the pathological and certain neurochemical changes in the brains of non-demented elderly subjects. They also exhibit diminished vitality and increased vulnerability which causes them to succumb following traumas, infections and metabolic disturbances often of a minor character. In the advanced stages of Alzheimer's disease these are liable to be followed by heightened mental confusion and then rapid decline and death. It is of interest in this connection that cognitive performance is correlated with life expectation even among non-demented subjects (Kay et al 1977). Finally the brains' neurons comprise a population of post-mitotic irreplaceable cells and organs as well as organisms so constituted are particularly liable to exhibit the structural changes and functional impairments correlated with the ageing process.

NEUROBIOLOGY OF SENILE DEMENTIA

Recent Developments in Relation to Structure and Neurochemistry and their Association.

The disorder found at highest prevalence among the dementias of middle and late life is Alzheimer's disease, an illness with a distinctive clinical picture and pathological changes that are also characteristic. There is a discrepancy between clinical diagnosis and pathology but 15% would accord better with the findings of European workers than the 30 - 40% cited by Dr. Brody.

The most important question that arises in relation to the dementias of late life concerns the reasons for the immense disparity between the aged person in his eighties or nineties who remains mentally intact and vigorous and the middle aged individual in his fifties who may suffer from an advanced and progressive dementia. This question can be most appropriately posed in relation to Alzheimer's disease because the pathological changes found in the brain in this condition are qualitatively similar in certain important respects to those to be found in the cerebral cortex of mentally well preserved individuals of advanced age.

At this point it may prove helpful to examine the historical background of recent developments. Until about 15 years ago the significance of the pathological changes described by Alzheimer was considered ambiguous. Senile plaques, tangles and the other pathological changes were judged to be non-specific, secondary and unimportant. However, quantitative assessments of dementia during life and measurements of the pathological changes after post mortem have shown that there was a significant and orderly relationship between them (Roth 1971, Roth et al 1967, Blessed et al 1968, Tomlinson et al 1968, 1970). Further enquiries demonstrated that these pathological changes could not be epiphenomenal to the cerebral degenerative process underlying Alzheimer's disease. Until quite recently (Terry 1977) doubts were raised as to whether there was any significant difference in neuronal out-fall between normal aged and demented subjects. Investigations in Cambridge have confirmed Terry's more recent view (Terry et al 1981) that there is a selective fall-out of larger neurones in the superior, middle and inferior frontal gyri, the cingulate gyrus and the superior and middle temporal gyri (Mountjoy et al 1983). Moreover, the findings showed that this fall-out had evolved in close parallel with the changes that have been described by Alzheimer. Neuronal counts have been shown to correlate with plaque counts in the middle and superior temporal gyri and with estimates of neurofibrillary change in a wider range of cortical areas (Mountjoy et al 1983)

The significant correlations between neuronal fall-out and both plaques and neurofibrillary tangles in the frontal and temporal regions are not isolated associations. A whole range of other changes converge in the same regions of the cortex. The most marked and widely distributed neurochemical lesion is the decrease in choline-acetyl-transferase activity (Perry et al 1977, White et al 1977, Rossor et al 1982, Davies and Maloney/1976). It has been reported to be significantly correlated with plaque counts in the cerebral cortex (Perry et al 1978). In the Cambridge investigations significant correlations have been found confined to the frontal and temporal gyri (Mountjoy et al 1984). ChAT activity is also correlated with cell counts but significantly so only in the superior frontal and superior temporal regions in cases of Alzheimer's disease of early onset (Mountjoy et al 1984). Significant correlations between the intrinsic transmitter GABA and cell counts among dements are limited to the superior temporal gyrus. The morphological and neurochemical changes are therefore not diffuse or random in distribution. They appear highly specific although the selective severity with which the frontal and temporal gyri are affected remains to be explained.

The recent shift in the focus of interest to sub-cortical structures stem stems from a number of fresh observations made in recent years. There are relatively few intrinsic cholinergic neurones in the cerebral cortex (Emson and Lindvall 1979). And most of the ChAT activity in the neo-cortex derives from nerve terminals whose origins in primates are in the cholinergic cells of the nucleus basalis of Meynert. The lesion responsible for the diminished ChAT activity in Alzheimer's disease must therefore be located in some part of this ascending projection. ChAT activity has been shown to be markedly reduced in the nucleus basalis not in adjacent structures and also in the septal nuclei, the sites of projection to the neo-cortex and hippocampus respectively (Rossor et al 1982). The demonstration by (Whitehouse et al (1982)) of reduced cell counts in the cholinergic cells of the nucleus basalis has strengthened the evidence suggesting that the cholinergic deficit observed in the cerebral cortex arises from damage to an ascending projection system.

A similar combination of structural lesions and neurochemical deficits have been brought to light in relation to the noradrenergic system within the brain. Here again the noradrenergic input to the cerebral cortex originates from the pigmented cells of the nucleus locus coeruleus and not from intrinsic neurons. A count of the entire cell population of this nucleus has demonstrated that there is a 70-80% fall-out among the younger groups of patients with Alzheimer's disease (Bondareff et al 1981). The presence of a noradrenergic deficit has been confirmed by significant reductions in the concentration of noradrenaline in the hippocampus and the cingulate mid-frontal and mid-temporal gyri (Mountjoy et al 1984) as well as reduction in the activity of the marker enzyme dopamine-β- hydroxylase in the cerebral cortex (Cross et al 1981).

New hypotheses regarding the causation of Alzheimer's disease in terms of neurotransmitter deficits would inject fresh impetus to enquiries in this field. Although further evidence has been adduced (Leathwood). that treatment with choline improves age dependent impairment of psychological performance in lower animals, the effects of such treatments in man have not for the present provided independent and convincing support for the cholinergic hypothesis.

Professor Gottfries has referred to the multiple deficits in the concentration of transmitters in the post mortem brain described by a number of investigators including his own group. In addition to a lesion of the cholinergic system, there are the well established structural and neurochemical deficits in the noradrenergic system (Bondareff et al 1981, Rossor et al 1984, Adolfsson et al 1979). Evidence has also been adduced in favour of diminished dopaminergic and serotoninergic activity. And the age related increase of monoamine oxidase B has been reported to be present in more pronounced form in patients with Alzheimer's disease (Gottfries et al 1983). However, treatment with dopamine-receptor agonists, the 5-HT precursor tryptophan and monoamine oxidase inhibitors have not proved any more successful in producing improvement in Alzheimer's disease than have attempts to remedy the cholinergic deficit.

It has been suggested that correction of the entire range of transmitter deficits brought to light during the past 7-8 years might yield better results. But no clear hypotheses can be

framed for the present in terms of this whole range of dysfunctio
and no firm predictions could be made regarding the effects of a cocktail with a large number of ingredients. Focussing attention on the cholinergic and noradrenergic deficits would be preferable to such a blunderbuss approach. In both instances the chemical deficits have been shown to be relatively wide spread in the cortex and each is associated with a well established and specific structural lesion in a sub-cortical nucleus.

A unifying theory for the origin of the neurochemical and structural lesions in Alzheimer's disease has been advanced by Professor Constantinidis It has its starting point in lesions which are established in the first instance in neurones in which GABA is the intrinsic transmitter. These neurones would be the first sites of neurofibrillary tangle formation causing both a decrease in GABA activity and possibly a diminutic in the concentration of somatostatin. It is not entirely clear why this second chemical deficit should follow. The main pr problem with this hypothesis is that whereas the diminution in respect of ChAT is to be found in the greater part of the cerebral cortex in Alzheimer's disease both of late and early onset, the other neurochemical deficits are far more localised. A significant diminution in GABA is confined to the cells of the frontal and temporal cortex and found only in cases of Alzheimer's disease of early onset. The reduction in respect of somatostatin is even more markedly circumscribed (Rossor et al 1984). A further problem is that it is the senile plaque not the tangle that is the first pathological lesion in cases of Alzheimer's disease. However, in advanced cases, tangles but not the deficit in respect of GABA are to be found in every part of the cortex.

Other Aspects of Aetiology and Pathogenesis

It is already evident that investment of all effort in theories based on transmitter deficits and ignoring other possibilities would be unwise. The primary lesions or disorder may prove to be in some unsuspected quarter. The philothermal response of polymorphonuclear leucocytes which have been reported by Dr Jarvik to be altered in their motile behaviour in Alzheimer's disease may reflect a more general change. It may for example extend as she suggests to neuroglia. If so, a new path for investigating the aetiology of Alzheimer's disease might be opened. However, the findings require replication and the mechanisms underlying the philothermal response remain to be determined.

The possibility remains open that some or all of the deficits in respect of neuro-transmitters are secondary to structural lesions. Dr Meier-Ruge has described another aspect of structural change when he reported that not only was there significant shrinkage of the cerebral cortex in Alzheimer's disease but the size of nerve cells showed a significant increase as compared with age matched controls Shrinkage, neuronal fall-out and biochemical deficit may be different stages in the evolution of one and the same aetiological process.

The Association with Down's Syndrome

The possible association with Down's syndrome is another clue to the aetiology of Alzheimer's disease that has been actively explored in recent years. Characteristic changes of Alzheimer type are present in the great majority of individuals with Down's syndrome over the age of 35 years. The dementia is inconsistent but no quantitative investigations have been undertaken for the present of the degree of mental decline during life or of the intensity of pathological change after death. It is not therefore known how strict a relationship obtains between them. The observations favouring a possible association were first advanced by Heston and his colleagues (Heston and White 1977) have now come from another quarter. Dr. Cohen and Eisdorfer have adduced evidence that advanced maternal age may be a risk factor common to Alzheimer's disease and Down's syndrome. More investigations are needed to exclude the chance of statistical artefacts. Heston has suggested that defective organisation of microfilaments and microtubules may be the pathogenic factor common to the two conditions. The basic aetiological causes must of course be different. But comparison and contrast with the aid of genetical, neurochemical and ultra-structural studies of Alzheimer's disease, Down's syndrome and the Parkinsonism-dementia complex that is indigenous in the island of Guam might generate fresh ideas regarding the aetiological basis of Alzheimer's disease.

EEG Findings

Although mild abnormalities are common, a severely abnormal E.E.G. with high voltage, synchronised slow wave discharges is exceptional in Alzheimer's disease. Dead cells seem to tell no tales. Only those in process of rapid destruction appear to do so. In Creutzfeldt-Jacob disease on the other hand there are characteristic medium to high voltage sharp wave discharges of generalised distribution with a regular period of 0.5-2 seconds. Epileptic fits occur in excess frequency in both diseases, albeit only in a small minority of cases. They are commoner in the earlier than in the later onset cases of Alzheimer's disease. The studies of Dr Traub et al have shed fresh light on these phenomena Their findings suggest that increased synchronisation reflected in the sharp-wave discharges of CJD and occasionally Alzheimer's disease are due to neuronal fusion, usually as a result of the viral infection in CJD giving rise to an increased number of electrotonic junctions. The fact that despite such increasing synchronisation epileptic fits are rare is attributed to the integrity of intrinsic neuronal inhibitory mechanisms. Slowing of inter-neuronal transmission may play its part here and increased latency of the P300 among other components of sensory evoked potential which reflects this, deserve more detailed exploration as a possible adjunct in clinical diagosis.

The Neurofibrillary Tangle

A problem of central importance in the neurobiology of Alzheimer disease is the structural character and origin of the neurofibrillary tangle. When present in profusion in the cerebral cortex it constitutes the most specific of the morphological changes found in Alzheimer's disease. It was demonstrated by Kidd twenty years ago(Kidd 1964) that tangles were composed of pairs of filaments twisted about each other to produce a helix. Smaller aggregates of paired helical filaments (PHF) are found in the swollen dendrites surrounding the central core of amyloid in the senile plaque. The nature of the relationship between these two structures is one of the unsolved problems of Alzheimer's disease. As there are elements common to them, it is possible that they represent different stages to the development of one and the same process. This is compatible with the presence of plaques alone in the cortex of normal aged people but difficult to reconcile with the fact that in the Guam-Parkinsonism-dementia syndrome, tangles are found without plaques.

The tangle has proved difficult to investigate for a number of reasons. As shown by Selkoe's group (Selkoe 1982) PHF are highly resistant to the usual reagents and proteolytic enzymes that seem capable of dissolving insoluble proteins making it possible to characterise their peptides. The cause of the insolubility of tangles is unclear. When this problem has been resolved more light will have been shed on the nature of the cellular elements that constitute paired helical filaments and tangles. Ordinary in situ immunochemistry has not succeeded in shedding light on the protein structure of PHF. A number of the anti-sera that stain tangles react also both with microtubular and neuro-filament preparations. Dr. Wisniewski has adduced evidence that the normal young brain contains polypeptide material which cross reacts immuno-chemically with paired helical filaments. He concludes from his findings that PHF result from post transcriptional modifications in the affected neurones rather than new protein formation.

However, the chemical structure of PHF is far from solved and purified homogenous preparations have yet to be prepared. Further investigations with the tools of molecular biology may provide answers to hundreds of questions in respect of Alzheimer's disease. Is the distinction between normal ageing of human brain and Alzheimer's disease essentially quantitative or qualitative? Are the transmitter deficits second to structural change or does the process begin with a neurochemical defect? If the analogy with Parkinsonism drawn by many investigators proves valid the structural change will prove to be primary but this will not necessarily preclude treatment that mitigates the symptoms of the illness particularly in its early stages.

ALZHEIMER'S DISEASE OF EARLY AND LATE ONSET

A recent enquiry has suggested that Alzheimer's diseases of early and late onset are separated by a line of demarcation. Difficult though it may be to define this boundary line with precision, the evidence suggests that, while there may be lines of continuity in respect of certain structural and neurochemical features there are qualitative distinctions in respect of others. If this is the case, neurobiological investigations of Alzheimer's disease will have to take account of the new classification which merely reinstates an older one on the strength of fresh evidence. For as Dr Brody pointed out, failure to do this may lead to important clues being missed through dilution of two biologically distinct entities.

The evidence favouring this diversity within the unified concept of Alzheimer's disease is derived from a number of sources. Comparisons with well preserved elderly subjects have demonstrated a significant fall-out of neurones in the higher cell classes in the frontal and temporal regions of patients with Alzheimer's disease of early onset. No such differences between cases of late onset and normal controls have been found (Mountjoy et al 1983). Plaque counts and estimates of neurofibrillary tangles have proved to be significantly higher in patients within the early onset group (Mountjoy et al 1983). A fall-out of 70-80% of the cells of the nucleus locus coeruleus has been found in the younger group of Alzheimer cases (Bondareff et al 1981). In patients of late onset the fall out is limited to 10-20% of cells and there is no clear demarcation from normal subjects.

In patients dying in the ninth or tenth decade there is a relatively pure cholinergic deficit confined to temporal lobe and hippocampus together with reduced concentration of somatostatin in the temporal cortex alone. By contrast in the younger group dying in their seventh and eighth decades there is a widespread and severe cholinergic deficit together with significant reductions in respect of noradrenalin, GABA and somastostatin (Rossor et al 1984).

Analogies have often been drawn in recent years between neurobiological deficits in Parkinson's disease and those in Alzheimer's disease. A combination of structural lesion and neurotransmitter deficits is found in both. In the case of Parkinsonism it has proved possible to compensate for the dopaminergic defect with the aid of agents such as Levo-dopa. No comparable form of treatment has been found in the case of the Alzheimer syndrome. But there are certain similarities in respect of the evidence relating to structural damage. A threshold effect has been demonstrated in the case of Alzheimer's disease in respect of intensity of plaque formation; those with average plaque counts above 12 per field prove to be demented in the majority of cases, those below it to be mentally intact (Roth et al 1967, Blessed et al 1968, Roth 1971)). There are reasons for assuming a similar effect in respect of tangles particularly as PHF elements are to be found within the plaque. Neuronal outfall has not yet been directly demonstrated to be subject to a definite threshold effect.

But there are highly significant inverse correlations between both plaque counts and tangle densities on the one hand and neuronal counts on the other. It would seem likely that the threshold effect in respect of plaques and tangles arises from the existence of some threshold limit at a more basic neuronal level; in the case of Parkinson's disease a threshold effect in respect of neuronal fallout has been firmly established. Approximately 80-85% of nigral neurons have to be lost and 80% of the dopamine content of the striatum needs to be depleted before frank symptoms of Parkinson's disease appear (Marsden 1983). Compensation in pre-synaptic mechanisms and by means of an increase in post-synaptic receptor sensitivity can for a time make good the dopaminergic deficit. But with the progressive march of degeneration and fall out in nigral neurons decompensation eventually occurs and symptoms of Parkinsonism then make their appearance. Unfortunately, the sequence of events has not yet been as clearly mapped in the case of Alzheimer's disease. Nor has any one neurochemical deficit been established as indubitably linked with the dementing syndrome.

Returning to the subdivision of Alzheimer's disease, it is noteworthy also that it is only in the younger group of patients that a significant correlation between ChAT activity and neuronal fall-out has been observed. It is found only in the superior frontal and temporal regions (Mountjoy et al 1984).

In investigations of a possible parallelism between Parkinsonism and Alzheimer's disease it may be most fruitful to focus on investigations on the younger group of cases; those in whom symptoms of dementia make their appearance before the age of 75 years. It would be logical to compare and contrast the findings in this group with those in Alzheimer's disease of late onset as well as control subjects.

SOCIO-MEDICAL ASPECTS AND THE ORGANISATION OF SERVICES

Professor Gilliand has described maintenance of autonomy of the aged person as the central purpose of the organisation of the Health and Social Services devoted to their care. In other papers during the session Professor Gommers, Airie and Schwed have provided examples of psycho-geriatric services which maintain a judicious balance between care by Health Services, by the family, and action to protect those responsible for the provision of care and support to aged relatives from undue stress.

The question posed by Dr Maddox as to how we are to take care of the caretakers is important for a number of reasons. Some twenty years ago it had already become known (Kay et al 1964 a & b) that for every patient with dementia living in a hospital or institution there were four individuals suffering from mental deterioration of comparable severity surviving in the community. This remains largely true at the present time. But we remain in ignorance of the skills and strategies utilised by the familial and social networks of elderly demented subjects to avert the institutional care of their relatives with senile dementia. Of course at advanced stages in the disease an excessive dependence and burden upon the family will often demand institutional care on an intermittent or lasting basis.

Dr Bergmann has pointed out we cannot assume that the right of the aged person to be cared for at home can automatically be accepted as some other persons' duty to care for him in a familial and domestic setting. Rapid social change and geographical mobility are probably eroding the old networks which previously sustained elderly people in non institutional settings. There are fewer pairs of willing and dedicated female hands at home. The increasing separation between the generations is one difficulty. For willingness to make sacrifices on behalf of elderly parents and relatives cannot be transmitted across large distances. There is a paucity of information about the rate at which these precious resources are being eroded. Nor is any systematic attempt being made to substitute other support systems and human relationships.

Many of those who provide care are themselves approaching or are already beyond the threshold of old age. Be this as it may no health and welfare service in the world can by itself take on the roles assumed at the present time by families and kinship networks within the community. The point has been repeatedly made that if only a fraction of those at present being cared for in the community were to become dependent within a short period upon the Health and Welfare services they would burst at the seams. The responsibility for the care of those suffering from dementia cannot be effectively shouldered by the family or the community alone. An imaginatively conceived partnership between them provides the only foundation for a realistic and humane approach.

Dr Gurland's comparative study methods of patterns of care in the U S and Great Britain posed important questions regarding the optimal setting for the long term care of psychogeriatric patients. In New York a shift from residence in mental hospitals to care in nursing homes has been in progress for a number of years. This preponderence of nursing home provision represents one of the conspicuous differences between the two cities. There is no need to review once again the deadening effect exerted by a chronic hospital ward upon the morale, personal integrity and motivation of people and old people in particular. For the choices open to them are even more limited to those available to the young. But there is an exaggerated emphasis in the recorded literature upon the site at which care should be given to the exclusion of the quality of life enjoyed by those to be served. A place in a residential home or nursing home is preferable to a bed in an overcrowded chronic ward. But in the course of time domestic accommodation is liable to become a repository for cases of moderate and severe dementia without benefit of the nursing care required by many disturbed, wandering and incontinent old people.

Valuable lessons would be bound to emerge from comparative studies of the patterns of care provided for psychogeriatric patients in different countries. A great deal of critism has been advanced against privately financed nursing homes in the United States, particularly where stringent supervision of the standards of care and accommodation has not been made mandatory.

The services in the Netherlands (1982) provide a model that merits wider investigation. Approximately 9% of those of 65 and over are accommodated in residential homes of a superior and specially designed homely character and a further 3% are housed in nursing homes in which the majority of chronic psychogeriatric patients are cared for. Hence 12% of the elderly are receiving institutional care and this takes place almost entirely outside the hospital system which is devoted in its entirety to the care of those with acute illness. Domiciliary services are provided in addition and on a generous scale. This must be a very expensive service but the standard of care and facilities provided is impressive. The quality of life that obtains in such institutional forms of care as compared with that in a home environment with all its deprivations and inconveniences is more important than any economic consideration. The choices and preferences of old people have also to be given weight. Policy makers should not make all decisions over their heads.

Policies in relation to the long term care of elderly psychogeriatric and chronically ill people have in the past been determined largely on the basis of tradition, sentiment and economic and political considerations. There is urgent need for policies informed by data regarding the quality of life in the different settings and systematic ascertainment of the wishes and aspirations of the elderly and their families.

PERSPECTIVES FOR THE FUTURE

The greatest stimulus to scientific investigation in this field is that vast disparity between those who end their lives with their minds intact and those who do so in a state of total oblivion, conferred most typically by advanced Alzheimer's disease. There must be definable and ultimately controllable factors underlying such differences. One leading objective of scientific endeavour in this field would be to try and narrow this gap. Clinical research has played a leading role in the advancement of knowledge of Alzheimer's disease in the last half century and it will continue to do so in the foreseeable future. There is a pressing need for sharpened tools of clinical observation and psychological measurement. Methods of evaluation sensitive to the earliest stages of Alzheimer's disase are of particular importance. They have to be rendered serviceable for epidemiological enquiries. The quality of "tedious dedication" upheld by Dr Brody as being of prime importance in this area is not found at high prevalence. But it has to be fostered because many years of effort may be needed to gain insight into aetiology and to achieve advances in treatment; the progress of recent years is no more than a promissory note.

Although no effective pharmacological treatments for senile dementia have emerged from recent enquiries further endeavours that draw inspiration from knowledge of all the neurochemical deficits that have been defined, are bound to be undertaken. There are no known means of preventing Alzheimer's disease. But if it is accepted that threshold effects occur both in respect of neuronal outfall and Alzheimer changes certain implications follow. Any cerebral disease or injury which destroys part of the brain's neuronal population may predispose the individual to the development of dementia. A certain amount of evidence supports this view. There are several examples of potentiation of the effects of age related decline in neurones by environmental insults causing further neuronal damage followed by dementia that might not have arisen in the absence of the insult (Roth 1980). In the case of the dementia of pugilists several years may elapse between the last cerebral insult during a contest in the ring and the first appearence of symptoms of mental deterioration. Neurofibrillary tangles are prominent among the pathological changes in this disorder. In Down's syndrome which is associated with a limited endowment of cerebral neurons, dementia occurs at an early age and tangles are again a characteristic feature. Dementia commonly follows head injury in late life whereas it is very rarely seen in the first few decades of life.

A similar hypothesis has been advanced in relation to the aetiological basis of Parkinson's disease (Calne and Langston 1983). It has been suggested that the condition arises as the result of a combination of age related decline of dopaminergic cells which cannot by itself give rise to the disorder and some as yet undefined exogenous toxin or viral infection similar in its effects to MPTP (1-methyl-4-phenyl-1,2,5,6-tetrahydropyridine) which produces selective damage to dopaminergic cells of the substantia nigra. The aggregation of these two types of neuronal damange eventually causes the dopaminergic cells of the substantia nigra to fall below the critical threshold of an 80% loss. Decompensation follows and Parkinsonian symptoms then make their appearance.

Concluding Remarks

The natural course of demented illness is one of progressive decline, but the statistics that depict this overall outcome subsume a large range of variation. The task of those engaged in the treatment and care of the individual with dementia is to try to defeat this prophecy rather than observe its fulfilment. They need to pay meticulous attention to every detail of health and nutrition, take steps to ensure that the individual's links with family and community are not severed, that his emotional suffering is relieved, and his dignity and morale sustained. We are all too liable to see mainly demented depressed or disabled old people and to forget that even after the age of 75, the majority continue to live where they have been, manage to sustain loves and friendships, and ailments notwithstanding, to expand their horizons. Knowledge is advancing and some of the factors underlying this variation are better understood; but it would be unrealistic to expect that the problems of dementia will have ceased to challenge society within one or two decades. Imagination and effort have therefore to be invested to provide the best possible means of care and support. This must have first priority in any plans made for services for those suffering from dementia. But some of the most significant advances in knowledge have issued from groups of workers noted for the excellence of the service and the care they devoted to demented patients.

References

Adolfsson R, Gottfries CG, Roos CE, Winblad B (1979). Changes in the brain catecholamines in patients with dementia of Alzheimer type. Brit J Psychiat 135;216-223.

Blessed G, Tomlinson BE, Roth M (1968). The association between quantitative measurements of dementia and of senile changes in the cerebral grey matter of elderly subjects. Brit J Psychiat 114: 797-811.

Bondareff W, Mountjoy CQ, Roth M (1981) Selective loss of neurones of origin of adrenergic projection to cerebral cortex (nucleus locus coeruleus) in senile dementia. Neurology 32: 164-168

Calne DB, Langston JW (1983). Aetiology of Parkinson's disease. Lancet 2: 1457-1459.

Copeland JRM, Kelleher MJ, Kellett JM, Gourlay AJ, Gurland BJ, Fleiss JL, Sharp L (1976). A semi-structured clinical interview for the assessment of diagnosis and mental state in the elderly: the Geriatric Mental State Schedule. I. Development and Reliability. Psychol Med 6:439-449.

Cross, AJ, Crow, TJ, Perry EK, Perry RH, Blessed G, Tomlinson BE (1981) Reduced dopamine- - hydroxylase activity in Alzheimer's disease. Br. Med J. 282: 93-94.

Davies P, Maloney AJF (1976). Selective loss of central cholinergic neurons in Alzheimer's disease. Lancet 2: 1403.

Emson PC, Lindvall O (1979) Distribution of putative neurotransmitters in the neocortex. Neuroscience 4:1-30.

Gottfries CG, Adolfsson R, Aquilonius SM, Carlsson A, Eckernas SA, Nordberg A, Oreland L, Svennerholm L, Wiberg A, Winblad B (1983). Biochemical changes in dementia disorders of Alzheimer type (AD/SDAT). In Press. Neurobiol Aging.

Hagnell O, Lanke J, Rorsman B, Ojesjo L (1981) Does the incidence of age psychosis decrease? A prospective, longitudinal study of a complete population investigated during the 25-year period 1947-1972: The Lundby Study. Neuropsychobiology, 7 (4): 201-211.

Heston LL, White J (1977) Alzheimer's disease, trisomy 21 and myeloproliferative disorders: Associations suggesting a genetic diatesis. Science 196: 322-323.

Kay DWK, (1962) Outcome and cause of death in mental disorders of old age: A long-term follow-up of functional and organic psychoses. Acta Psychiat Scand. 38: 249-276.

Kay DWK, Beamish P, Roth, M (1964) Old age mental disorders in Newcastle upon Tyne I.- A study of prevalence. Brit J Psychiat 110: 146-158.

Kay DWK, Beamish P, Roth M (1964) Old age mental disorders in Newcastle upon Tyne. 11 - A study of possible social and medical causes. Brit J Psychiat 110: 668-682.

Kay DWK, Bergmann K (1966) Physical disability and mental health in old age. J Psychosom Res 10: 3-12.

Kay, DWK, Bergmann K (1980). Epidemiology of mental disorders among the aged in the community. In Birren JE, Sloane RB (eds):

"Handbook of Mental Health and Aging":Prentice-Hall Inc.
Kay DWK, Roth M, Hopkins B (1955) Affective disorders arising in the senium I: Their association with organic cerebral degeneration. J Ment Sci 101: 302-316.
Kay DWK, Bergmann K, Foster, EM, McKechnie AA, Roth M (1970). Mental illness and hospital usage in the elderly: a random sample followed up. Comp Psychiat 2: 26-35.
Kay DWK, Britton PG, Bergmann K et al (1977). Cognitive function and length of survival in elderly subjects living at home. Australian and New Zeal J Psychiat 11: 113-117.
Kidd M (1964) Alzheimer's disease - an electromicroscopical study. Brain 87: 307-320.
Marsden CD(1983). Basal gangalia disease in neurotransmitters and CNS disease. A Lancet Review: 21-27.
Mountjoy CQ, Roth M, Evans NJR, Evans HM (1983) Cortical neuronal counts in normal elderly controls and demented patients. Neurobiol of Aging, 4: 1-11.
Mountjoy, CQ, Rossor MN, Iversen LL, Roth M (1984). Correlation of cortical cholinergic and GABA deficits with quantitative neuropathological findings in senile dementia. In Press. Brit Med J.
Netherlands National Report on Policy of Aging (1982). National Report for the United Nations World Assembly on Aging, pp 32.
Perry EK, Perry RH, Blessed G, Tomlinson BE (1977) Necropsy evidence of central cholinergic deficits in senile dementia. Lancet 1: 189.
Perry EK, Tomlinson, BE, Blessed G, Bergmann K, Gibson PH, Perry RH (1978) Correlation of cholinergic abnormalities with senile plaques and mental test scores in senile dementia. Br Med J 2: 1457-1459.
Rossor MN, Garrett NJ, Johnson AL, Mountjoy CQ, Roth M, Iversen LL (1982) A post-mortem study of the cholinergic and GABA systems in senile dementia. Brain 105: 313-330.
Rossor MN, Iversen LL, Reynolds GP, Mountjoy CQ, Roth M. (1984) Early and late onset types of Alzheimer's disease are neurochemically distinct. In Press.
Rossor MN, Svendsen C, Hunt SP, Mountjoy CQ, Roth M, Iversen LL (1982). The substantia innominata in Alzheimer's disease: an histochemical and biochemical study of cholinergic marker enzymes. Neurosci Lett 28: 217-22.
Roth M (1971) Classification and aetiology in mental disorders of old age. Some recent developments. In Kay DWK and Walk Brit J of Psychiat Special Publication, no. 6: Headley Bros. London.
Roth M (1980) Ageing of the brain and dementia: an overview.

In Amaducci L, Davison AN, Antuono P (ed) Ageing, v. 13 Raven Press.
Roth M, Kay DWK (1956). Affective disorders arising in the senium. II - Physical disability as an aetiological factor. J Ment Sci 102 (246): 141-150.
Roth M, Tomlinson BE, Blessed G (1967). The relationship between measures of dementia and of degenerative changes in the cerebral grey matter of elderly subjects. Proc R Soc Med (Lond) 60: 254-259.
Selkoe DN (1982). Molecular pathology of the aging human brain. Trends in Neuroscience 5: 332-336.
Terry RD, Fitzgerald C, Peck A, Millner J, Farmer P (1977) Cortical cell counts in senile dementia. J Neuropathol Exp Neurol 36-633.
Terry RD, Peck A, DeTeresa R, Schechter R, Horoupian DS (1981). Some morphometric aspects of the brain in senile dementia of the Alzheimer type. Ann Neurol 10: 184-192.
Tomlinson BE, Blessed G, Roth M (1968). Observations on the brains of non-demented old people. J Neurol Sci 7;331-356.
Tomlinson BE, Blessed G, Roth M (1970). Observations on the brains of demented old people. J Neurol Sci 11:205-242.
White P, Carrasco LH, Williams IEI, Bowen BM (1977). Neocortical cholinergic neurons in elderly people. Lancet 1: 668-670.
White P, Hiley CR, Goodhardt MJ, Carrasco LH, Keet JP, Williams IEI, Bowen BM (1977). Neocortical cholinergic neurons in elderly people. Lancet 1: 668-670.
Whitehouse PJ, Price DL, Struble RG, Clark AW, Coyle JT, DeLond MR (1982) Alzheimer's disease and senile dementia. Loss of neurons in the basal forebrain. Science 215: 1237-1239.

Index